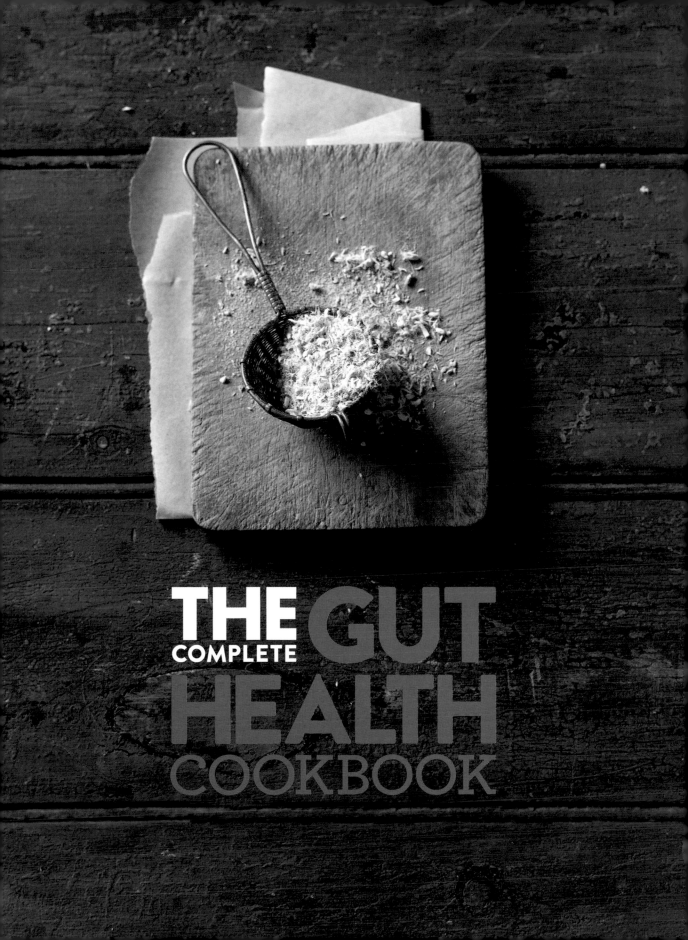

THE
COMPLETE GUT
HEALTH
COOKBOOK

This book is dedicated to YOU and the trillions of bacteria that live in and on YOU. Look after them and they will look after you!

THE COMPLETE GUT HEALTH COOKBOOK

Everything you need to know about the gut and how to improve yours

PETE EVANS

with HELEN PADARIN

weldon**owen**

A NOTE FROM THE AUTHORS

This book is about how digestive health leads to overall good health. It explains some of the emerging science of good gut health and some of the medical problems that may stem from or be associated with poor gut health. It is important to note that much of this science is in its early stages, though we have endeavored to provide references to some of the best studies that are available at this point in time (see References, page 332). We believe that a good diet of unprocessed food is one of the best ways to deal with poor gut health, and that the paleo diet, which is based on nutrient-dense ingredients that have had little or no processing, is a great way to eat if you want to improve your gut health and, by extension, your overall health. These opinions are based on our own experiences, those of the thousands of people who write to Pete about their diet via his online sites, and Helen's clinical experiences and those of many of her colleagues. Nutritional science is constantly evolving. For example, less than a decade ago many doctors were urging us to eat more carbs and less fat; now the message is reversed. It is our hope and expectation that the principles of the paleo diet will soon be mainstream and the subject of numerous studies. We are not saying that a paleo diet is a cure for disease or presenting the paleo diet as gold-standard science at this stage; we are saying it is an excellent plan for avoiding some of the ingredients that have a demonstrated negative effect on our health, and incorporating ingredients with proven benefits.

CONTENTS

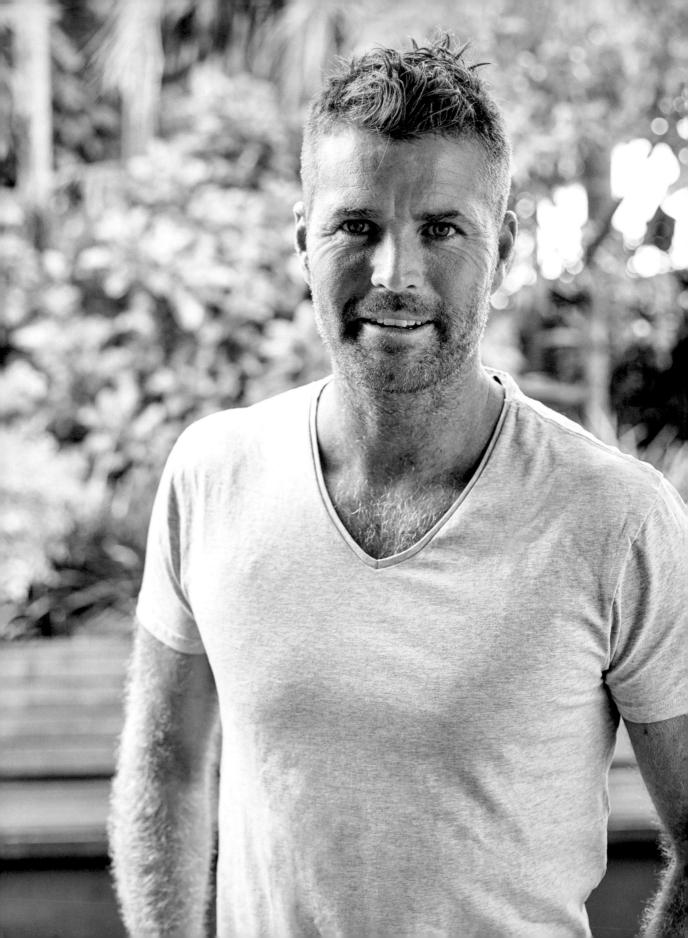

INTRODUCTION

First off, I want to thank you for deciding to pick up this book. As the title suggests, it is all about good gut health and how to achieve it, following the simple but powerful premise that wellness stems from a balanced digestive system. I cannot stress enough that without a healthy gut, it will be quite difficult to achieve optimum health. I am sure you have heard the saying "you are what you eat"; but, in fact, that is not entirely true, and we really should be saying "we are what we absorb."

For this book, I have teamed up once again with my dear friend, nutritionist and naturopath Helen Padarin, who has dedicated her life to helping others with chronic health problems reclaim their health. Helen is one of the most committed and passionate people I have had the good fortune to cross paths with and learn from. Her positive results bring tears to my eyes, because what she is teaching her patients is basic common sense, and should be more widely known and accepted.

Together, Helen and I aim to bring this common-sense approach to a mainstream audience. As well as Helen's clear overview of the basics of a healthy gut, we are proud to share some delicious new recipes designed to promote gut health and well-being. From super-charged broths, warming soups, simple dinners, snacks, and vegetable dishes, to wonderful teas and beverages and a few easy treats for celebratory occasions, we have you covered. We have even slipped in a few recipes for simple home remedies using bath salts and essential oils.

We provide the information you need to become a shining example of true health, so that you can not only motivate yourself but also show your friends and family that there is a simple, utterly delicious, and extremely achievable solution that is sustainable for you, the planet, and coming generations.

I suffered, as a lot of people do, from poor digestion, nasal issues, and dry, flaking skin for pretty much all of my life until I discovered paleo. I was amazed and at the same time frustrated that such a straightforward method for improving health – through easy-to-adopt dietary and lifestyle changes – was not readily known. We're so quick to use pills, potions, and injections – short-term solutions that only mask the problems and never deal with the underlying concerns, which, in my case, were caused by the foods I was eating and the beneficial foods I was not including in my diet.

When I first heard about fermented vegetables I was shocked that as a chef I had not learned about them through my training and my own pursuit of my craft. Bone broths were something that I was taught at culinary school, but only as a base for sauces or soups; never once was it mentioned that these nutritional powerhouses have the ability to heal in such a delicious way. I have seen the effects on my children. Their bloating issues and constant illnesses have been virtually non-existent since we have adopted the paleo way of life. I have also seen my own mother reap the benefits from including nourishing and balancing bone broths and fermented vegetables in her diet.

Helen and I have included a basic meal plan for you, but, like all things, please use your good sense and view it as a guide only. After a week or two you may not feel the need to eat three meals a day and will be quite content with one or two nutrient-dense meals, or sometimes you may feel like fasting, which is completely normal. For those who like to stick to a plan while they adjust to their new lifestyle, we hope you find what we have laid out is an easy, delicious, and achievable program to follow for the years ahead. The idea is that we help you build your culinary repertoire so that you ultimately create your own dishes by tweaking and adapting our recipes or your own according to the simple formula we spell out in this book.

Anyone who has seen me talk on stage can attest to the fact that I am very pushy about getting the correct information about paleo out to people. Eating the paleo way is primarily about healing the gut and helping it thrive. At its heart it is about embracing real foods and eliminating any that may upset the gut and cause inflammation in our bodies. So what foods do we embrace? You'll be pleased to know that there is an abundance of natural and delicious foods to include in your diet. Here are our recommendations:

* Eat up to a palm-sized portion of animal protein at every meal. Focus on sourcing protein from animals that have had a natural diet, such as grass-fed beef, wild-caught seafood, free-range and pasture-raised poultry and pork, and wild game. (Children and pregnant or breastfeeding women may increase their protein intake.)
* Enjoy an abundance of organic vegetables, with a preference for the least starchy varieties.
* Include good-quality fat from avocados, olives, nuts, seeds, eggs, and animals in your daily diet.
* Include bone broth in your daily diet for good gut health. You can drink bone broth straight up, or add it to soups, curries, or braises.
* Add a spoonful of fermented vegetables to every meal if possible. Start off with a teaspoon a day, then work your way up to about a tablespoon or two per meal. (Do not heat as it destroys the beneficial bacteria.)

When making any dietary changes, always consult your health professional to make sure they feel it is safe for you, taking into account your overall health and any existing medical conditions that you may have. Luckily, more and more doctors are promoting this way of life for their patients, and that is wonderful to see.

We have also gone a step further with this book by offering AIP (Autoimmune Paleo) alternatives to as many recipes as we can (look out for the AIP markers on recipes), and Helen shares a wealth of information on AIP on pages 69–71. For further reading on AIP, I suggest Sarah Ballantyne's book *The Paleo Approach*.

As always, I want to encourage you to see that the paleo way of life is an adventure – as all of life is – and the best way to implement it is with an open mind, a curious palate, and a thirst for knowledge. Of course, to experience the full health benefits, you must cook with love and laughter, and be organized, prepared, and willing to give our dietary plan a red-hot go by embracing it 100 percent for at least ten weeks. Over the first month or so you may experience lethargy, grumpiness, headaches, different sleep patterns, etc. It will be rough for some, but stick with it; the rewards when you come through the other side are enormous.

I hope you love this book, use it often, and lend it to others, and I look forward to hearing and sharing your stories of success!

Love,
Pete xo

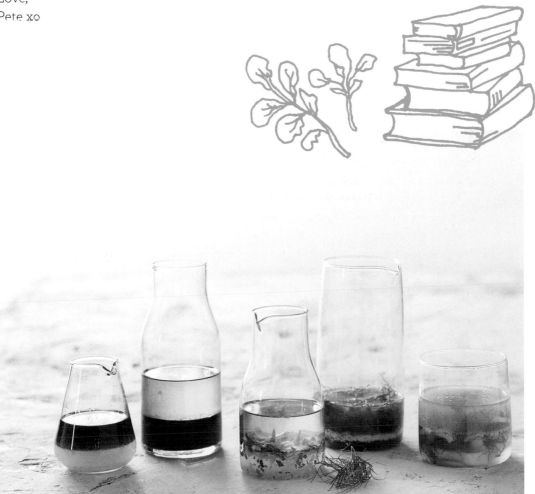

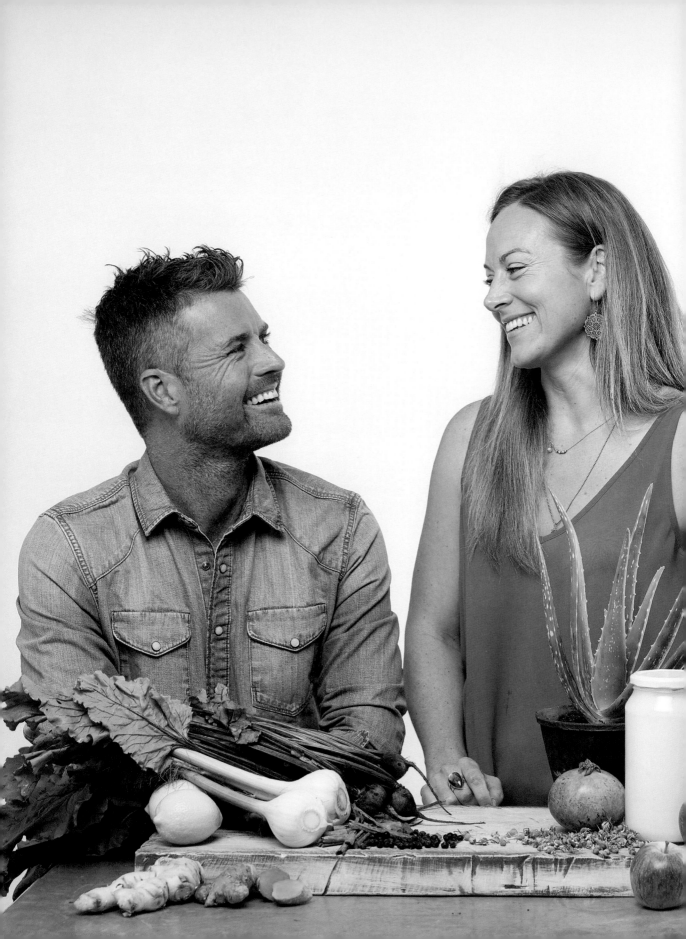

PART ONE

GUT HEALTH GUIDE

EVERYTHING YOU NEED TO KNOW ABOUT GUT HEALTH AND HOW TO IMPROVE YOURS

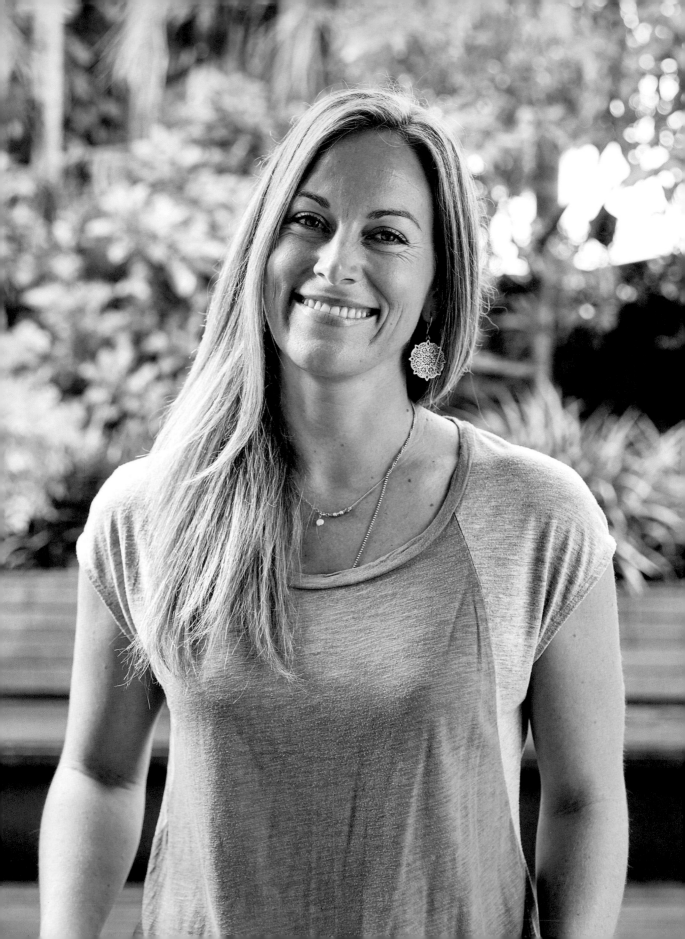

MY STORY: HELEN PADARIN

The first thing I remember being taken to the doctor for as a young child was constipation (a nice fact to share so publicly!). Not a fun doctor's visit. Knowing what I know now about the link between gut health and asthma and eczema I believe my gut issues started from day one. When I threatened to arrive into the world three months early, my loving mum was given corticosteroid medication to speed up the maturity of my lungs. While this possibly saved my life, it also left me on slippery footing as far as my (and my mum's) microbiome (the collection of bugs in and on us) went. So, in my early days I developed eczema – head to toe covered in it – and by the time I was eighteen months old, asthma came along too. Add to that a few allergies (I would break out in hives just from touching raw egg white, and you could put me in a room that a cat had been in and watch my eyes tear up and swell) and it is clear my immune system – and therefore my gut – was out of balance.

My eczema cleared up in early childhood, but my allergies, asthma, and the onset of recurrent infections followed me through my teens. Tonsillitis and bronchitis were regular visitors. At fourteen I had pneumonia and at seventeen I had shingles. In my mid-to-late teens depression arrived, which was undiagnosed and I kept it to myself for a good decade before sharing with my family how I'd been feeling.

At around twenty, while studying naturopathy and nutrition, I learned that I had polycystic ovary syndrome (PCOS). This helped explain my very painful (to the point of vomiting) and often heavy periods, and my blemished skin. I decided to opt for a natural approach. I changed my diet to include more protein (I had been vegetarian for a few years) and reduce my starches to help balance my insulin levels (did I mention my low blood sugar crashes?). I took herbs to help regulate my estrogen, progesterone, and androgens and had acupuncture from a fantastic practitioner. Within a few months, all signs and symptoms of PCOS had disappeared.

Around this time, I was still having oats for breakfast. After a lifetime of slow bowel habits, I didn't mind that by the time I finished my last mouthful of oats every morning I was running to the loo. I had not yet connected the dots between which foods were causing constipation and which were creating urgency. And it wasn't until I started seeing patients with celiac disease that I began to think, hmm, that's like me! I had never really thought too much about it – despite my studies – because that experience was all I knew. It was my normal. I asked one of the GPs I worked with to run celiac serology on me, and, despite being on a fairly low-gluten diet, my anti-gliadin antibodies were elevated. So, I decided to go gluten free to see how I'd feel. Wow! What a revelation!

No more bloating after meals; my mood lifted; and my midafternoon fatigue disappeared. My mind felt less foggy. Low moods still came at times, and to a lesser extent occasionally still do, but it's very different now. The moods no longer own me. I am not consumed or defined by them. If they come up I can sit back and observe them. "Oh, well that's interesting. What's going on to create these feelings?" Most often for me it's not enough quiet time or enough play and movement. It is also food choices. In the early years I was not so strict about avoiding gluten, but as time went on, the way it and other nutrients affected my gut became clearer. So, the temptation and desire to eat any of these trigger foods dissipated. The short-term gratification of consuming them wasn't worth the impact on the happier, healthier me.

As I worked out what did and what didn't work for me, my diet gradually evolved. I began eating fermented vegetables and following the Body Ecology Diet. I also investigated the Specific Carbohydrate Diet (SCD), which eventually led me to bone broths and the Gut and Psychology Syndrome (GAPS) diet. All the diets and ways of eating used for healing the gut and restoring healthy gut flora that I read about had a few things in common: they eliminated grains, sugars, and legumes, minimized starches, and had at least a period of eliminating dairy, and then reintroduced only fermented dairy, if any at all.

So, by chance, my diet and lifestyle ended up being paleo. One of the things that guided me into paleo was working with many individuals with gut disorders. This is an exciting area of research and we're getting a better and better understanding of this very intimate link between the gut, the immune system, and the brain.

You may be wondering, is eating the paleo way going to heal me? When healing any condition, we need to keep in mind that health is multifaceted. It is, of course, very heavily influenced by what we eat, but it is also influenced by our genetics and our epigenetics – everything that happens in life that affects whether our genes are "switched on" or not. This includes previous illnesses, environmental toxin exposure, stressful or traumatic life experiences, our thoughts and emotions, and even what kind of people we surround ourselves with – all affect our health and well-being.

While changing your diet is an important foundation from which to build your health, it may not be enough to get well. If you suffer from a chronic condition – such as irritable bowel syndrome, Crohn's disease, or ulcerative colitis, or even chronic health conditions involving other body systems – it is *really* important that you find a supportive health practitioner to guide you through the healing process. The more chronic your condition, the more important it is for you to get professional help.

Think of this book as one of the resources to help in your journey to achieving and maintaining good gut health. In the following pages, Pete and I give you all the background information, practical guidance, and wholesome recipes you need to start understanding this fundamental factor in our overall health and well-being. Personally, I'm excited to help you make the transition from surviving to thriving.

Love,
Helen

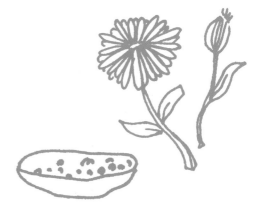

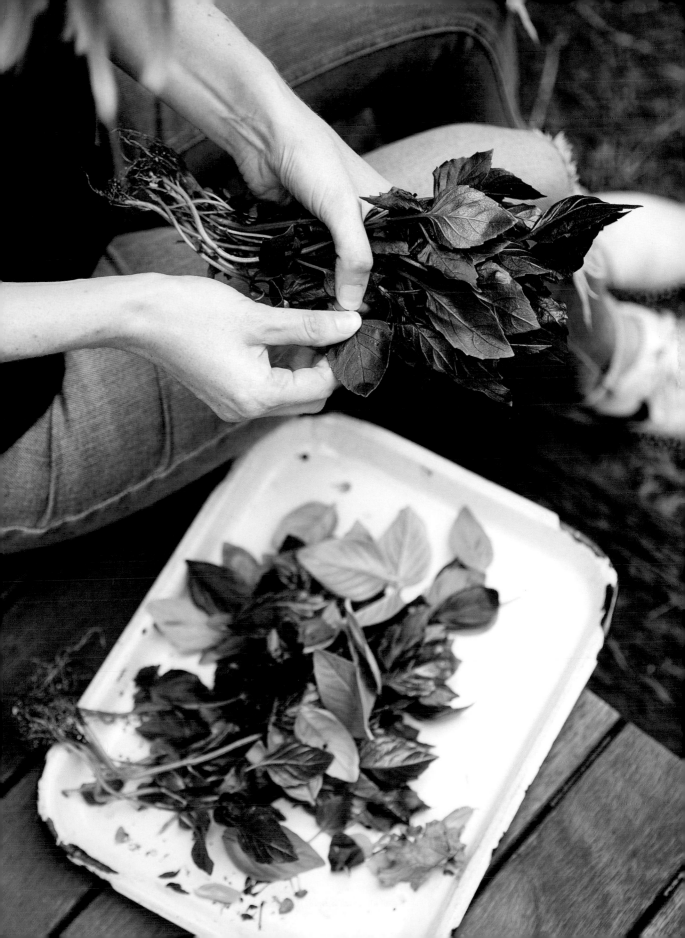

DIGESTION, LEAKY GUT, AND BUGS

To understand gut health, we need to discuss not just the parts involved, but also the function – that is, the anatomy and the physiology.

A Cook's Tour of Digestion

The term "gut" most often refers to the digestive tract, from the stomach through the small intestine and large intestine (colon) to the anus. If it was unfolded and laid out flat, the surface area of the average human digestive tract would span half a badminton court! But, of course, the digestive tract starts at the mouth, and involves accessory organs, including the salivary glands, liver, gall bladder, appendix, and pancreas.

Digestion starts before food gets to your mouth. In fact, it begins in your brain. At the mere thought of food, you will have a physical response – salivating over something you imagine to be delicious, or feeling nauseous about something repulsive. The sight, smell, and sound of food also elicit the same responses, which are an important first step in priming your gut – getting your digestive juices (acids and enzymes) to flow in preparation for the coming meal.

The brain also regulates the hormones around satiety and hunger. For example, the better nourished your cells become, the less frequently you'll need to eat and the more sensitive your leptin receptors will become (leptin is the hormone that signals to your brain that you are full. Better leptin sensitivity equals increased satiety). When your stomach shrinks, because it's empty, you produce what's referred to as the hunger hormone: ghrelin. Once your stomach is full and the walls of your stomach are stretched, secretion of ghrelin stops.

Once you take a bite of your food, mechanical and chemical digestion begin to occur in your mouth. Mechanical digestion happens in the form of chewing to break down your food into small particles and provide a greater surface area for chemical digestion to get to work on. Chewing also mixes the food with saliva to make it slippery and easy to swallow, so it can pass through the esophagus to the stomach. Chemical digestion in the mouth arises in the form of salivary enzymes, predominantly amylase, which starts to break down carbohydrates in food.

Once food is swallowed, it travels through your esophagus and into your stomach, where further chemical and mechanical digestion occurs. Cells in the lining of your stomach produce hydrochloric acid (HCl), which has a pH of roughly 2. That's acidic enough to burn your finger! The

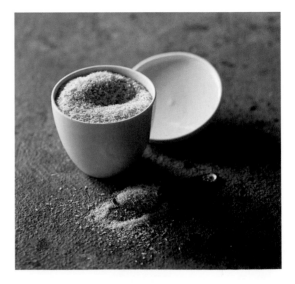

CELL RENEWAL – CONSTANTLY BUILDING A NEW YOU

The cells lining the surface of the intestine are in a constant state of renewal and are replaced every 2–8 days. The ones that secrete antimicrobial agents last a little longer. Each time they renew, the food choices you make either improve the renewal process or damage it.

Cells lining the stomach last 5 days.

Liver cells are replaced roughly every 300–500 days.

Oxygen-carrying red blood cells last 4 months.

White blood cells (our immune system) are replaced at startlingly high rates. Neutrophils last for just a few hours, while lymphocytes are replaced at a rate of 10,000 cells every second!

The surface layer of the skin is replaced roughly every 2 weeks.

The average age of a muscle cell is 15 years.

Head hair lasts roughly 6–7 years.

duodenum. It's really important that this chyme is quite acidic, because the more acidic it is, the more bicarb ions are released by the pancreas to buffer the acid. The more bicarb that is produced, the more digestive enzymes the pancreas releases into the small intestine. These enzymes include amylase (for carbohydrates), proteases (trypsin, chymotrypsin, and carboxypeptidase for proteins) and lipases (for fats), as well as enzymes that break down RNA and DNA (ribonuclease and deoxyribonuclease) so that the "identity tags" are taken from your food molecules in order to be rebuilt as your own cells with your own DNA (that is, your own "identity tags").

When chyme empties into the small intestine, receptors in the cells of the intestinal wall detect how much fat and protein are in the mix. When protein and fat are detected, the cells produce a hormone (cholecystokinin or CCK) that enters the bloodstream, travels to the gall bladder, and triggers the gall bladder to contract and release bile acids. (Bile acids are produced in the liver and sent to the gall bladder for storage until required.) Bile emulsifies fat molecules, making them smaller and easier for pancreatic lipases to get to work on.

If your gut was unfolded and laid out flat, it would span half a badminton court.

Once the chyme has been worked upon by pancreatic enzymes and bile, the small intestine begins to absorb the nutrients. The small intestine, with a diameter of roughly 1 inch, has varying lengths from person to person, but averages 20 feet. It has a wrinkly wall lined with finger-like projections called villi, which themselves

stomach lining also produces protective mucous to form a barrier between the acidic contents and the stomach wall. Stomach acid is particularly important for breaking down proteins and is also essential for the absorption of an array of minerals, including calcium, magnesium, and iron. To make sure food is well combined with the acid, the muscles of the stomach wall squeeze and churn to get a good mix.

Depending on the meal, within 30 minutes to 2 hours the mix of food and acid (called chyme) leaves the stomach and enters the first part of the small intestine – the are covered in smaller projections called microvilli that increase the surface area of the small intestine by 60–120 times. This surface area provides a greater capacity to absorb nutrients.

After traveling along the 20 feet of your small intestine, what's left of your meal passes through your ileocecal valve and arrives in your large intestine. At this point there is actually little left that you can digest yourself. This is where, given the right pH, your gut flora get to work, breaking down fibers that we humans cannot digest. As a result, the gut microbes produce a range of nutrients as by-products, including short-chain fatty acids, amino acids (such as tryptophan, tyrosine, and phenylalanine) and vitamins (such as biotin, B vitamins, vitamin K), as well as coenzyme Q10. These microbes in our gut are nutrient-producing factories, so you want to keep a healthy collection of them. Without the right ones, we can get undesirable acid production, changing the pH of the large intestine to be more acidic (it should be neutral or only slightly acidic), producing more gas (hello bloating!), and resulting in a deficiency of the key nutrients that help to keep the gut wall in mint condition.

TRANSIT TIME & RETENTION TIME

Transit time is how long it takes for the first part of a meal to exit your bowels. The ideal transit time is 15–17 hours. This is easy to measure by taking something like a tablespoon of activated charcoal powder (see page 92) in water, which results in unmistakable black stools.

Retention time is the time it takes for the entire contents of a single meal to pass through your gut. So, from when you

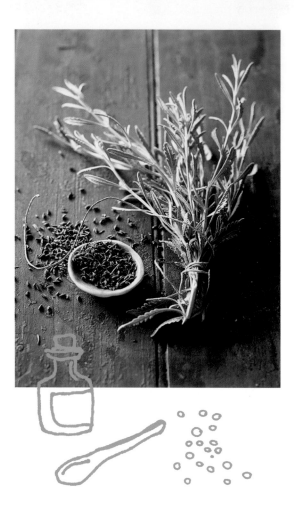

swallowed the charcoal in water to the last time you see the charcoal in the toilet bowl.

Ideal retention time is 55–72 hours. Less than this indicates that there may be irritation, inflammation, or infection, resulting in food moving through too fast so that it doesn't provide adequate time for digestion and absorption of nutrients. On the other hand, if transit and retention times are too long, this may indicate issues with liver or pancreatic function or poor gut motility, resulting in reabsorption into the bloodstream of compounds that the body is trying to eliminate. Slow transit and retention times create a double-up of work for the liver, and may result in constipation, skin, or lung problems.

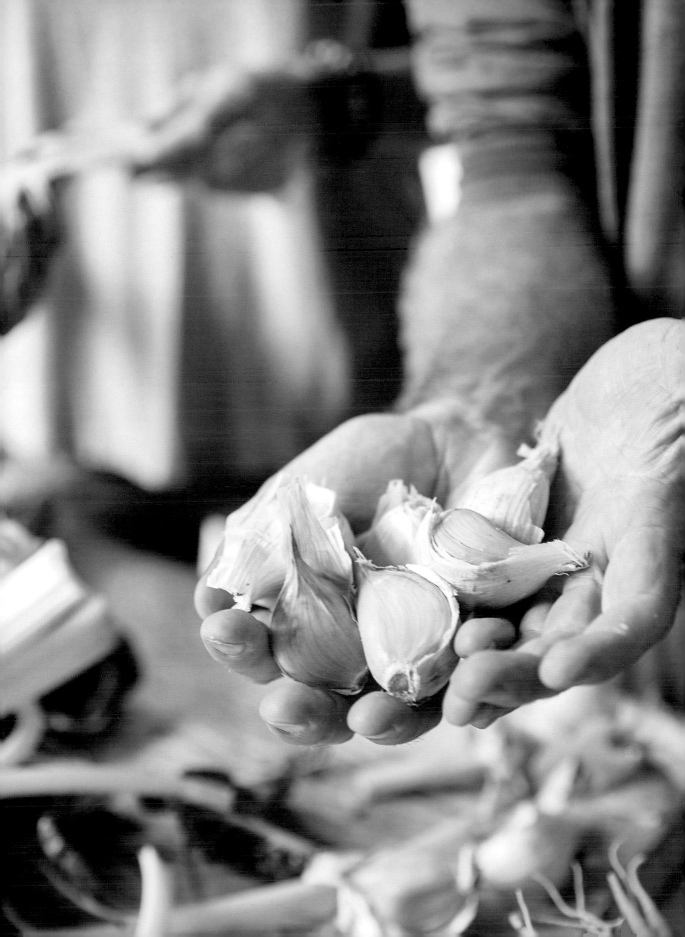

A Bug's Disrupted Life: What is Dysbiosis?

"Gut flora," the "human microbiome" and "gut bugs" are all names given to the population of microbes (bacteria, yeasts, parasites) living in the gut. These tenants we play host to outnumber our own cells 10 to 1. That's right: there are 10 times as many of them living in and on us as there are human cells. We are actually more bug than human. And we need them. Without these bugs, we wouldn't be here. So essential to our existence are they, that the microbiome is now being considered by many as another organ of the human body. They help to regulate our immune function, metabolize cholesterol and hormones, produce neurotransmitters, make health-giving short-chain fatty acids, vitamins, and amino acids, and digest fibers for us. However, with the wrong mix of bugs in the gut, a multitude of things can go wrong. Disrupted or imbalanced gut flora – an undergrowth *or* overgrowth of good bacteria – is called dysbiosis (literally "disruption of life"!). When dysbiosis occurs, the normally life-giving, health-promoting populations of bugs can end up becoming a source of stress and injury themselves. Overgrowths of opportunistic bacteria and yeasts produce waste products that, among other things, alter the pH of our intestines and our tissues, increase intestinal permeability (leaky gut), and affect our ability to sleep, think, and defend ourselves from infection.

There is increasing evidence (see pages 24–27 and references at the end of the book) that gut bug balance may be implicated in a range of disorders, including inflammatory bowel disease, thyroid disease, rheumatoid arthritis, allergies, asthma, obesity, depression, anxiety, and more. And it's a two-way street. Disorders of different systems and organs can also disrupt our gut flora.

Disrupted gut flora is called dysbiosis (literally "disruption of life"!). When dysbiosis occurs, the normally life-giving, health-promoting bugs can end up becoming a source of stress and injury themselves.

Leaky Gut

No, it's not a case of your belly button springing a leak! Let me explain by first showing you what happens in a healthy gut. Imagine food is like a string of pearls. As the string of pearls moves through your digestive tract, thanks to both mechanical and chemical digestion, the strands become much shorter.

Once in the small intestine, your "string of pearls" has now been broken down into single, double, or triple pearls – no long strands are left. These pearls can then fit through the *very* tightly joined gaps between the cells lining your small intestine (the gaps are so tight they are called tight junctions – no awards for creativity there!) or through the cells themselves. On the other side of the small intestinal cells are tiny, tiny blood capillaries and lymph vessels (part of your immune and detox systems). The blood capillaries take up the nutrient (the pearl), and so begins its journey first to the liver, and then around the rest of the body to where it's needed.

So that's a tight gut. A leaky gut – officially termed "intestinal hyperpermeability" – occurs when there are *leaky* junctions instead of tight ones. The gaps between the cells lining the intestine get ever so slightly wider. This small increase in gap size results in a much broader range of compounds – from partially digested food (think strands of five or ten pearls), to microbes and toxins – being able to pass through. This then puts the immune system on red alert, as it identifies these larger molecules as invaders, resulting in an inflammatory response. Inflammation is important – we need it to heal our tissues. When we have leaky gut, however, inflammation becomes chronic and results in tissue damage. Having a leaky gut means you may potentially end up with inflammation in any part of your body, depending on your personal and family history, your environment, and your genetics. You may get inflammation in your big toe (gout), it could be in your fingers (arthritis); it could be in your brain (depression or dementia); or it could be the trigger for an autoimmune cascade, resulting in conditions such as Hashimoto's thyroiditis (an underactive and/or overactive thyroid), multiple sclerosis, diabetes, lupus, psoriasis, rheumatoid arthritis, and more. Migraines and seasonal allergies such as hayfever are commonly linked to leaky gut, and syndromes such as chronic fatigue and fibromyalgia are also believed to involve a leaky gut.

SO HOW DOES A GUT GET LEAKY?

A number of factors cause increased permeability of the gut wall, including stress, lack of sleep, some medications, toxins, and health conditions such as giardia infections, celiac disease, and inflammatory bowel disease. When it comes to diet, foods that are particularly high in starches, especially processed ones, and sugars can disrupt our gut bugs. And when our gut flora is out of balance, the protection normally provided by gut bugs is compromised, and so the integrity of the gut wall may be breached.

POTENTIAL SIGNS AND SYMPTOMS OF A LEAKY GUT:

* Allergies, including hayfever
* Asthma
* Bloating
* Brain fog
* Burping
* Chronic or recurrent headaches
* Constipation, diarrhea, or alternating between the two
* Difficulty gaining weight
* Difficulty losing weight
* Fatty liver
* Fluid retention
* Food intolerances
* Gas
* Heartburn/reflux
* Hives
* Increased visceral (abdominal) fat
* Joint pain
* Migraine
* Muscle pain
* Period pain
* Skin rashes

What does a leaky gut look like?

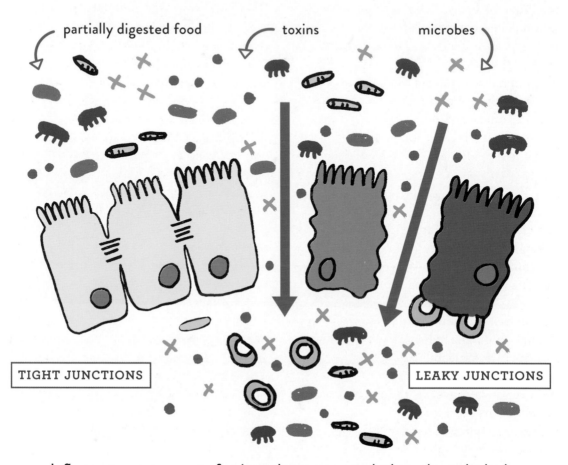

partially digested food

toxins

microbes

TIGHT JUNCTIONS

LEAKY JUNCTIONS

Inflammatory response to foreign substances spreads throughout the body

A leaky gut occurs when there are leaky junctions instead of tight ones between the cells lining the intestine. This results in a much broader range of compounds — from partially digested food to microbes and toxins — being able to pass through. This then puts the immune system on red alert, as it identifies these larger molecules as invaders, resulting in an inflammatory response.

ATTENTION DEFICIT HYPERACTIVITY DISORDER (ADHD)

ADHD involves impaired or diminished attention combined with impulsivity and hyperactivity. Food choices, food additives, and gut and bowel problems may all be implicated in the expression of ADHD.

AUTISM

Autism is a developmental disorder most commonly diagnosed by three years of age. Once thought to be a psychiatric disorder, current research shows that autism is a whole-body disorder, resulting in neurological (cognitive, behavioral, and developmental) symptoms. Whole-body issues that may relate to features of autism involve problems within the gut, immune dysregulation, and disruptions in metabolic pathways and mitochondrial function.

AUTOIMMUNE DISEASES

There are dozens of autoimmune diseases and many are on the rise. These include rheumatoid arthritis, Hashimoto's thyroiditis, multiple sclerosis, psoriasis, lupus, and type 1 diabetes. While each of these disorders is named according to the organ or system it affects, its expression involves dysregulation of the immune system. Gut microflora play crucial roles in regulating immune function, and a leaky gut can often predispose one to autoimmune activity due to absorption of molecules into the bloodstream that otherwise would not be allowed entry. The absorption of these foreign molecules mounts an inflammatory response that can drive autoimmune activity.

BRAIN FOG

Brain fog is a very common experience for those with inflammatory bowel symptoms and bacterial or yeast overgrowths in the gut. Inflammation and by-products from microbial overgrowth affect cognitive function, resulting in cloudy thinking.

CHRONIC FATIGUE SYNDROME (CFS)

CFS is a poorly defined condition due to the large array of symptoms that can be present in different individuals. Onset is often after exposure to a virus. At its core, it is characterized by a persistent profound fatigue and is usually accompanied by other symptoms such as headaches, depression, anxiety, and tender lymph nodes (the latter in particular indicating that an immune response is at play). As we've discussed, the immune system both inside and outside of the gut is heavily influenced by gut flora and gut permeability, so addressing gut health provides a crucial foundation on which to provide further interventions for CFS.

CROHN'S DISEASE AND ULCERATIVE COLITIS

These inflammatory bowel diseases (IBD) are most prevalent in the Western world, although developing countries experiencing an increasing rate of industrialization are now also exhibiting higher rates of IBD. IBD is largely autoimmune in nature and, as such, is a result of immune dysregulation. Immune system regulation is managed in large part by permeability of the gut barrier and the microflora in the gut. Low vitamin D levels due to lack of sun exposure are also thought to be contributing factors, due to the regulatory role vitamin D plays in the immune system.

DEPRESSION

Depression is a state in which one feels an overwhelming sadness, hopelessness, disconnection, and unworthiness. It is often accompanied by poor concentration, inactivity, insomnia, and sometimes suicidal tendencies. Immune cell activation in the brain, leaky gut, and dysbiosis are all important factors to consider when treating depression.

DIABETES

A serious disease in which the body is unable to properly control blood sugar levels due to either lack of production of insulin by the pancreas (type 1 diabetes) or decreased sensitivity to insulin (type 2 diabetes). Type 1 diabetes is certainly autoimmune in nature. Type 2 diabetes is largely metabolic and potentially also has autoimmune implications. Treatment for both conditions is heavily influenced by dietary and lifestyle choices. Healing the gut wall and restoring healthy gut flora can be a powerful way to help regulate immune function and improve metabolic features in both forms of diabetes.

DIVERTICULITIS

Diverticulitis is an inflammatory disease of the bowel that occurs when pouches in the bowel wall, called diverticuli, become inflamed. The diverticuli are often formed in the first place due to weakness in the muscular wall of the colon, which can be brought about by a history of chronic constipation. Inflammation often occurs as a result of debris or bacteria becoming trapped in the pouches. Restoring digestive function and gut wall integrity and improving bowel flora all have a big impact on reducing the effects of diverticulitis.

ECZEMA

An inflammatory skin condition characterized by redness, itching, weeping, crusting, and scaling. The link between early-in-life disturbances to gut flora and onset of eczema has been well established (for example, being born by caesarean section increases the risk of developing eczema, due to lack of exposure to mom's microbiome in the birth canal). Using diet to optimize gut flora and function can help with eczema, even in adulthood.

FIBROMYALGIA

Fibromyalgia is a syndrome characterized by widespread muscle pain, joint stiffness, and severe fatigue, making even simple daily tasks overwhelming and exhausting. Anxiety and/or depression are commonly present as well. It is more prevalent in people who have celiac disease, irritable bowel syndrome, and non-celiac gluten sensitivity.

HAYFEVER

An allergic reaction with symptoms of sneezing, watery eyes, and sometimes a cough. Tiredness and trouble concentrating may also be experienced when hayfever is present. As most of the immune system resides in the gut and immune regulation is linked to populations of gut flora, addressing the health of both may improve the allergy response, and this is certainly something I regularly see in clinic.

IRRITABLE BOWEL SYNDROME (IBS)

IBS is a functional gastrointestinal disorder, meaning that as far as modern medicine is concerned, there is no physical abnormality contributing to the condition. Common symptoms are abdominal bloating, abdominal cramps, and nausea, along with diarrhea and/or constipation. Common contributing factors to IBS include dysbiosis, stress, and insufficient production of digestive acids or enzymes. Supporting digestion and restoring gut flora can help improve the quality of life for many who suffer what can be a quite debilitating illness.

MIGRAINES

Migraine incidence is often associated with

gastrointestinal disorders. As with all health conditions, other factors may certainly be involved, but in my clinical experience great benefit to migraine sufferers is seen when issues surrounding the gut and inflammation are addressed.

MULTIPLE SCLEROSIS (MS)

MS is a chronic autoimmune disease in which the protective coating of the nerves in the central nervous system (the myelin sheath) is destroyed. The myelin sheath speeds up the rate at which information travels along nerves. Where the myelin is destroyed, patches of scar tissue (plaque) form, further disrupting nerve communication. The resulting symptoms are affected movement (including tremors and, eventually, the inability to walk), neurological sensations, and loss of bodily functions. Evidence suggests that the gut microbiota affects the development and function of microglia (the immune cells in the central nervous system), and that gut microbes can affect antibody development against myelin (meaning the immune system attacking the myelin sheath). Researchers are currently looking into the questions around gut flora's effects on neurological tissue and function.

POLYCYSTIC OVARY SYNDROME (PCOS)

PCOS is a metabolic disorder affecting multiple systems, but predominantly influencing women's hormone regulation. Symptoms include painful periods, acne, menstrual pain, and possibly infertility. PCOS is commonly associated with metabolic conditions such as insulin resistance, diabetes, and cardiovascular disease, and is also linked to leaky gut. Zonulin, a marker for leaky gut, is increased in women who have PCOS and correlates with insulin resistance and menstrual disorders. This indicates that gut permeability may play a role in the process of PCOS. A recent study has shown that women who have PCOS and have higher levels of zonulin have fewer menstrual cycles. Reducing zonulin and gut permeability may play an important role in addressing PCOS.

PREMENSTRUAL TENSION (PMS)

PMS occurs in the lead-up to some women's menstruation, when there is a state called estrogen dominance – in which the amount or activity of estrogen outshines that of progesterone. This can result in symptoms of breast tenderness, breast swelling and/or cysts, changes in mood, fluid retention, low energy, and headaches. Estrogen dominance can also result from exposure to estrogens found in certain plastics, pesticides, fragrances, and cosmetics. It can also result from the body's inability to eliminate excess estrogen, which in turn is potentially affected by constipation and disruptions in gut flora.

PSORIASIS

Psoriasis is an autoimmune disorder affecting the skin and, in severe cases, the joints. It causes raised red scaly patches to appear on the skin, most commonly on the knees, elbows, and scalp. It can itch, burn and/or sting, and is often associated with altered gut flora as well as other serious chronic inflammatory conditions, including inflammatory bowel diseases, diabetes, depression, and heart disease.

ROSACEA

Rosacea is a chronic inflammatory condition resulting in redness of the skin on the face (especially the nose and cheeks) caused by dilation of capillaries (tiny blood vessels). It can also present with acne-like pimples. Rosacea often occurs in combination with gastrointestinal disorders such as small intestinal bacterial overgrowth (SIBO).

THE GUT, THE BRAIN, AND THE IMMUNE SYSTEM

All systems in the body are intricately connected, so it's impossible to talk about gut health without discussing the immune system and the brain, in particular.

The following fascinating facts will help you understand just how intimately intertwined the gut, brain, and immune system are:

① About 80 percent of your immune system is in your gut (in the gastrointestinal associated lymphatic tissue – known as GALT). Current research is teaching us more and more about how the kind of bacteria, yeasts, and parasites you have living in your gut affect how your immune system responds to different triggers (such as potential pathogens or allergens).

② You have more neurons in your gut than you do in your brain. This collection of neurons is known as the enteric nervous system. It's how you get "gut feelings."

③ You have more immune cells (microglia) in your brain than you have brain cells.

> *You have more neurons in your gut than you do in your brain.*

THE VAGUS NERVE

The vagus nerve is a long and wandering nerve that originates in your cerebellum and brain stem, and regulates the "rest-and-digest" (parasympathetic) and "fight-or-flight" (sympathetic) functions of your digestive system and visceral organs. It is essentially the translator between your gut and brain – with messages going both ways.

To aid good digestion, we want our nervous system to be in rest-and-digest mode. Here are some quick tips for soothing the nervous system and getting the vagus nerve ready to make digestion happen:

Gargle. Gargle each day for 30 seconds, or as long as you can. Have a little break. Repeat. Repeat this process three times.

Meditate. Whether it's for 1 minute or 1 hour. Research shows that even mini-meditations have an astounding impact on nerve function.

Breathe. We often forget to do this properly! Slow down your breathing for 10 breaths. Close your eyes if you like. Breathe in slowly for a count of 4, hold for 1 second then exhale completely for a count of 6. Repeat 10 times. Remember to breathe into your abdomen first, then let your breath fill your chest.

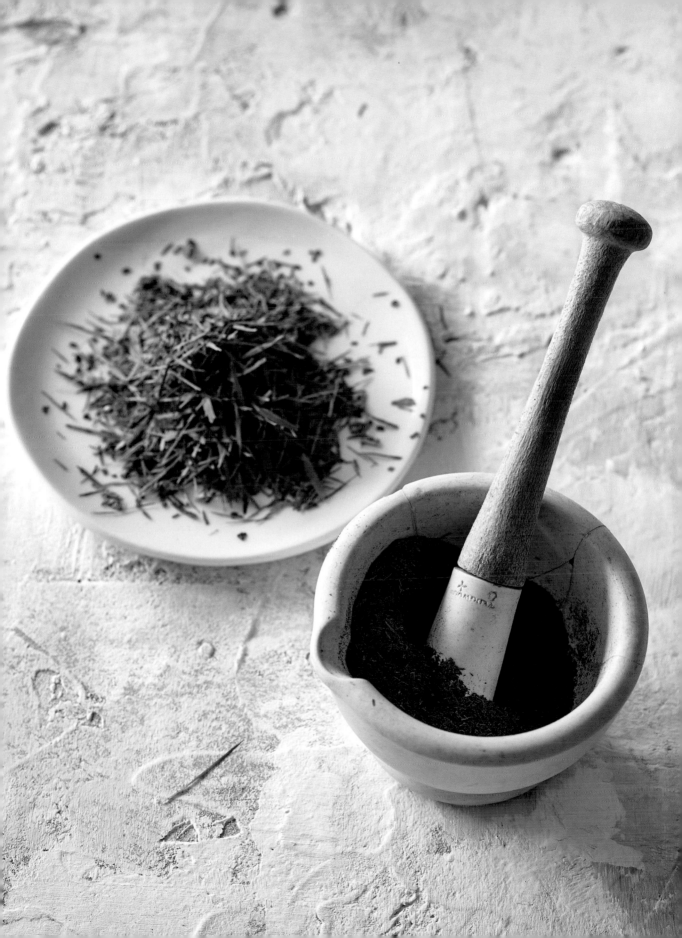

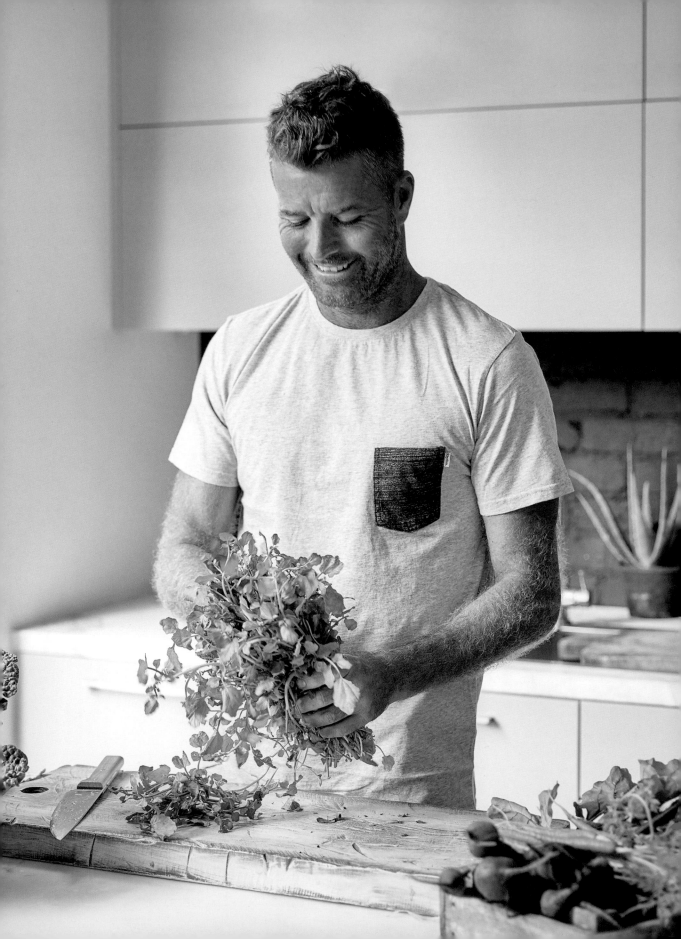

GUT DISRUPTERS

A number of factors influence the leakiness of your gut and your overall digestive function. These factors may affect people to differing degrees, depending on health status, genetic issues, stress levels, and environmental situation. Once again, it is important to note that this is an emerging area of science and the research in some areas is still in its infancy.

FACTORS THAT MAY CAUSE DIGESTIVE TRACT DAMAGE:

* Alcohol
* Antacids
* Antibiotics
* Artificial sweeteners such as sucralose (Splenda)
* Burn injuries
* Chemotherapeutic drugs such as Methotrexate
* Coffee
* Dysbiosis (gut flora imbalance)
* Environmental toxins
* Gluten
* Herbicides and pesticides (including cupric sulphate and glyphosphate)
* High-starch diet
* Lack of sleep
* Lectins
* NSAIDs (nonsteroidal anti-inflammatory drugs) such as aspirin, ibuprofen, diclofenac, meloxicam, naproxen

* Organ dysfunction
* Over-training
* Parasite infections and pathogens
* Partially digested food particles
* Processed dairy
* Steroid medications
* Stress
* Sugar
* Vitamin A deficiency
* Zinc deficiency

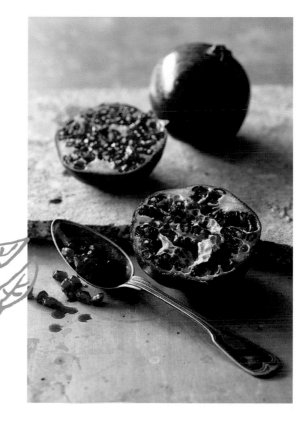

UNDERSTANDING GUT HEALING

The great thing about improving your gut health (and overall well-being) is that it's never too late to start. The journey of healing, particularly if a condition has been around for a long time, is a gradual process. Healing is not a race. It happens one step at a time, and requires patience and awareness. Nourish and hydrate your body, provide yourself with the greatest self-care, and allow your body to do the rest.

Personalized healing (n = 1)

Awareness is a big part of the journey. Some of us in our rushed lives become disconnected from our bodies (and minds – both the one in our head and the one in our gut!), then one day suddenly notice significant symptoms. More often there have been niggling signs along the way before full-blown symptoms and diseases come into play. This is your body's very wise pain messenger. If you don't listen to the more subtle messages, pain will start to yell "Hey you! I've been trying to tell you something, but you haven't been listening, so I'm going to say this in a way you can no longer ignore!" So, rather than scold your pain and suppress it, learn to befriend it. It is your teacher. As you begin to change your food choices and lifestyle, you will start to notice what suits you and what doesn't. That is your guide. Follow it.

In clinical studies, "n" indicates the number of people involved in the trial. If you see a paper stating n = 1574, that means there were 1574 people in the study. It is often considered more important to have larger numbers of people in a study. And sure, there's some value in that; however, it also means the results are based on an average of 1574 people (or however many people are in any given study). That means recommendations given as a result of the study are based on that average. But, obviously, clinical trials, no matter how thorough, cannot account for all our individual variables The most significant clinical trial you can do is your own: n = 1. Your observation of yourself and how you respond to any given food, herb, nutrient, activity, or medication. No two people are identical. Even though a particular food is theoretically good for you, it may be that you have a sensitivity or reaction to it. In that case, there's no point in forcing it.

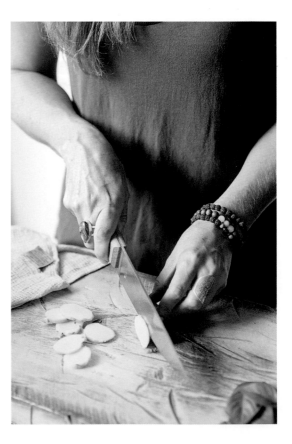

DAILY HABITS FOR GUT HEALTH

Quiet time. Quiet time energizes us and enables us to function more efficiently and with more enjoyment. Pick the quiet time that sings to you – meditation, gentle walking in nature, chi gong, tai chi, gentle yoga, deep-breathing practices. Aim for 10 minutes daily. If you do 20 or 30 minutes, fantastic!

Drink good-quality filtered and remineralised water. As well as removing undesirable substances, most water filters remove the good stuff too – including minerals that act as electrolytes to facilitate water absorption. Remineralised water is filtered water with the beneficial minerals added back in.

Remember, you are made up of about 75 percent water, and need water for nearly all your body functions – for example, to make enzymes and digestive acids to carry nutrients into cells and toxins out. Drink 64 fluid ounces (8 cups) per day, or ½ fluid ounce per pound of body weight.

- Start each day with a glass of warm water, mixed with the juice of ½ lemon and a tiny pinch of "dirty" sea salt (sea salt that is a bit grayish in color, damp in texture, and high in minerals).

Chew your food, chew your smoothies, swish your liquids. It's amazing how something this simple can transform your digestion. Aim for twenty chews per mouthful.

Eat in a calm state and a calm environment so that you're in rest-and-digest mode.

Move. Our bodily systems, including our digestion, work like pumps. Movement helps these pumps to function.

- Activities that twist, bend and stretch the abdomen are particularly great for facilitating the pumping of the digestive system. If you're fatigued or chronically ill, keep in mind you may need to keep your movement gentle and avoid anything high-intensity.

Get 8 hours of sleep a night. This allows for tissue repair and replacement, and for healthy hormone and neurotransmitter production. The rhythm and flow of a good night's sleep every night will greatly help the rhythm and flow of your digestion and bowel habits.

Write down what brings you joy without the need for another person. Whatever it is that lifts your spirit, brings a sparkle to your eye, or makes you talk really fast! Then schedule a joy time at least once a week.

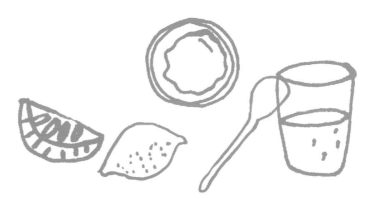

TESTIMONIALS

"I have always had a "funny tummy," but a few years ago it got noticeably worse. I saw a series of doctors and was eventually diagnosed with irritable bowel syndrome. Not really satisfied with that diagnosis, I started making dietary changes to see if I could find the trigger causing the constant trips to the bathroom. I gave up sugar, then gluten, then lactose, but nothing seemed to make any difference.

In early 2015, I joined The Paleo Way program. I read stories of other people on the program healing their irritable bowel, but 6 weeks into the program I was still spending way too much time in the bathroom. After doing some research and stalking Helen Padarin's Q&A on Facebook, I decided to make an appointment. I met Helen with a healthy dose of scepticism and a desperation to not have my bowel in charge of my life any more. After some testing, Helen diagnosed me with gut dysbiosis and a parasite. Helen convinced me to go 100 percent paleo and ditch the dairy and lingering grains. She also put me on a regime of supplements to kill off the "bad" bacteria in my gut and replace them with "good" bacteria. It was magic. I started feeling better within a few weeks. My urgency to visit the bathroom many, many times per day disappeared. I am now "normal" for the first time in my life.

There have been several other benefits to enjoying improved gut health, too. I have lost 24 pounds. I no longer experience the red face associated with rosacea. I no longer have stomach cramping and discomfort after I eat. I'm no longer bloated. I no longer go through a box of tissues every few weeks from a near-constant runny nose. Best of all, I feel like I am in control for the first time in a long time, instead of having my "funny tummy" in control of me."

CHRISTY, AGE 45

"I was diagnosed with mild ulcerative colitis at the age of 21. As I hailed from a family of doctors, I was immediately put on medications as part of the conventional treatment. Unfortunately, the drugs never did much for me and a year later I was diagnosed with severe ulcerative colitis with cancerous cells. I was shocked, as I was doing everything according to my doctors' instructions.

In my quest for a better life and a cure, I met the most renowned doctors in Sydney and Delhi. However, I was repeatedly told the same thing: that ulcerative colitis isn't curable and as I was not responding well to medication I would have to get a colectomy.

Fortunately, my search for an alternative treatment lead me to Helen Padarin's website. I liked what I read about her approach to healing the gut through nutritional interventions. Under Helen's guidance my symptoms subsided within weeks, and within months I could carry on with my life like a normal healthy person. After two years following her protocol I had no symptoms whatsoever of ulcerative colitis.

It's now been six years and I would have to say I have the strongest digestion amongst all my friends and family. Touch wood!"

CHANDNI, AGE 30

" Growing up in an Italian family, my life has always centered around food – the preparation, the sharing, and the family events fill up my memories. My weight has always been concentrated around my middle area, and I was constantly bloated and lethargic. I just got used to it and this was my kind of normal. Gut health was not a topic anyone knew anything about.

Six years ago, after having my son, I was eventually diagnosed with ulcerative colitis. I remember crying on the way home from the doctor with the realization that I would be on medication for the rest of my life. So began the process of flare-up and treatment, flare-up and treatment. I have never believed in long-term medication, so this was an adjustment I was not happy about. The specialist had nothing to offer me other than more or stronger medication that would eventually impact my liver and kidneys. This was not a road I was prepared to go down.

It wasn't until three years ago, after some pretty major life-changing events, that I started to investigate just what gut health meant and the impact that it could have on all areas of my life and my health. At one point a specialist mentioned that the inflammation in my body was greater than I had anticipated. I had no idea that it was an autoimmune disease or even what an autoimmune disease was. And so began the path that has changed not only my own health, but that of all my family.

There is no going back; this is my life now. The results and impact on my health have been phenomenal. I'm not perfect and some small imperfections occasionally slip past the lips, but I know this is the best thing for me. My only struggle and loss that I feel is for my son, and our Italian culture. It was such a major part of my growing up that I don't want it to be lost forever, so I endeavour to adapt as many favorites as I can, and keep the tradition alive in our family. **"**

ANNA MARIA, AGE 42

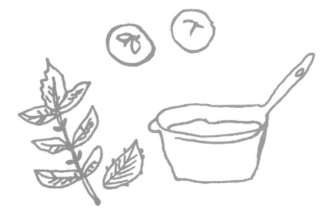

A NATUROPATHIC APPROACH TO HEALING YOUR GUT

When you have a troubled gut, there's rarely a single cause. Indeed, there's often a whole range of factors, which all overlap. In order to heal your gut, you need to look at all of the factors involved in gut wellness. Rather than seeing it from the perspective of "what do I need to do to treat IBS?" or "what do I need to do to ease my bloating?" or "how do I eliminate my brain fog?" look at it like this: what do I need to do to have a healthy gut? A visit to a qualified health practitioner with experience in this area is the best place to start. Regardless of the label given to your symptoms, most of the time the requirements to heal are pretty similar (if not identical). The emphasis put on particular aspects may vary, but all aspects need to be given attention. So let's look at what they are.

1. Address acute inflammation

This is number one, because if there is an acute state of inflammation going on, it's not the time to be focusing on causes. Just ask anyone who is having a flare-up of Crohn's disease or ulcerative colitis. There's no point trying to clean the house while it's on fire. Put the fire out first, then start the clean-up. This is achieved by a combination of eliminating the most common dietary triggers of inflammation and by utilizing foods, herbs, and nutrients to help dampen the inflammatory response. Some people may also require medication. It's always best to consult with your healthcare professional to address this acute stage of inflammation.

2. Improve gut wall integrity

This is the wound-healing aspect. Once the fire is out, we can focus on the rebuild. When there's irritation or inflammation in the gut wall, it's much like having a wound in the gut. It could be microdamage – only visible under a microscope – or it could be quite significant and visible, as ulcers are when a scope is sent down your tube to investigate. The cells in the gut wall are responsible for the production of mucous, digestive enzymes, and immune compounds. These cells need to be in good condition to absorb nutrients into the bloodstream and block absorption of toxins. By putting some initial attention into providing support to heal this one-cell-thick layer of lining, you'll be in a better place to improve your digestion, absorption, inflammation control, immune function, and overall gut health.

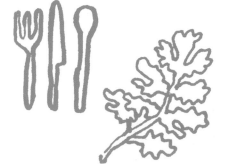

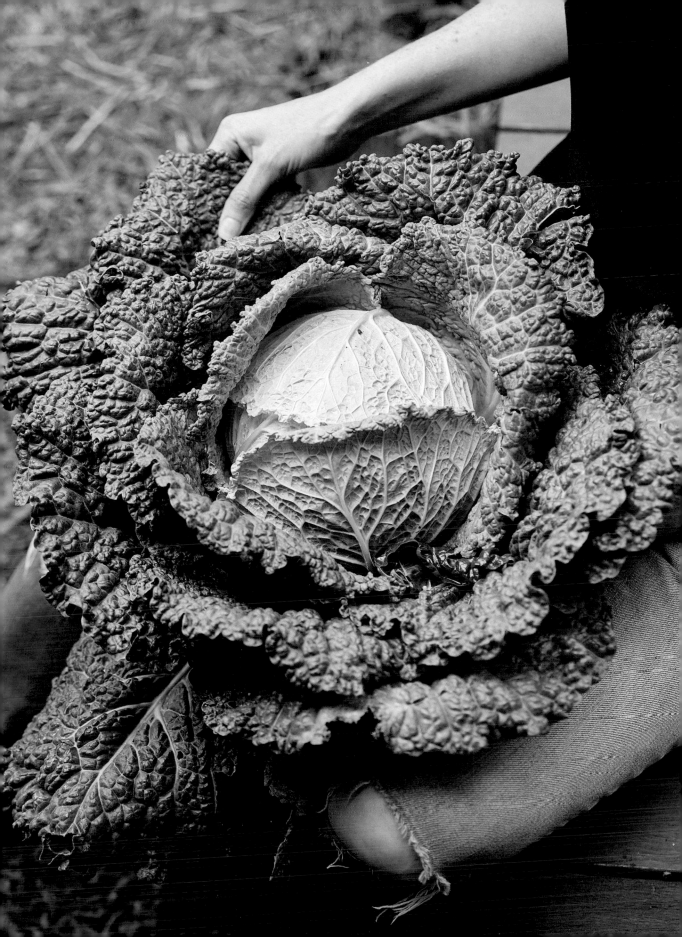

3. Support the function of digestive organs

Digestion, of course, is not just about the gut. It is very much about the accessory organs of digestion, including the brain, the liver, the gall bladder, and the pancreas.

THE BRAIN

Digestion, as we've seen, starts in the brain. The mere thought or smell of food can result in your mouth watering and your stomach acid production kicking into gear, ready for the arrival of morsels to process. For this to occur, you need to make sure your brain is sending and receiving the right messages of rest and digest – what's called the parasympathetic response of the autonomic nervous system. When we are in a state of fear, anxiety, anger, stress, or worry, our nervous system is in fight-or-flight mode (sympathetic response). The brain thinks we're in danger, so the priority is to run, not to digest. Energy and blood are sent to areas of the body that will help to get us out of danger, quickly. That means pupils dilate, heart rate increases, and blood flow to skeletal muscles increases (while blood flow to abdominal organs decreases). In prehistoric times, these episodes would have been short-lived. But with our stressed-out modern lifestyles it is easy to get stuck in fight-or-flight mode for long periods of time.

In rest-and-digest mode, your body produces salivary enzymes, digestive acids, and pancreatic enzymes, and readies your gall bladder to expel bile as needed.

The more patients I see, and the more I repair my own digestion, the more I understand how stress affects digestion. When we are stressed, our bodies produce stress hormones that, among other things, drive our cravings for sugar and prevent us from burning our fat stores. Mindfulness is one practice that can help.

HOW TO EAT MINDFULLY

Pay attention to your food. What does it taste/smell/feel/sound like? Make eating a meditative practice.

Be grateful. Before tucking in, take a moment to be grateful for the food you have.

Turn off the screen. Vision takes up an extraordinary amount of energy. Switch off your TV/phone/tablet/computer so that your mind (and eyes) can focus on your food.

THE LIVER AND GALL BLADDER

Our livers are amazing organs that perform hundreds of roles in the body, including neutralizing toxins, manufacturing proteins and hormones, controlling blood sugar, assisting blood-clotting, and fighting infection. The liver is also an important digestive organ because it produces bile, which is stored in the gall bladder. When you eat a meal with fat in it, a hormone response triggers your gall bladder to contract, squirting bile into your small intestine. Bile is responsible for emulsifying fats, or turning big globules of fat into tiny droplets – kind of like dishwashing detergent. Being in tiny droplets increases the surface area of the fat on which the pancreatic enzymes can work, making for a better digestion job. If the duct that carries bile from the liver to the gall bladder and to the small intestine gets blocked, bile backs up into the liver and gets into the bloodstream, causing yellowing of the skin and eyes (jaundice).

When the gall bladder is removed, there is no storage site for bile. That means the liver needs to work on demand to produce bile. When you consider the number of roles the liver plays, this is no small ask. As a result, it is very common for those with no gall bladder to develop deficiencies of essential fatty acids and fat-soluble vitamins. It is advisable if you have had your gall bladder removed to take a bile salt supplement with each meal, and a liver support herbal supplement daily to help prevent deficiencies down the track.

How to love your liver and gall bladder

To support your liver, clean up your food and your environment. The less overloaded your liver is from having to process toxins, the more effectively it will function. Following the principles in this book of eating easy-to-digest, nourishing, toxin-free food is the way to go. Ditch the sugars, grains, and dairy. No more artificial colorings, flavorings, preservatives or flavor enhancers. The term "natural" is a very loose one and often hardly resembles the natural substance at all, so I recommend you steer clear of any "naturally" flavored foods too.

In our environment, the greatest source of controllable toxin exposure comes from what we put on our bodies and what we use in our households. Many fragrant chemicals used in our skincare, beauty, hygiene, and household cleaning products are known toxins, carcinogens, or immune and hormone disrupters. Avoid products that are scented with anything other than pure essential oils. Reducing your toxin exposure will enable your liver to focus on digestion and burning fat for energy, rather than always playing catch-up trying to protect us from toxic chemicals.

When we are in a state of fear, anxiety, anger, stress, or worry, it means our nervous system is in fight-or-flight mode. The brain thinks we're in danger, so the priority is to run, not to digest.

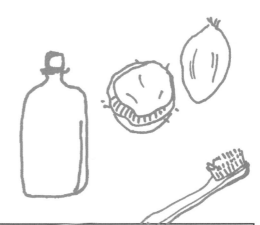

DIY CLEANING

Overhauling your household cleaning products doesn't have to be expensive. Many cosmetic and household cleaning agents can be made at home with basic ingredients. Use extra-virgin olive oil, coconut oil, or even tallow as a moisturizer, or melt the oils to mix with a little beeswax or cacao butter to make a beautifully smoothing moisturizer. Make toothpaste out of baking soda, coconut oil, and a couple of drops of peppermint oil, or use activated charcoal powder for a super-bright, white-toothed smile. Most household cleaning can be done with water, baking soda, white vinegar, or lemon juice. Instead of perfumes, use your favorite essential oil blends and use essential oils in a diffuser to fragrance your home.

THE PANCREAS

Your pancreas has several important functions. Its endocrine (hormone) related functions are involved in regulating blood sugar levels. Its role in digestion is to produce digestive enzymes. To do this, the pancreas needs minerals, trace elements, bicarbonates, and vitamins. Deficiencies in any of these nutrients can result in suboptimal pancreatic enzyme production, which can then affect your ability to absorb nutrients, and so it becomes a vicious cycle. Pancreatic enzymes work well only when the pH of the small intestine is on the slightly alkaline side. Small intestinal bacterial overgrowth (SIBO), poor food choices, smoking, alcohol, drugs, some medications, and candida overgrowth can lead to the small intestine being too acidic. Signs and symptoms of pancreatic insufficiency are many and varied and may include bloating, alternating constipation and diarrhea, foul-smelling stools, food visible in stools, gas, cramping, and fatigue.

One of the best ways to support your pancreatic enzyme function is to drink mineral-rich water (a good-quality filter and remineralizer is a must-have for all households wanting to achieve optimum health). You can increase the minerals in your water by adding a tiny pinch of "dirty" sea salt (sea salt that is a bit grayish in color, damp in texture, and high in minerals). In the short term (for a few weeks, unless done under the guidance of a healthcare practitioner) dissolve ¼ teaspoon of aluminium-free baking soda in water and take 30–40 minutes after meals.

Once again, stress is a big factor in determining digestive function, including that of the pancreas. More stress equals less pancreatic enzyme production. So follow the guidelines on page 28 for soothing your nervous system to promote great digestion.

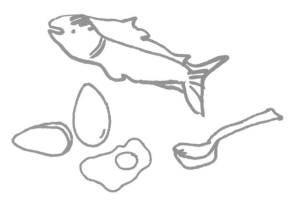

4. Restore healthy gut flora

Gut bugs – of which you have roughly 37.2 trillion (give or take a few trillion) – perform an incredible array of roles in your body. To remain well, we need to have the right balance of these microbes.

Over the last decade, research into the human microbiome has resulted in an ever-increasing understanding of the impact of gut flora on our health. Most of the microbes in our gut reside in our large intestine – the bowel – where, in a healthy state, the environment is relatively alkaline. If the pH (acidity) of any part of the gut changes, this affects which microbes thrive, and can result in dysbiosis. When the overgrowth is located in the small intestine, this is referred to as small intestinal bacterial overgrowth (SIBO). In the large intestine it is just referred to as dysbiosis.

Restoring healthy gut flora is not just a matter of killing overgrowths and putting the good guys back with probiotics. We need to address the environment within the gut. It's exactly like real estate. If you have a good property in good condition, you'll attract good tenants, who will in turn look after your property. This is why it's called a symbiotic relationship. When we look after our bugs, they look after us. When digestion is working well and the pH (acidity) of the digestive tract is appropriate for the location, and when we eat nourishing foods and have a healthy level of stress (not too much!), we foster the growth of beneficial bacteria.

5. Make healthy food choices

Our food choices affect all aspects of gut healing. Food can add to inflammation or help to ease it. Food can damage the gut wall or heal it. Food can add toxins to the body or can facilitate the clearing of toxins. Food can result in the depletion of our nutrient status or it can provide a nutrient boost. Food can contribute to the creation of stress or it can help minimize stress. We are what we eat, so it makes perfect sense to choose the best-quality foods so that our bodies can build the best-quality cells. Eating a paleo diet means you'll be consuming foods that are nutrient-dense, toxin-free, easy to digest, and so likely to be the least inflammatory. Perfect!

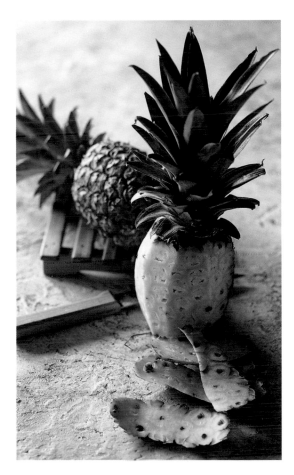

6. Detoxify

Detox plays an important role in keeping your gut lining in great condition and your gut flora in beautiful balance. Even though it is all the rage now, detoxing is often misunderstood. There is a staggering amount of chemicals in our food, air, water, workplaces, playgrounds, and homes that did not exist a century ago. They affect our hormones, immune systems, neurotransmitter production, cell replication, fat storage, and more. While our ancestors didn't need to detox or drink green juice, we're not living in our natural state and so we do need to pay extra attention to assisting our bodies clear out the mess.

But – and there's a big but – detox needs to be done in a *gentle* manner, at a rate that is suitable for any given individual, and at a suitable time in the healing process for that individual. While a gentle "surface level detox" in the beginning of a wellness journey can be a good start, encouraging too much detox early on can be a bad idea. Because your liver, bowels, kidneys, lungs, skin, and lymphatic system all play major roles in detoxification and elimination, if you try to detox too heavily you could overdo it. Side effects of detoxing include irritability, headaches, fatigue, cravings, and sometimes even skin rashes. Changes in bowel habits can also be experienced. If you experience any of these symptoms, get plenty of rest, make sure you're having 64 fluid ounces (8 cups) of water daily, and check out pages 78–79 for tips on what to do if you experience detoxification symptoms. If symptoms are quite severe, you may need to slow down your approach and/or consult with your health practitioner so you can be guided appropriately.

> ### THE LYMPHATIC SYSTEM
> Your lymphatic system is a network of vessels, similar to your blood vessels, that run through your body. Instead of channels for blood flow, they are for lymphatic fluid. Most people are aware of lymph nodes in the neck, groin, or under the arms that can become swollen or tender when an infection is present. Aside from playing a central role in immune function, the lymphatic system picks up waste and toxins from your cells and transfers them to the blood so that they can then be neutralized and filtered by the liver and kidneys.

So, before detoxing you need to make sure the routes of elimination are open. That means:

Skin:
* You're sweating and shedding.

Bowels:
* You're having complete, well-formed movements, 1–3 times daily.

Kidneys:
* Your urine is clear and colorless.

Lungs:
* You make times during the day to take 10 conscious breaths or do restorative practices that deepen breathing.

Detox needs to be done in a gentle manner, at a rate that is suitable for any given individual, and at a suitable time in the healing process for that individual.

ASSISTING DETOXIFICATION

For your bowels:

✳ Eat plenty of fiber-rich foods to act as a broom for your colon. In the early stages of gut repair, this may mean a focus on well-cooked vegetables and small amounts of fermented veggies. As time goes on you can gradually increase the amount of raw veggies you have in your diet.

✳ Drink plenty of water.

✳ If diet and adequate water intake are not enough, try one of the following boosters, followed with another glass of water:

  • Mix 2 tablespoons of freshly ground flaxseeds in a glass of water. Grind them at home in a coffee or spice grinder or high-speed blender. If you have any left over, store for up to a week in an airtight glass container in the fridge (the fragile omega-3 essential fatty acids will oxidize otherwise). Up to 2 times daily.

  • Mix 1 heaping teaspoon of slippery elm powder QUICKLY in a glass of water and drink immediately (the longer you leave it, the thicker it gets). Up to 3 times daily. For first-time users, start with ½ teaspoon and gradually increase (to prevent bloating).

  • Mix 1 tablespoon of psyllium husk in a glass of water. Up to 3 times daily. For first-time users, start with ½ teaspoon and then gradually increase (to prevent bloating).

✳ Used at appropriate times, colonic irrigation and/or enemas can also be fantastic for cleansing the colon. Note: they are not appropriate if your bowels are in an acute state of inflammation, or you're having a flare-up of a chronic condition. You'll need to work on getting the inflammation down first. Your health practitioner can help with this.

✳ Drink liver-loving herbal teas: dandelion root, burdock, yellow dock. There are herbs such as cascara and rhubarb that have quite a strong laxative effect, but I do not recommend these for regular use.

For your lungs:

✳ Practice deep breathing. Slowly inhale into the abdomen for a count of 4, hold for 1 second, exhale for a count of 6. Repeat 10 times. Do as many sets as you like during the day. (Pranayama – yogic breathing practices – are fantastic for this.)

✳ Do some exercise – whether it be gentle and nurturing walks, yoga, chi gong or a high-intensity blast, exercising gets you breathing better. As a general rule, the higher your stress (whether it be physical, mental, or emotional), the lower intensity your exercise should be.

✳ Drink herbal teas such as licorice root, mullein, hyssop, or marshmallow root or leaves. Licorice root is what's called a demulcent and marshmallow is a mucilage; both are soothing mucous-membrane tonics with particular benefit for the lungs. Mullein and hyssop are expectorants, which means they help make it easier to cough up phlegm or mucous.

For your kidneys:

* Drink enough fluid so that your urine is colorless. Having a 32-fluid ounce (8-cup) glass water bottle is a great way to monitor how much you are drinking during the day. Aim for 64 fluid ounces (8 cups), or ½ fluid ounce per pound of body weight.
* Drink herbal teas such as clivers (cleavers), dandelion leaves, or nettle.

For your skin:

* Get a good sweat on. Again, just gentle exercise if you're fatigued, stressed, or chronically ill.
* Try dry skin brushing before showering to lift off dead skin cells (this is a traditional naturopathic way of stimulating lymph flow).
* Drink herbal teas such as red clover, calendula, echinacea, or burdock.

For your liver:

* Eat clean: unprocessed whole foods free of additives.
* Eat sulfur-containing veggies (e.g., brassicas), which support liver detoxification. Broccoli, broccoli sprouts, Brussels sprouts, cauliflower, bok choy, cabbage, kale, collard greens, arugula, watercress, horseradish, mustard greens, and turnips all fit the bill. Glucosinolates (of which there are more than 100 types) and isothiocyanates (including sulforaphane, which has been associated with decreased cancer risk in some studies) are the star phytonutrients in this family. Onions and garlic have a similar collection of detoxifying sulfur compounds.
* Eat beets – they provide betaine-rich liver support.

* Every morning on rising, squeeze the juice of ½ lemon into a glass of warm water with a small pinch of "dirty" sea salt. Have 1–2 glasses of this before anything else. This is the best way to start your day, rehydrating and alkalizing your system all in one go.
* Drink black roasted dandelion coffee or these herbal teas: dandelion root (unroasted), St. Mary's thistle, or burdock.

For your lymphatic system:

* Dry skin brushing – as mentioned opposite, this is a great stimulator of lymphatic flow.
* Get plenty of exercise. Lymph vessels rely on the contraction of skeletal muscles to pump through lymphatic fluid. So to move your lymph, move your body. It can be as simple as going for a walk 20 minutes before lunch or after work.
* Infrared saunas. Patients with fibromyalgia, chronic pain, and some autoimmune diseases have experienced improvement in symptoms and/or less lymph node tenderness after infrared saunas. Note: this treatment is not suitable in pregnancy or for those with recent myocardial infarction or unstable angina. Check with your health professional before starting infrared sauna therapy.
* Drink herbal teas such as clivers, calendula, echinacea, burdock, or ginger.
* Get regular massages. It's a great way to move your lymphatic fluid and also to calm the nervous system, which will help you digest better in its blissfully relaxed state.

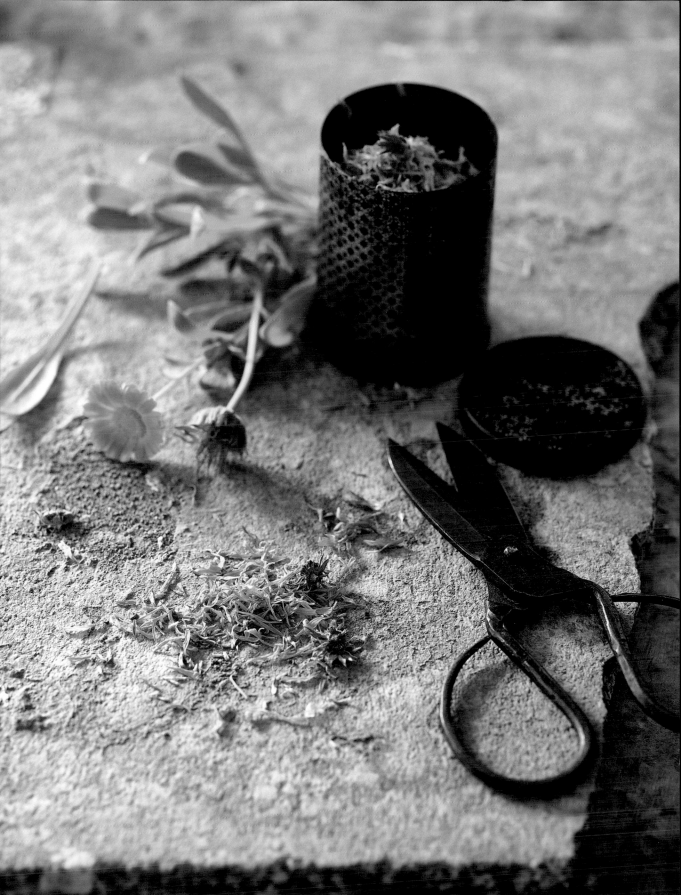

A BRIEF LOOK AT FASTING

There are many ways to fast. Done correctly, fasting in an appropriate way can really speed up the healing process, particularly in the case of digestive disorders. So, while we're not covering this topic in detail, here is a little information to enable you to explore further.

Digestion, as you've learned by now, is a big process that requires a lot of energy, not just from the gut itself, but from the nervous system, stomach, liver, gall bladder, and pancreas, too. Giving your digestive system a holiday from having to digest all the time means energy can be put towards healing instead. Cells of the stomach and gut wall repair, the pancreas gets to reset, and the liver gets to focus on the clean-up job, rather than having to process new incoming material. This is a big deal.

Fasting first and foremost gives your gut a break, whether it's for one day, one week or one month. If there is inflammation in the gut and you continue to eat foods that aggravate, it's like brushing sandpaper over a graze. Eating healing foods, on the other hand, can provide excellent soothing and nourishing support. This is the premise for utilizing exclusive enteral nutrition (EEN, or 100% liquid nutrition) in individuals with inflammatory bowel disease. EEN reduces the amount of work the gut has to do to be able to digest and absorb nutrients, resulting in beneficial outcomes that include higher rates of gut wall healing, altered gut microbes, improved vitamin D status, improved weight gain, and better quality of life after treatment. Fasts, such as the broth fast on page 75, also give the digestive system a break. Bear in mind the broth fast provided here differs from EEN: we have simply suggested a short broth fast, followed by the introduction of broth-based soups and then eventually meals, to cover your nutritional needs. For a real-food version of EEN, your nutritionist can provide a full spectrum of nutrients required for optimal health.

As a result of the liver's having more time to focus on the detoxification process, when people fast they can go through a "detox crisis," which basically means you may feel worse for a few days – or up to a few weeks – before feeling better. Some practitioners and coaches may say, that's great, keep going! I say, step back a little, we're going too fast.

PREPARING TO FAST:

1. Eliminate junk food, caffeine, and alcohol from your diet.
2. Increase your intake of water to 64 fluid ounces (8 cups) per day (or ½ fluid ounce per pound of body weight) to make sure your cells and tissues are sufficiently hydrated for nutrient and waste product exchange.
3. Eat whole foods – small amounts of protein, small to moderate amounts of fat, and mostly plants, with a big emphasis on greens (raw if you can digest them in comfort, otherwise cooked, steamed, or simmered in broth, or made into broth-based soups).

Do the above for a couple of weeks before embarking on a fast. The best way to promote detoxification is to first make sure you have the nutrients you need to carry out the metabolic processes. Ditching the processed stuff, drinking water, and eating real food in the lead up to a fast will help achieve that.

Broth fast

This is a super-nourishing way to fast. It's also an excellent fasting option in cooler weather. Fasting with bone broth or broth with very well cooked vegetables (overcooked really) is great for those with super-sensitive guts. A huge intake of minerals and an excellent supply of easy-to-assimilate protein in the form of collagen makes the healing process very effective. Simply have broth or broth-based soup for all meals and snacks during the day (for a sample broth fast see page 75).

Dealing with cravings

Cravings are not meant to be a battle of willpower. Just like pain, a craving is your body telling you that something is going on that needs attention. When you resolve the physiological issue that creates the craving, the craving will go away with little to no mental battle required.

COMMON CAUSES OF SUGAR CRAVINGS:

① **Gut dysbiosis**
As you now know, there is evidence that microbes may communicate with your brain via the vagus nerve and by producing neurotransmitters. They say to your brain, "feed me sugar" or "feed me starch." That's because sugars and starches are the favorite food source of opportunistic microbes, and they want to be fed. The most profound way to end these sweet cravings is to restore healthy gut flora (see page 48).

② **Blood sugar dysregulation**
Sugar cravings hit hard, so great is your body's instinct for survival (that's really what it's about – your body is in a fight-or-flight state and is trying to keep you alive). Chronic stress, combined with high-sugar diets and low activity levels, leads many of us to obesity and conditions such as hypoglycemia, insulin resistance, and leptin resistance – all of which lead to sugar cravings, with the aim to get glucose into cells quickly. To help resolve these cravings, make sure you have protein and fat in all of your meals, while minimizing starch and sugar intake. Additionally, you may require some supplementation of nutrients involved in blood sugar regulation or herbs that help improve insulin and leptin sensitivity (see page 48).

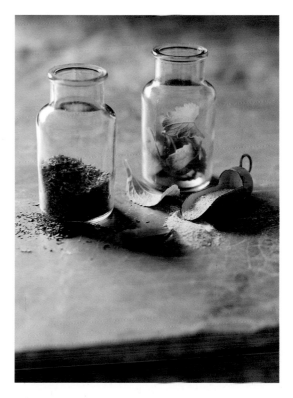

TIPS TO OVERCOME SUGAR CRAVINGS

Here are some quick steps to take to help eradicate cravings while you are dealing with the longer-term underlying issues:

* Drink a glass of water. Wait 5 minutes.
* Have 1–2 teaspoons of fermented veggies (the amount depends on how much you are used to consuming), or a shot of Coconut and Ginger Kefir (page 296) or Beet, Ginger, and Turmeric Kvass (page 301). This approach helps if the cravings are caused by gut flora overgrowths.
* Take 1 teaspoon of glutamine powder directly under the tongue. Let it sit there and dissolve for about 30 seconds before washing down with a glass of water.

Just like pain, a craving is your body telling you that something is going on that needs attention.

If your sweet cravings are particularly for chocolate, start supplementing with a good-quality magnesium powder (such as magnesium glycinate or magnesium citrate) providing 300–500 mg magnesium per day for a month. You should find your chocolate cravings ease or go away completely.

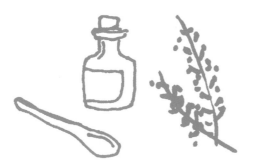

Nutrient supplements for blood sugar regulation:

* Chromium
* Activated B vitamins
* Biotin
* Zinc
* Magnesium

Herbs and foods to help improve insulin sensitivity:

* Cinnamon (2–4 teaspoons daily)
* Goat's rue
* Fenugreek
* Gymnema
* Turmeric
* Olive leaf extract
* Berries (strawberries, bilberries, cranberries, blackberries)
* Berberine-containing herbs (golden seal, oregon grape, barberry)
* Spirulina
* Black cumin

Many of these can be consumed as a tea, or for a higher therapeutic dose, ask a herbalist for a formula made of the tinctures of these herbs. Cinnamon and turmeric can be included readily in many drinks, smoothies, and meals. Add spirulina to smoothies.

Herbs and foods to improve leptin sensitivity:

* Piperine (one of the active constituents in black pepper)
* Curcumin (the active ingredient in turmeric)
* Pectin (found in fruits and vegetables, and in supplement form)
* Acetyl-L-carnitine (in supplement form)

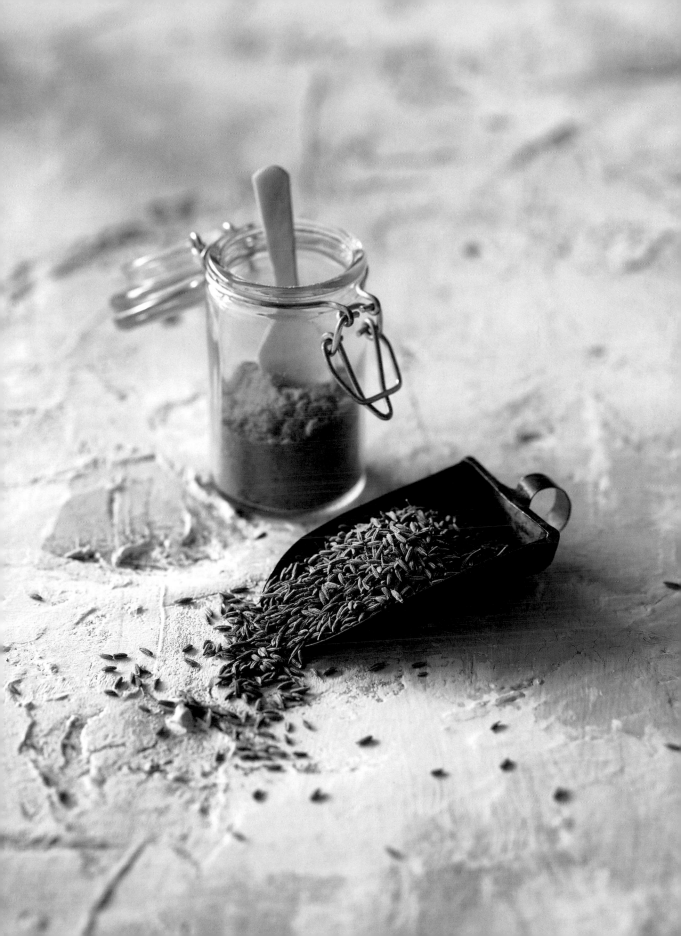

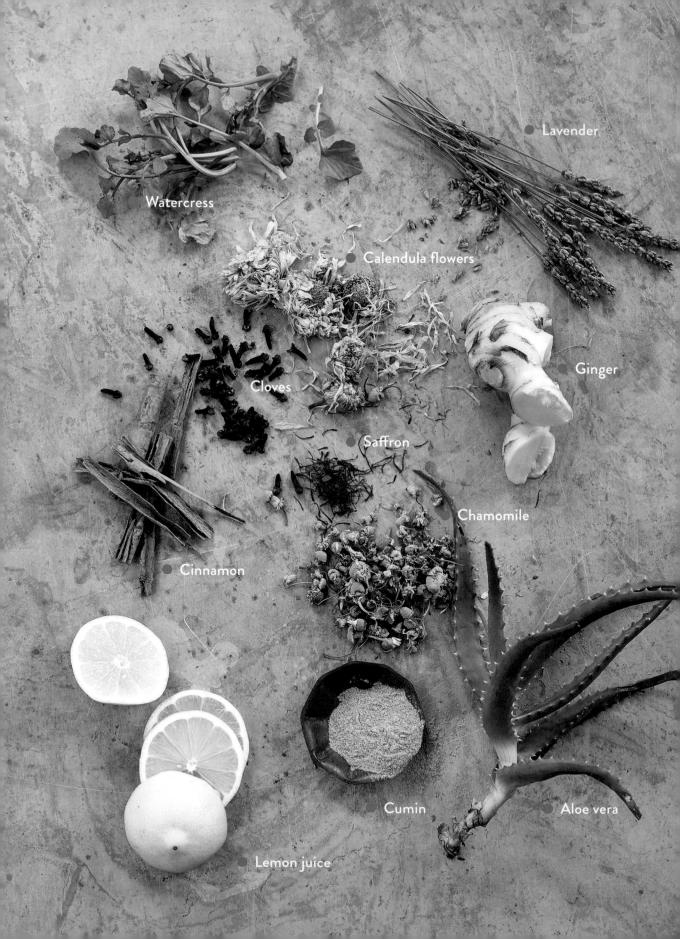

FOODS TO HEAL THE GUT

The following is a list of the star ingredients that may help if you're serious about improving and maintaining your gut health. In my practice, we see a good response when clients work these ingredients into their diet.

STAR INGREDIENTS FOR GUT HEALTH

STAR INGREDIENT	STAR QUALITIES
APPLE CIDER VINEGAR	Must be raw (unpasteurized) and unfiltered. This fermented tonic stimulates the production of digestive acids and bile, and often provides relief if you're experiencing discomfort after a meal. Dilute 1–3 teaspoons in a glass of water to drink, use in salad dressings, or pour over cooked veggies mixed with a little extra-virgin olive oil to stimulate digestion.
ALOE VERA	Aloe vera has anti-inflammatory and antioxidant properties. Each of these actions play an important role in gut repair. Studies also show that when taken before using NSAIDs, aloe vera reduces the impact of these drugs on the liver. So whether it's gingivitis, esophagitis, stomach or duodenal ulcers, or irritable or inflamed bowels, aloe vera can provide excellent healing relief. Add the inner gel of the leaf to smoothies, or use a preservative-free aloe vera juice as a tonic. Aloe vera can lower blood sugar levels, so those on diabetic medication should use with caution and under the guidance of their health practitioner.
BONE BROTH	A traditional food used for centuries, bone broth is incredibly rich in minerals, glycine, proline, and glutamine. Glutamine is the most important amino acid for healing the gut wall. Exceptionally easy to digest, bone broth provides a nourishing, nutrient-dense delivery system that soothes the gut lining, stimulates digestion, and requires very little energy to assimilate.
CALENDULA FLOWERS	Calendula (marigold) is useful in healing the lining of the gut wall. It has antioxidant and anti-inflammatory properties, and being a bit bitter, stimulates bile production. It is soothing for conditions such as gastritis/heartburn as well as colitis. Calendula tea can be used as an enema to soothe the bowel wall.

STAR INGREDIENT	STAR QUALITIES
CARDAMOM	Cardamom is a beautifully warming and calming spice. Its antispasmodic activity means it's great for helping to relieve intestinal cramping and gas pains.
CHAMOMILE	Chamomile is a wonderful anti-inflammatory herb. It's related to meadowsweet, which is what aspirin was originally created from. It has mild pain-relieving properties and is great for easing intestinal cramping. It is also mildly bitter, so stimulates digestion and bile production.
CINNAMON	One of nature's most powerful medicines, cinnamon has antimicrobial (against fungi/yeasts, bacteria, and viruses), antioxidant, and anti-inflammatory properties. It's great for relieving intestinal cramps and is a warming digestive stimulant. It is also useful for improving insulin sensitivity and regulating blood sugar levels.
CLOVES	A superfood indeed, cloves have the highest ORAC (antioxidant score) of all foods. Cloves stimulate digestion and have anti-inflammatory and anti-parasitic properties. You'll notice if you chew on a clove your tongue and gums may go numb – it's actually an anaesthetic, and is a great remedy for toothache. It is also great for relieving nausea, bloating, and intestinal cramping.
COCONUT OIL	Lauric, capric, and caprylic acids in cold-pressed extra-virgin coconut oil have antimicrobial, antifungal, and antiviral properties.
CUMIN	Cumin is a digestive stimulant, antispasmodic and carminative (relieving flatulence) – great for improving digestion and reducing digestive discomfort. It's particularly useful for stimulating pancreatic enzyme production. Research shows black cumin is helpful for pancreatitis and may help decrease the risk of pancreatic cancer. It also improves insulin sensitivity.

STAR INGREDIENT	STAR QUALITIES
DANDELION LEAVES	Dandelion leaves are a diuretic, so are great for relieving fluid retention. As a prebiotic, they're useful for supporting the growth of beneficial bacteria in the gut. Often seen as a weed, this is actually a valuable nutrient-dense green packed with folate, vitamin K, and magnesium. Add the leaves to green juices, smoothies, soups, and salads.
DANDELION ROOT	Dandelion root is a bitter tonic that stimulates digestive acids in the stomach and increases bile production in the liver. Due to the effects on the liver, it can be useful in helping to improve bowel habits if constipation is a problem. Dandelion root can be made into a tea, or the roasted root can be made into a "dandelion coffee." The powdered root can also be added to smoothies.
ENZYME-RICH FRUITS	Enzyme-rich fruits such as pineapple, papaya, and kiwi fruit can be useful to help stimulate digestion and break down proteins. They should only be consumed on an empty stomach about half an hour before enjoying your meal. Drizzle with some lime juice to add to the digestive-stimulating properties. If you have any candida issues or need to avoid fruit completely due to bacteria overgrowth or parasitic infection, then wait until there is improvement in your gut flora before including this as a digestive aid.
FENNEL SEEDS	Soothing fennel seeds are great to assist with bloating, gas, and gastrointestinal cramping.
FERMENTED FOODS	Along with bone broths, fermented veggies rule the gut-healing food world. These amazing foods are rich with live, active enzymes and probiotics. The tart flavor helps to stimulate digestive acids and there are many immune-supportive and anti-carcinogenic acids in fermented foods to further help with gut health. The key is to start with very small amounts, and slowly increase.

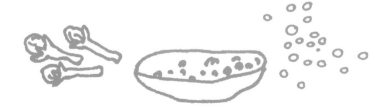

STAR INGREDIENT	STAR QUALITIES
FLAXSEEDS	Flaxseeds are rich in anti-inflammatory omega-3 fatty acids as well as other anti-inflammatory lignans. Flaxseeds also have a demulcent (gelling and soothing) property. It's important to always buy flaxseeds whole, not already ground. Grind them at home in a coffee or spice grinder or blender. If you have leftovers, store them in an airtight glass jar in the fridge or freezer. Omega-3 essential fatty acids oxidize and become inflammatory very quickly when exposed to heat, light, or oxygen. To relieve constipation, mix 2–4 tablespoons of freshly ground flaxseeds in a glass of water and drink. Follow with another glass of water. Do this 1–2 x daily as needed.
GINGER	Another of the world's best spices, ginger is a potent anti-inflammatory. Studies have shown combinations of ginger and turmeric to be more effective than NSAIDs at reducing inflammation. Ginger is also an excellent warming digestive aid, soothes gas pains in babies, and can be great for relieving nausea.
GUBINGE/ KAKADU PLUM	An Australian native, gubinge is the world's best-known food source of vitamin C. Gubinge is packed full of bioflavonoids as well, making this super tart fruit an excellent anti-inflammatory and immune support. It's most commonly available as a powder, which can be mixed into water or smoothies.
KUDZU	Kudzu root has been used for centuries in Chinese medicine for a range of conditions, including alcoholic liver disease, high blood pressure, and sugar dysregulation, and it is still used in healthcare today – often for chronic alcoholism. It is a rich source of flavonoids and has been shown to reduce permeability of the gut wall. It also has a calming effect on the nervous system. It can be used in herbal teas or as a thickener for soups and sauces.

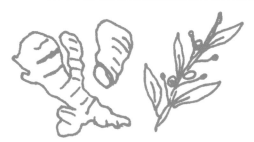

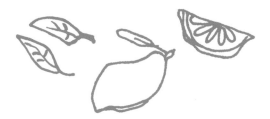

STAR INGREDIENT	STAR QUALITIES
LAVENDER	Lavender seems so old fashioned, but over the years it has become one of my favorite herbs as it has so many applications. It is fantastic for easing stress, anxiety, depression, and nervousness. This helps emotionally, of course, but also helps the gut – by putting the nervous system into the rest-and-digest mode we need for optimum digestion. It is also directly useful for digestion because (as a bitter herb) it stimulates the production of digestive acids and bile, it can ease stomach and intestinal cramps, and it is effective against streptococcus – a type of bacteria that commonly overgrows in the bowel when things ain't right. Use the essential oil topically (apply to the soles of the feet before bed for a great sleep), use the dried herb in herbal teas or Helen's Lavender Panna Cotta (see recipe, page 277), or see a herbalist for a therapeutic-strength tablet or tincture preparation.
LEMON JUICE	So simple, yet so good. One of the best ways you can start your day is to drink a glass of warm water with the juice of ½ lemon and a tiny pinch of "dirty" sea salt. The citric acid from the lemon and the minerals from the salt help stimulate digestive acids and bile flow, and also improve the rate of absorption of the water. You'll notice that with lemon and salt in your water, it won't sit in your stomach for a while, as it does if you drink just plain water. It often works to get the bowels moving, too, and is good for picking up energy levels if you're feeling a bit flat. A great alkalizing, liver-loving start to the day.
LICORICE ROOT	Licorice root is a demulcent – a slippery, soothing anti-inflammatory agent for mucous membranes, including those that constitute the gut wall. Licorice root also supports adrenal gland function and liver function. Note: it's best to avoid licorice root if you have high blood pressure, as licorice can raise blood pressure in some individuals.

STAR INGREDIENT	STAR QUALITIES
MARSHMALLOW ROOT	Another beautifully soothing demulcent herb (pop it in some hot water and you'll soon see just how slimy it gets!), this root is great for soothing flare-ups of inflammatory conditions of the mouth, stomach, intestines, and bowels (and the lungs and bladder, too, for that matter). Use it to make tea or jellies or buy the powdered root to add to smoothies.
ORGAN MEATS	In days gone by, these meats were saved for pregnant and breastfeeding women or the chiefs and warriors of a village or tribe. And for good reason: the nutrient density of organ meats far outweighs that of the muscle meats we are so used to eating these days. Organ meats are the most concentrated source of pretty much every vitamin, mineral, essential fatty acid, and essential amino acid, including vitamins A, D, B1, B2, B6, folate, and B12, zinc, selenium, calcium, magnesium, iron, and iodine. Organ meats also tend to be easier to digest than muscle meats, and ethically encourage a no-waste policy when sacrificing animals to nourish us.
OYSTERS	Oysters are without doubt the best source of zinc – a mineral that is crucial for over 500 enzyme pathways in the body (including those in digestion), as well as for the production of neurotransmitters and hormones. Zinc is also a mineral that is deficient in many people's diet. It is virtually impossible to heal the gut without adequate zinc. Remember to check out the source of your oysters and make sure they come from clean waters.
PEPPERMINT	Tried-and-true peppermint is fantastic for relieving gas and cramping pains in the gut. The essential oil can be diluted and massaged into the abdomen, or use dried leaves or fresh leaves to make an uplifting gut-soothing tea. Peppermint is a great cooling agent when you have feelings of heat or burning in your gut.

STAR INGREDIENT	STAR QUALITIES
POMEGRANATE	Pomegranate is a bit like a "polypill" – one of those mythical pills that has countless benefits – but better, because it's a whole food without any side effects. Pomegranate is a potent antioxidant and anti-inflammatory fruit. It is gastroprotective (i.e., protective of the mucosal lining of the gastrointestinal tract) and liver protective, and can help treat bleeding gums and gingivitis. It is antifungal and antibacterial against pathogens such as clostridia, yet helps promote the growth of beneficial bacteria in the gut. Pomegranate peel has been used in naturopathy to assist in the treatment of ulcerative colitis. And, in fact, when I was traveling in India years ago, locals told me to eat pomegranate – especially the white pith – if I experienced traveller's diarrhea!
RAW MEATS	A specialty in many fine restaurants in the form of steak tartare or carpaccio, fresh and well-stored raw meats from a grass-fed organic source are actually a very easy-to-digest way of consuming meat. No oxidized fats, damaged proteins, or lost nutrients. Eat meat raw only if you can completely trust the source – it's not worth gambling your health on meat that may be contaminated with pathogens.
SAFFRON	In herbal medicine, saffron is used to help treat depression, anxiety, and Alzheimer's disease. Its calming and uplifting effect helps the nervous system get into rest-and-digest mode, which improves digestion. Saffron suppresses lipopolysaccharide (LPS) – a toxin released by gram-negative bacteria such as *H.pylori*, which often overgrow in states of dysbiosis – and can thereby reduce the damage caused by the toxin in the gut. Saffron is also a potent free-radical scavenger, providing important antioxidant support to promote gut healing.

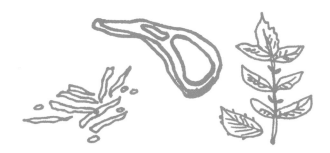

STAR INGREDIENT	STAR QUALITIES
SLIPPERY ELM	A soothing demulcent and bulking agent, slippery elm is great for both constipation and diarrhea. If there is diarrhea, slippery elm will absorb the excess water in the bowels, creating more formed stools. If there is constipation, it will absorb more water into the bowels and, in doing so, soften the stools, making them easier to pass. Slippery elm is a good "mop-up" agent, working as a sort of a broom for the intestines, with anti-inflammatory activity to boot.
SPEARMINT	Similar to peppermint, spearmint is a slightly gentler, not-so-cold herb to help ease digestive discomfort from gas and bloating. And it tastes delicious, too. Perfect in herbal tea blends.
SPROUTED BROCCOLI SEEDS	Sprouted broccoli seeds are very high in sulforaphane, an isothiocyanate that has been associated with decreased cancer risk in some studies. It's easy to grow your own sprouts in 4–7 days.
STEWED APPLE	Stewed apple is a lot easier to digest than raw apple. It's rich in soluble fiber and immune-enhancing polyphenols, and may aid gut function (including mucosal immune tolerance, i.e., improving tolerance/resilience of the immune activity in the mucosal lining of the gut wall). Peel the apples, but stew the peel as well, as most of the phenolics and pectin are found in the peel. Remove the peel once cooked for better texture and easier digestibility.
TURMERIC	What's not to love about turmeric? It helps stimulate bile production and is a potent anti-inflammatory (shown to be more effective at reducing inflammation when combined with ginger than NSAIDs) and antioxidant. It's also been shown to help protect against some neurological conditions such as Alzheimer's disease, and, let's face it, who doesn't want to protect their brain?
WATERCRESS	Watercress is a digestive stimulant and, thanks to its isothiocyanates content, has powerful antioxidant and detoxifying properties, too. It can be used in soups, salads, and smoothies.

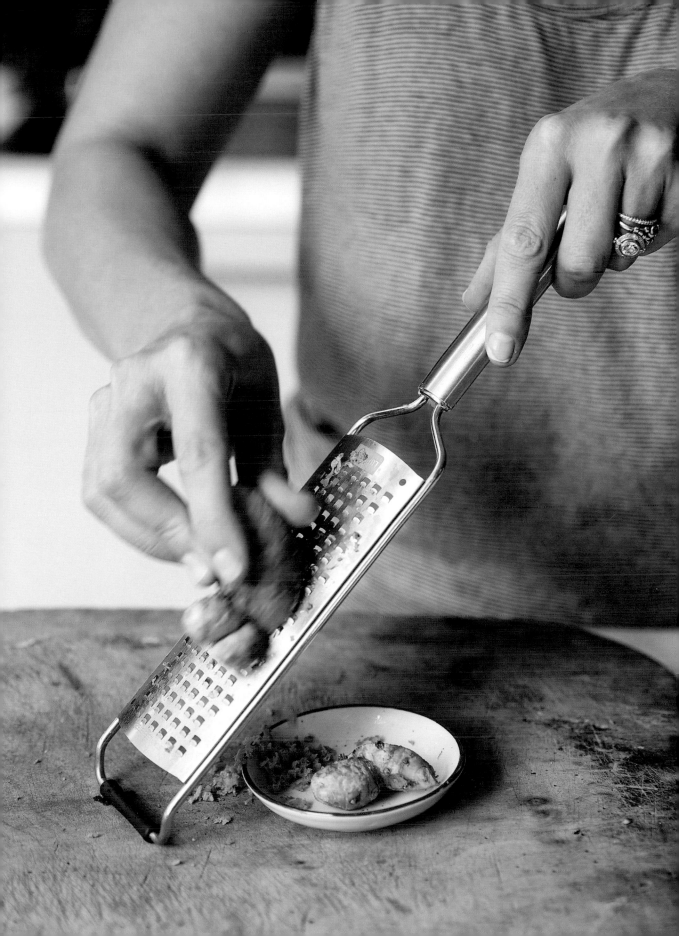

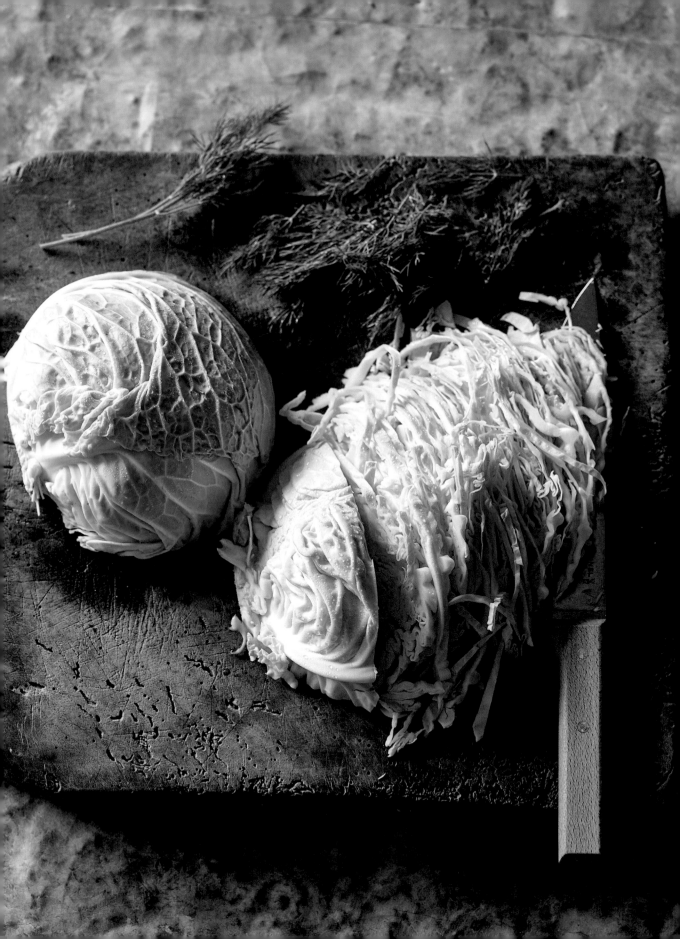

WHY FERMENTING IS FABULOUS

Along with bone broths, fermented foods are the most significant additions you can make to your regular diet in terms of gut health. As little as ten years ago, people wondered what on earth I was on about. Thankfully, fermenting is making a comeback. This is not some new fad to jump on. If it is, then beer, wine, and cheese are all fads, too – as these all came about through the process of fermentation.

In many ancient societies, fermenting foods was a way to preserve them for the sparse winter months. These cultured or fermented foods were revered for having healing properties. The word "kefir," for example, is Turkish in origin and translates to "feel good." Unfortunately, in most Western cultures the advent of refrigeration spelled the end of fermented foods. We now have the science to help us understand why fermented foods like kefir make us feel good and why we should include them in our diet. Throughout the fermentation process, an abundance of enzymes is produced, which improve digestion and liver function.

Not only do fermented foods improve digestion on the enzyme front, they also improve digestion on the acid front. Sour or tart foods (which ferments are) stimulate receptors on your tastebuds that send messages to your brain and then back down to your stomach to produce more hydrochloric acid (HCl). As discussed earlier (in A Cook's Tour of Digestion, see pages 16–18), the more HCl you produce the better you break down your proteins and absorb your minerals and vitamin B12. Remember, a good production of stomach acid has a cascade effect that results in the pancreas producing more of its digestive enzymes, further improving the digestive procession. For these two reasons, many people find fermented foods can be a really simple way to reduce bloating and improve bowel habits.

You may absorb 50–300 times more vitamin C from fermented cabbage than from raw or cooked cabbage!

The next boon for fermented foods is their nutrient content. Because the friendly bacteria – predominantly lactobacilli – partially digest the food, the nutrients are easier for your body to absorb. Not only that, microbes are actually vitamin producers – especially B vitamins, biotin and vitamin K. They also produce a number of amino acids, such as tyrosine (important for thyroid function), and even more nutrients, such as coenzyme Q10, which is essential for energy production. As a result, we get more vitamins and minerals from fermented foods than we do from raw or cooked foods. For example, you may absorb 50–300 times more vitamin C from fermented cabbage than from raw or cooked cabbage!

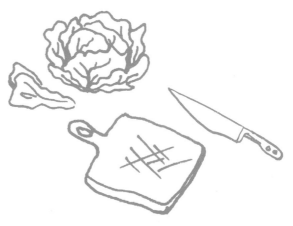

INTRODUCING FERMENTED FOODS INTO YOUR DIET

Before you get too excited and eat a bucketful of fermented veggies to get that good gut and youthful glow happening, read this. These are really powerful foods. You're sending in troops of beneficial bugs ready to fight off opportunistic bugs in your gut, a load of enzymes, and a whole heap of active nutrients.

So start with a teaspoon a day (or even just ½ teaspoon if you are particularly sensitive). If you're feeling fine on that for a couple of days, then gradually increase. But if you increase and you feel a bit bloated or as though you have a little hangover, then just reduce the amount back down again. Work towards having 1–2 tablespoons with each meal.

In the art of fermentation, it is understood that the degree to which you react to a fermented food is often an indication of the degree to which you need them. That means, the better health you're in the faster you'll be able to increase the amount of fermented veg you can have. The more inflammation and toxicity you have from chronic ill health or long-term unhealthy lifestyle practices, the more slowly you need to go with increasing the amount you have. So it could take you anywhere from a week to a couple of months or more to get to a tablespoon or two per meal. Another reason some people may react to fermented veggies is if it results in an overgrowth of the beneficial bacteria in the gut (yes, you can have too much of a good thing). Or if you have histamine intolerance, in which case – with the help of a health practitioner – focused gut work, gut flora restoration, liver detoxification, and methylation support is required to improve the situation.

DO FERMENTED VEGGIES AND LOW THYROID FUNCTION MIX?

If you have low thyroid function you may have heard that you should avoid foods from the brassica family, such as cabbage, broccoli, cauliflower, kale, etc. These contain goitrin, which can interfere with iodine uptake in the thyroid (the thyroid needs iodine to make thyroid hormones). The truth is, you would literally need to eat paddocks full of these veggies in order to elicit a goitrogenic effect. And, for the majority of people with thyroid problems, it's actually important to include the brassica family in the diet as they contain fantastic sulfur compounds that greatly assist detoxification. Since the thyroid gland is so sensitive to environmental toxins, we need to make sure we're including detoxifying foods in the diet. Of course, as always, we need to remember the importance of bioindividuality, and if you have a thyroid issue and you do feel worse for eating brassicas, then by all means avoid them until a later date when your thyroid is functioning better (at which point, try reintroducing them with the support of your health practitioner). However, if you feel good on them, keep them in.

Anyway, you can still enjoy the benefits of fermented foods whether or not you're eating brassicas. The sky is the limit in terms of veggie combos to ferment. Beet, ginger, and turmeric kvass, cultured carrot sticks, fermented cucumbers, coconut yogurt, and coconut water kefir are just some examples of brassica-free ferments.

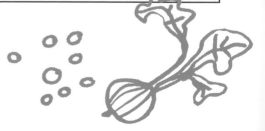

THE BEAUTY OF BONE BROTH

A beautiful bone broth provides an incredible source of nutrition and is one of our kitchen essentials. Exceptionally high in minerals and collagen, glutamine, glycine, and proline, broth is an amazing healing food for the gut lining and forms the base for many recipes in this book. In addition to gut-healing properties, bone broth helps to stimulate digestion, so while it is normally wise to avoid drinking with meals, ½ cup of bone broth with your meals can actually improve digestion.

As it's been slow-cooked, bone broth is a great source of easily absorbable protein (it has a "protein-sparing" effect thanks to all the glycine, which means you can get away with having less protein in your diet, while still reaping the benefits of a higher protein diet). Broth requires very little digestion, making all the nutrients easy to absorb.

Making your own bone broth is super simple and a super cheap way to pack a lot of nutritional punch into your meals.

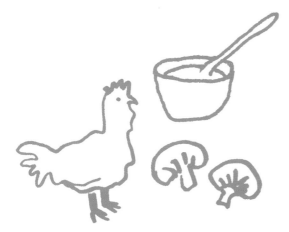

Bone broths have been used to promote health and healing for generations by many different cultures. There's a reason why chicken and veggie soup is a traditional remedy for flu. In vitro (test tube) studies indicate that chicken broth may have antiviral and immune-boosting activity. In 2000, scientists at the University of Nebraska Medical Center in Omaha studied the effect of chicken soup on the inflammatory response. They found that some components of chicken soup inhibit neutrophil (a type of white blood cell) migration that may have an anti-inflammatory effect and could temporarily ease the symptoms of illness.

Some people are a bit squeamish about slowly simmering a pot of bones for 24 hours. As a former vegetarian I can relate; however, there are a few things that have really shifted my perception over the years. For starters, I believe it's important to source animal products such as eggs, meat, gelatin, and bones from animals that have been well-treated. I also believe that it is important to minimize waste and to acknowledge and appreciate the animals we use to nourish and heal us. With this in mind, using all parts of an animal that has been sacrificed for our nourishment is a way of honoring and respecting that animal. In traditional cultures, the bones and organs were the most highly regarded parts of the animal – not the fillets and breasts. And for good reason: these parts have far more nutrition and are easier to digest than muscle meats – an important factor when we're aiming to heal the gut.

Making your own bone broth is super simple and a super cheap way to pack a lot of nutritional punch into your meals. It also means you can happily avoid using stock cubes, powders, and cartons, which often contain MSG and other undesirable food additives.

You can drink your broth as is, simply seasoned with sea salt and black pepper (perhaps with some dried Italian herbs or some turmeric and cumin in there, too). Or you can create hearty, nourishing soups and stews using the delicious gut-healing recipes in this book. You can even add a shot of broth to smoothies or homemade ice blocks. Yum!

I recommend making a big batch of broth and freezing a portion or two, so that you always have some on hand when times are busy and you need an emergency meal. I like to use a slow cooker (ceramic dish, not Teflon) as I can happily leave it on overnight and during the day while I'm out at work; however, you can use a stockpot on the stovetop as well.

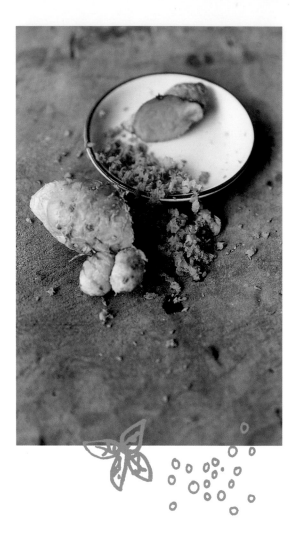

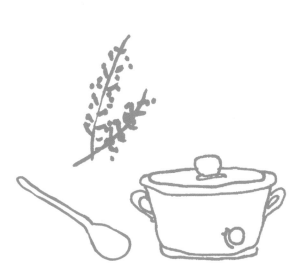

HOW TO INTRODUCE BONE BROTH INTO YOUR DIET

Most people will happily introduce slow-cooked bone broths into their diet without any hassle. For some, though, particularly those with histamine intolerance, it may be necessary to start with small amounts of broth cooked for as little as half an hour. The best way to do this is to dilute a shot of broth in some soup made using filtered water, and then slowly increase as gut flora begins to improve and liver function and metabolic pathways of detoxification are supported.

Where to exercise caution (contraindications)

Remember the principle of n = 1? It is important that food and therapeutic choices be suitable for you. The following are some clear contraindications for different approaches to gut healing.

Allergies and sensitivities

* If you have any known food allergies, omit these foods. Sensitivities are harder to determine, because the symptoms can take up to 72 hours to manifest, in which time you've eaten a whole host of different foods. If you've cleaned up your diet and the symptoms persist, then it may be worth considering food sensitivity testing through a reputable pathology service. This will let you know which foods to avoid and which foods to rotate, for example, once every 4 days, until your gut and gut flora have healed. When you have restored your gut health, you may find many or all of your sensitivities, and possibly even your allergies, disappear.
* People with yeast sensitivity should avoid kefir and kombucha, as they are yeast and bacterial ferments. I recommend that everybody start on bacterial ferments, such as fermented veggies or Beet, Ginger, and Turmeric Kvass (see recipe, page 301), and then graduate to coconut water kefir and lastly to kombucha.
* If you have had a fecal microbial analysis done and you have an overgrowth of lactobacilli in your gut, you may need to avoid ferments initially, until some balance has been restored to your gut flora.

Diabetes and thyroid issues

* Those on diabetes or thyroid medication should have fortnightly check-ins with their doctor in case dosages of medication need to be altered as a result of dietary and lifestyle changes.

Cancer recovery

* For individuals with cancer, it is best to avoid bone broths due to their high glutamine content. Research has shown that cancer cells may use glutamine as an energy source.
* For the same reason, glutamine powder, used for gut repair and sugar cravings, should also be avoided by individuals with cancer.

Seizure disorders and ADHD

* An extremely small subset of individuals with seizure disorders, ADHD, or aggressive behaviors may have trouble with high-glutamine foods. For those who do have these problems, small amounts of broth cooked for no more than 2 hours is a good place to start, as there is less glutamine content.

Histamine intolerance

* Individuals with histamine intolerance may need to delay the introduction of both fermented foods and bone broths until they have achieved a degree of liver support, gut repair, and gut flora restoration that allows them to consume foods high in histamines.

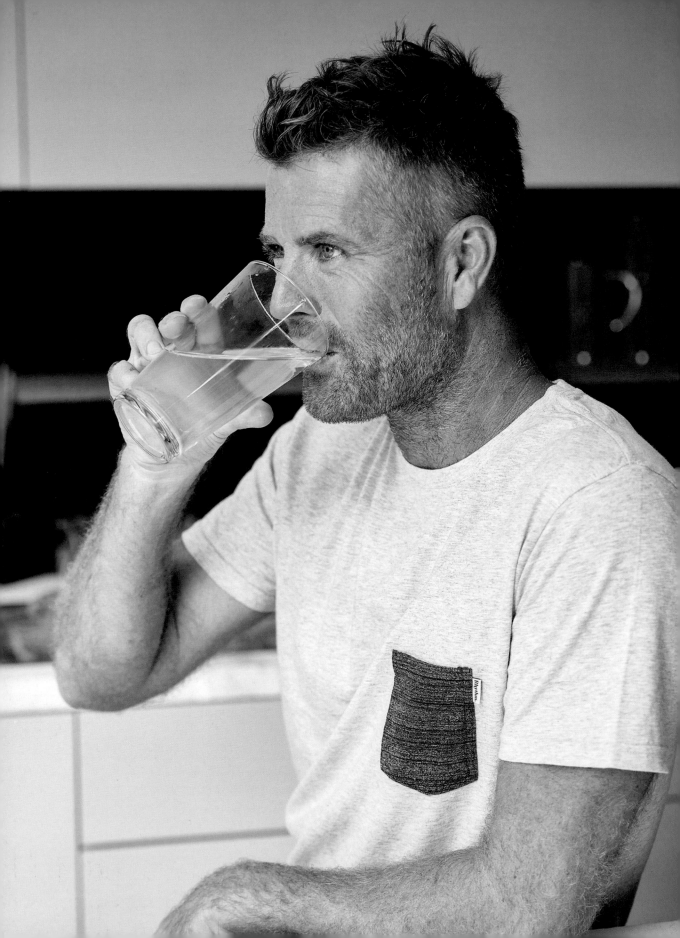

KITCHEN GARDEN FARMACY

Your own backyard or kitchen windowsill can be a rich source of medicinal herbs, spices, and teas, many of which have excellent antimicrobial properties (i.e., the ability to kill off or keep under control a range of unhelpful bacteria, yeasts, fungi, and parasites). Here are some to try:

Herbs, spices, and teas with antimicrobial properties:
* Basil
* Bay leaves
* Chamomile
* Chile
* Cinnamon (sticks and ground)
* Cloves
* Cumin
* Fennel seeds
* Garlic
* Ginger
* Green tea
* Horseradish
* Lavender
* Lemon balm
* Lemongrass
* Mustard seeds
* Nutmeg
* Oregano
* Parsley
* Rosemary
* Tamarind
* Thyme
* Tulsi (holy basil)
* Vietnamese cilantro

Herbs and spices that stimulate digestion:
* Bay leaves
* Chamomile
* Cloves
* Ginger
* Lavender
* Lemon balm
* Parsley

Herbs and spices that ease bloating and gas:
* Cardamom
* Chamomile
* Cinnamon (sticks and ground)
* Dill
* Fennel seeds
* Ginger
* Lavender
* Lemon balm
* Peppermint
* Spearmint

Herbs, plants, and spices that soothe the gut wall:
* Aloe vera (inner leaf juice)
* Calendula flowers
* Cardamom
* Lemon balm
* Licorice root
* Marshmallow root

How to blend tea

I just love opening packets of high-quality dried herbs and inhaling their aromas. I find the sensory experience of blending tea soothing and calming – and that in itself, as you now know, can improve digestion.

The beauty of herbs is that they tend to work more effectively when blended with other herbs than when used on their own. That's not to say single herb teas aren't great – they are a wonderfully simple elixir in themselves. However, if you can, find a combination of two to six herbs that you can blend together.

When it comes to blending your own teas there are no rules, so you can mix to your heart's – and tastebuds' – content. Here are a few tips for combining herbs for tea:

1. Start with the best-quality ingredients. There are great online suppliers of organic dried herbs that are a far cry from the dusty herbal tea bags in supermarkets and health-food stores.

2. Typically, you need less of the root and seed herbs than you do of the leaves or flowering tops. Roots and seeds tend to have a stronger flavor.

3. If you're using a combo of not-so-tasty herbs, then add some yummy ones. Good taste enhancers include fennel seeds, peppermint, spearmint, cinnamon, and licorice root.

4. Mix your herbs together in a large glass bowl to ensure an even blend, then store your unique herbal tea concoction in a glass jar with an airtight lid to seal in the freshness.

5. Use 1 heaping teaspoon of the tea blend per cup of boiling water. You can make your tea in a teapot or coffee plunger, and there are also tea ball infusers available.

6. Allow your tea to steep and infuse its goodness for at least 5 minutes – longer if you're using roots and seeds as part of your blend (10–15 minutes in that case). As roots and seeds are more dense, they take longer to absorb the water and release their active constituents.

7. You can leave your tea to steep overnight and then fill your water bottle with the infusion in the morning, so you can drink it throughout the day.

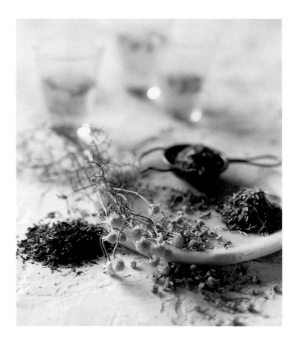

MAKING TEA WITH FRESH HERBS

You can also make tea blends using fresh herbs. Dried herbs are generally about four times more potent in flavor than fresh herbs, as their water content has been removed. So, when using fresh herbs to make tea, you may need to use more than you would typically for your dried herb blends. One big advantage of using fresh herbs is the added vitality. Pick up little handfuls of your desired herbs – mint, nettle, lemon balm, sage, thyme, rosemary, chamomile, lavender, or anything else you have growing organically – and pop them in a teapot or coffee plunger and steep for 5–10 minutes before drinking.

Fresh ginger and turmeric make a wonderfully flavorful and warming herbal tea. Grate at least 1 teaspoon of each, add boiling water, and allow to steep for 5–15 minutes before drinking. You can always make your tea stronger or weaker to suit your taste. Dried licorice root can be added for some sweetness.

AUTOIMMUNE PALEO PROTOCOL

AIP is a version of paleo that is being used by practitioners such as Dr. Terry Wahls (of the Wahls Protocol™) and Dr. Sarah Ballantyne to alleviate the symptoms of some autoimmune diseases. I use this when indicated with patients in my own practice, to good effect.

AIP is a step up from "regular" paleo as it eliminates the most common immune-reactive foods from your diet for a period of time. Once symptoms have settled down (this could take anywhere from four weeks to a year), you can then reintroduce foods that are allowed on the regular paleo diet – nuts, eggs, seeds, and nightshades. Reintroductions are done one at a time, with adequate time in between to note any flare-up in symptoms. Further gains can be made by having food sensitivity testing done and avoiding any foods that cause adverse reactions. This process needs to be undertaken with the guidance of a skilled healthcare practitioner. Following AIP principles can have dramatic effects in turning health around; however, usually diet alone is not enough. Once an autoimmune illness is manifest, it may have been preceded by years of dysbiosis and inflammatory damage, and these underlying issues will need some therapeutic support with either herbal medicine, nutritional supplementation, or lifestyle practices. It is a commitment, for sure, but one that can be life-changing.

Below is an expanded list of the basic rules of AIP. So, if you want to steer your gut healing towards AIP, you can use the information provided here as a guide for shopping and modifying your recipes. We have also provided a handy key throughout the book showing which recipes are AIP friendly and which can be easily made so.

FOODS TO EMBRACE

* Animal fats: bacon fat, beef tallow, duck fat, lard
* Avocado
* Coconut products: cold-pressed extra-virgin coconut oil, creamed coconut, coconut cream, coconut aminos, coconut milk (if canned, ensure it has no additives like guar gum and carrageenan and is not in BPA-lined cans), shredded preservative-free coconut
* Fermented foods: fermented veggies, coconut yogurt, kombucha, water kefir, coconut kefir, coconut water kefir
* Fish and shellfish – wild is best, farmed is fine for shellfish (not fish or shrimp)
* Fruits: limit to ½–¾ ounces fructose per day

* Glycine-rich foods (organ meat, gelatin, bone broth, and anything with connective tissue, joints, or skin)
* Grass-fed meats
* Green tea
* Herbs and spices (all fresh and dried non-seed herbs are allowed):

  • Basil leaves
  • Bay leaves
  • Cassia
  • Chamomile
  • Chervil
  • Chives
  • Cinnamon
  • Cloves
  • Cilantro (leaves and roots only)

- Curry leaves
- Dill fronds
- Fennel (fronds only)
- Galangal
- Garlic
- Ginger
- Horseradish
- Lavender
- Lemon balm
- Lemon verbena
- Lemongrass
- Mace
- Marjoram leaves
- Onion powder
- Oregano leaves
- Parsley
- Peppermint
- Rosemary leaves
- Saffron
- Sage leaves
- Spearmint leaves
- Tarragon leaves
- Thyme leaves
- Turmeric

* Himalayan salt or "dirty" sea salt (to improve your intake of important trace minerals)
* Non-seed herb teas: flowers, roots, leaves
* Organ meat and offal
* Poultry in moderation due to high omega-6 content (omega 6 is inflammatory unless balanced out by omega 3, so if you're eating lots of fish – which is high in omega 3 – you'll be fine)
* Vegetables of all kinds (except nightshades – see Foods to Avoid), as much variety as possible and the whole rainbow:
  - Green vegetables
  - Colorful vegetables and fruit (red, purple, blue, yellow, orange, white)
  - Cruciferous vegetables (broccoli, cabbage, kale, turnips, arugula, cauliflower, Brussels sprouts, watercress, mustard greens, etc.
  - Sea vegetables (excluding algae like chlorella and spirulina, which are immune stimulators)

* Vinegars: unpasteurized apple cider vinegar, coconut vinegar, red wine vinegar, balsamic (that has no added sugar).

Out of the foods to embrace, put a special emphasis on eating more of the following:

* Fish and shellfish – wild is best (aim for at least 3 x per week, the more the better)
* Organ meat and offal (aim for 5 x per week, the more the better)
* Vegetables of all kinds (except nightshades – see Foods to Avoid), aiming for 8–14 cups per day.

FOODS TO AVOID

* Alcohol
* All processed foods (i.e. additives, preservatives, emulsifiers, thickeners, colorings, flavorings, flavor enhancers)
* Alternative sweeteners such as xylitol, stevia, and mannitol
* Artificial sweeteners such as sucralose, aspartame, etc.
* Chocolate
* Dairy
* Dried fruit
* Eggs
* Grains
* Gums such as guar gum, tara gum, gum arabic
* Herbs and spices from seeds:
  - Anise
  - Annatto
  - Black caraway
  - Cayenne

- Celery seed
- Coriander seeds
- Cumin seeds
- Curry powder (usually a mix of ground coriander, cumin, fenugreek and other spices)
- Dill seeds
- Fennel seeds
- Fenugreek
- Mustard seeds
- Nutmeg
- Paprika
- Poppy seeds
- Red pepper flakes/chile powder
- Sesame seeds

Use the following spices with caution (it's best to eliminate them for the first 4–8 weeks):

- Allspice
- Black, white, green, pink peppercorns
- Caraway
- Cardamom
- Juniper
- Star anise
- Vanilla pod

* Legumes and beans
* Nightshades (a couple of these you might only ever encounter in supplements or traveling in tropical locations or outback Australia):

- Ashwagandha (*Withania somnifera*)
- Bell pepper
- Bush tomato
- Cape gooseberry (also known as Inca berries or ground cherries – not to be confused with regular cherries)
- Chiles (including jalapeños, habaneros, chile-based spices, cayenne pepper)
- Cocona
- Eggplant

- Garden huckleberry (not to be confused with regular huckleberries)
- Goji berries (wolfberry)
- Kutjera (desert raisin)
- Naranjillas
- Paprika
- Pepinos
- Pimientos
- Potatoes (not sweet potatoes)
- Tamarillos
- Tomatillos
- Tomatoes

* Vegetable oils (canola, corn, cotton seed, cooking oil, generic vegetable oil, grapeseed, peanut, rice bran, safflower, soy, sunflower, as well as fake butter substitutes and margarine)
* Nuts and nut oils (e.g., walnut and sesame oil)
* Seeds: flaxseeds, chia, pumpkin, sunflower, sesame and herbs and spices from seeds (see list opposite)
* Sugar, including coconut sugar, rice malt syrup, rapadura, etc.
* Tapioca

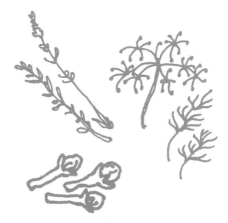

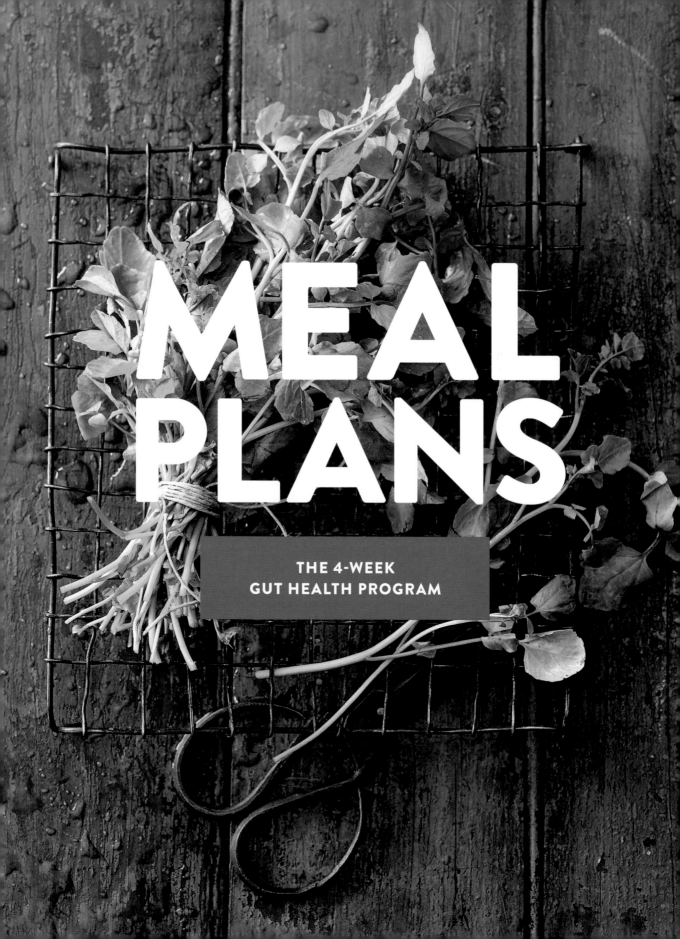

MEAL PLANS

THE 4-WEEK
GUT HEALTH PROGRAM

So now is the time to put your newfound knowledge to use. Giving yourself a good 4 weeks to focus on healing your gut is an excellent start to reclaiming your health and well-being – it's long enough to get some fantastic results, yet short enough to be achievable.

Prep

The week leading up to your 4-week program is your time to prepare as much as possible.

What to do:

* Make up 3 batches of bone broth (making different varieties will give you a range of flavors to enjoy) and freeze in 1- or 2-cup portions (for recipes, see pages 116–124)
* Make up 2 batches of fermented vegetables (again, so that you have some variety of flavor) (for recipes, see pages 94–111)
* Make up 1 of the following recipes and store in portions in the freezer (you will need these in the first and second week):

  * Ham Hock Soup (page 153)
  * Hunter Soup (Bigos) (page 156)
  * Hearty Oxtail Soup (page 160)
  * Thai Pumpkin Soup with Braised Beef Cheek (page 171)

If you still have space left in your freezer, purchase the following:

* Organic chicken livers (buy 1–2 pounds and freeze in 4-ounce portions)
* Extra bones for making additional batches of bone broth.

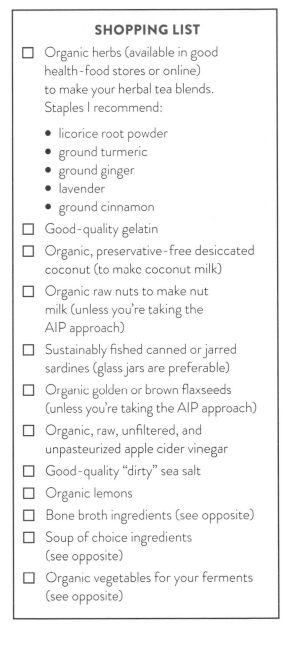

SHOPPING LIST

☐ Organic herbs (available in good health-food stores or online) to make your herbal tea blends. Staples I recommend:

  * licorice root powder
  * ground turmeric
  * ground ginger
  * lavender
  * ground cinnamon

☐ Good-quality gelatin

☐ Organic, preservative-free desiccated coconut (to make coconut milk)

☐ Organic raw nuts to make nut milk (unless you're taking the AIP approach)

☐ Sustainably fished canned or jarred sardines (glass jars are preferable)

☐ Organic golden or brown flaxseeds (unless you're taking the AIP approach)

☐ Organic, raw, unfiltered, and unpasteurized apple cider vinegar

☐ Good-quality "dirty" sea salt

☐ Organic lemons

☐ Bone broth ingredients (see opposite)

☐ Soup of choice ingredients (see opposite)

☐ Organic vegetables for your ferments (see opposite)

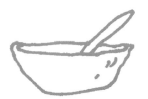

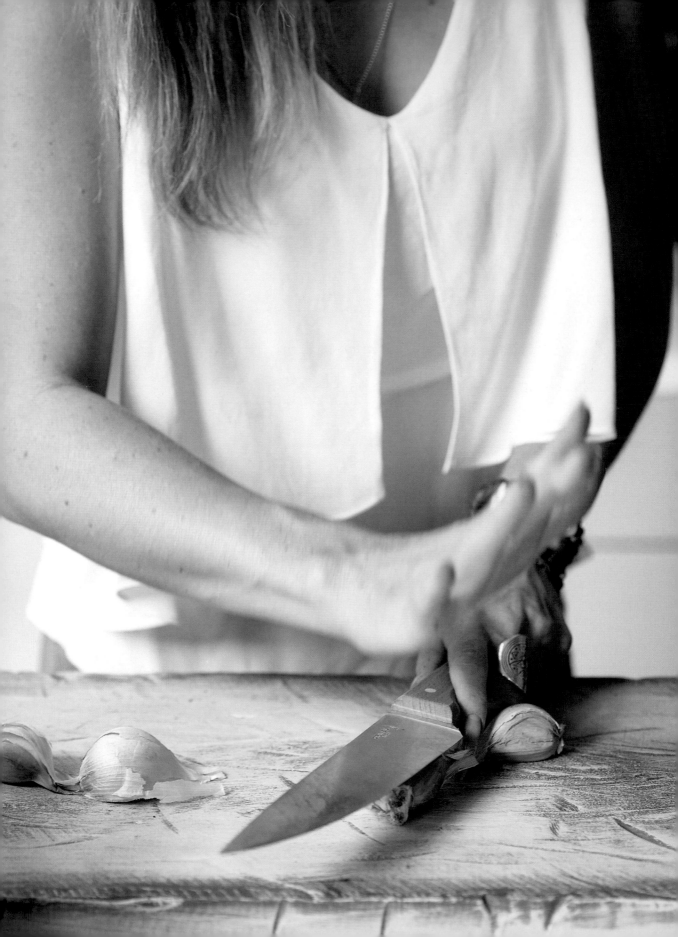

DAYS 1–3

The first 3 days are to reset and give your gut a break, and involve a broth fast (see page 47). That means 3 days of super-simple fish, chicken, lamb or beef broth.

I recommend that you do this on a Friday, Saturday, and Sunday, as you may feel tired and a little unwell (headaches and fatigue are common) as your body ramps up detoxification processes – especially on days 2 and 3. Even if you are used to having fermented foods, avoid them during these 3 days, with the exception of Beet, Ginger, and Turmeric Kvass (page 301) – 1 shot 1–3 x daily on an empty stomach (e.g., 10–20 minutes before broth, rather than with or after broth).

If you find you are experiencing the detox symptoms mentioned, you can:
* Drink the Charcoal Mop-up (page 290) between broths (1–3 daily). This is the best option for fast relief if you are feeling really poorly.
* Drink the Gut and Liver Cleanse Tea (page 289), 1–3 cups daily.

If you're feeling good on the simple broths on days 1–3, you can continue this for the remainder of the week, and wait until week 2 to bring in the slow-cooked soups.

DAYS 4–7

While still focusing on soups, now is the time to bring solids (well-cooked vegetables and slow-cooked meats) into the picture. The best four recipes to choose during this time and going into week two are the slow-cooked soups:
* Ham Hock Soup (page 153)
* Hunter Soup (Bigos) (page 156)
* Hearty Oxtail Soup (page 160)
* Thai Pumpkin Soup with Braised Beef Cheek (page 171)

If you suffer dysglycemia (spiking high or low blood sugar levels with symptoms such as dizziness, confusion, mood changes, and uncontrollable cravings if you go more than an hour or two without food) or have diabetes, then be sure to have regular meals during the day, especially breakfast. This will help get your cortisol and insulin better regulated while nourishing your cells with the nutrients they're needing. You will start to find that gradually your blood sugar levels become better regulated and you will naturally be able to last longer between meals. It is better to allow this process to occur naturally, rather than force extended periods between meals. The better nourished your cells become, the less frequently you'll need to eat and the more sensitive your leptin receptors will become (leptin is the hormone that signals to your brain that you are full; better leptin sensitivity equals increased satiety).

WEEK 2

Introduce a very small amount of fermented veggies. I'm talking really small: ½ teaspoon per day. If you feel bloating or discomfort, then drop back to ¼ teaspoon of the *juice* from the fermented veggies. If you're feeling good, slowly increase by ½ teaspoon every 3–4 days until you are eventually having 1–2 tablespoons with each meal. If you increase the amount and feel bloated or gassy, reduce to the lower amount and wait another week before increasing again. Remember: n = 1. Listen to your gut.

Continue with a mix of broth-based and slow-cooked soups, while also choosing from these shorter-cooked soups with super-tender veggies:

* Zucchini Soup with Fresh Mint (page 147)
* Healing Garlic Soup (page 150)
* Creamy Mushroom Soup (page 159)

During the first 4 weeks, leave out the nuts sprinkled on top. These little toppings are for later down the track when your gut is in better shape.

WEEK 3

Soups are still the feature at this stage – pick from any of the previously mentioned soup recipes that appeal to you, avoiding any ingredients you know you are sensitive to. You can also bring in a daily Green Smoothie (see recipe, page 295), keeping the mango to a minimum – just enough sweetness to make it enjoyable. If you can't get hold of a mango, use ½ banana or ½–1 cup organic frozen berries instead. Remember to drink your smoothies on an empty stomach, to chew them, and to wait at least half an hour before having anything else.

WEEK 4

Again, soups are the main feature, but you can now introduce one solid/main meal a day. A good guideline is two soup meals (e.g., dinner and either breakfast or lunch) and one main meal (e.g., breakfast or lunch) or a light meal/snack.

If your blood sugar levels are stable (you are not having crashes in energy or mood and no spikes in cravings) but you're not feeling hungry, then don't force yourself to eat a meal. Your body will tell you when you're hungry. If you eat when you are not hungry, you create extra stress on your gut (which won't be primed with acids and enzymes to digest food) and on your pancreas and adrenals, which produce insulin and cortisol. If you are not hungry, don't eat just because it's a defined mealtime. This is not about starving yourself – let's make that very clear. If you are hungry, eat appropriately – do not enforce fasting, especially if your blood sugar regulation isn't tiptop. Fasting will force your hormones into a stress response.

TREATS

If you really can't overcome a sweet craving, then we have a selection of treat recipes that are low in natural sugars and yet also contain anti-inflammatory gut-healing ingredients. I really encourage you to leave these for after your 4 weeks if you can, and to enjoy them only on occasion, not as a regular treat. As always, take note of how you feel when you consume them.

WEEK 5 AND BEYOND

Gut healing takes time – months or even years. It's a gradual process. The more aligned you can keep your diet and lifestyle, the sooner you'll get results. Use these 4 weeks wisely, sticking to the plan 100 percent. These 4 weeks are a great opportunity to observe how you feel on different foods. Keep this in mind when choosing your foods going forward.

Chances are that you will benefit from having the support of a health practitioner – either an excellent naturopath or integrative doctor – who can help with the nitty gritty details of repair. For example, it may be a huge benefit, and even necessary, to have a fecal microbial analysis done to help you determine the health of your gut flora. Blood tests to check nutritional biochemistry and immune and inflammatory markers can also be exceptionally useful. So, if your zinc is low, you may indeed need a supplement. Getting advice on the right form of zinc to take and the appropriate dosage will get you better bang for your buck.

If you are hungry, eat appropriately – do not enforce fasting, especially if your blood sugar regulation isn't tiptop.

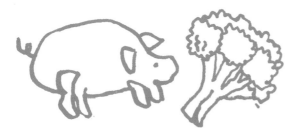

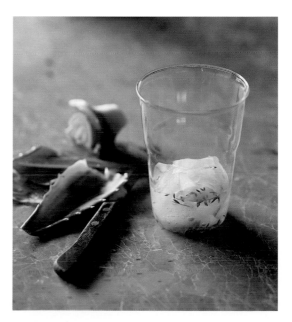

Here is a handy list of naturopathic remedies that I often recommend and which you can use at home to ease minor ailments. As always, see a health professional if conditions persist or worsen.

SYMPTOMS	OPTIONS	HOW AND WHEN
CANDIDA/THRUSH	Helen's Chai-biotic (page 284)	2–3 cups daily
COLD AND FLU SYMPTOMS	Coconut and Turmeric Kefir with Ginger and Cayenne (page 298)	1 shot 2–3 x daily
	Beet, Ginger, and Turmeric Kvass (page 301)	1 shot 2–3 x daily
	Coconut and Ginger Kefir (page 296)	1 shot 2–3 x daily
	Gut and Liver Cleanse Tea (page 289)	1 cup 2 x daily
	Tea tree and lavender essential oil blend	Pop in a diffuser or a bowl of hot water to inhale
CONSTIPATION	Gut and Liver Cleanse Tea (page 289)	Between broths/meals
	Warm Flaxseed Porridge (page 177)	As a snack or light meal
	Stewed Apple with Licorice Root and Flaxseed Meal (page 178)	As a snack or light meal
	1 tablespoon slippery elm or psyllium husk	Mix into a glass of water and drink immediately. Best on an empty stomach. 1–3 x daily
ESOPHAGITIS	Gut-Soothing Tea (page 283)	1 cup 2–3 x daily
FATIGUE	Bath with Enliven-Me Bath Salts (page 319)	20-minute soak, or even a 10-minute footbath, if time is short
FEELINGS OF ANGER OR FRUSTRATION (COMMON WHEN GOING THROUGH DETOXIFICATION)	Counseling	
	Gut and Liver Cleanse Tea (page 289)	2–3 cups daily
	Bath with Sweet Dreams Bath Salts (page 320)	20-minute soak
	Rose essential oil	Add to a bath, or dilute in a carrier oil and apply to the skin

SYMPTOMS	OPTIONS	HOW AND WHEN
GAS	Peppermint and chamomile massage oil blend	In a gentle circular motion on the abdomen, stroke up on the right-hand side, down on the left
HEADACHES	Gut and Liver Cleanse Tea (page 289)	1–3 cups daily
	Charcoal Mop-up (page 290)	1 glass 1–2 x daily if headache appears to be from detoxification
	Bath with Sweet Dreams Bath Salts (page 320)	20-minute soak to get a good dose of magnesium
	Peppermint and chamomile massage oil blend or rosemary essential oil	Apply a couple of drops of the blend (in a carrier oil such as cold-pressed jojoba, macadamia or olive oil, rosehip oil or organic tallow) to the fingertips and massage into the temples
INDIGESTION	Digestif Tea (page 286)	20 minutes after broths/meals
	Fire Tonic (page 302)	1–2 tablespoons in water 10 minutes before broths/meals
IRRITABLE BOWEL SYMPTOMS	Gut-Soothing Tea (page 283)	1 cup 2–3 x daily
MOUTH ULCERS	Gut-Soothing Tea (page 283)	1 cup 2–3 x daily
NAUSEA	Peppermint essential oil	1 drop on a tissue, inhale
	Ginger, chamomile, peppermint, and/or fennel tea	1 cup as needed
REFLUX	Chamomile and Licorice Tea (page 292)	1 cup as needed
	Fire Tonic (page 302)	1–2 tablespoons in water 10 minutes before meals
SKIN BREAKOUTS	Gut and Liver Cleanse Tea (page 289)	2–3 cups per day
	Bath with Epsom salts	20-minute soak as many days in the week as you can manage. Footbaths help, too

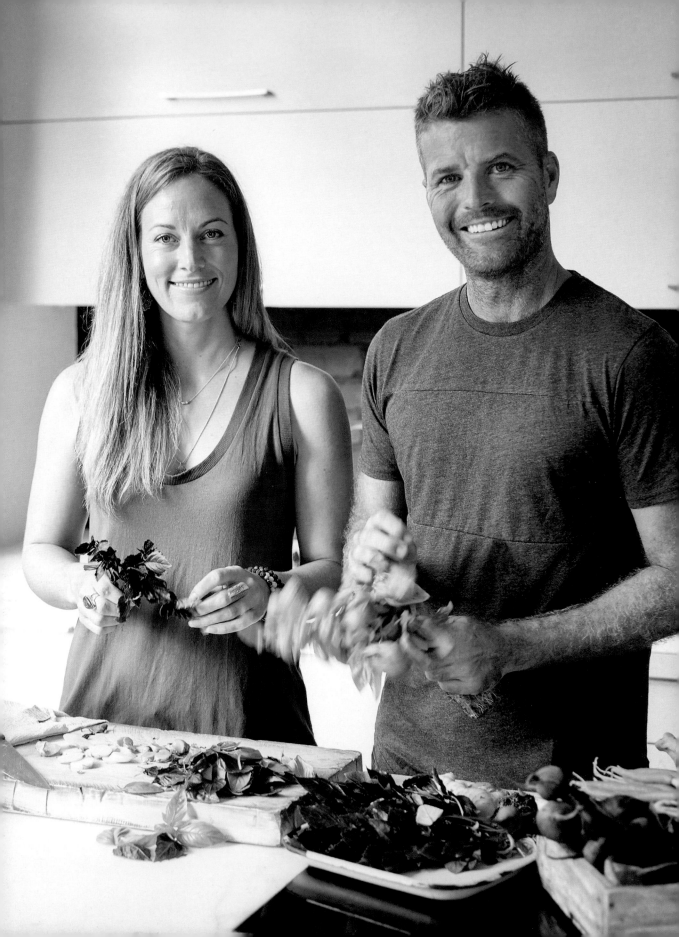

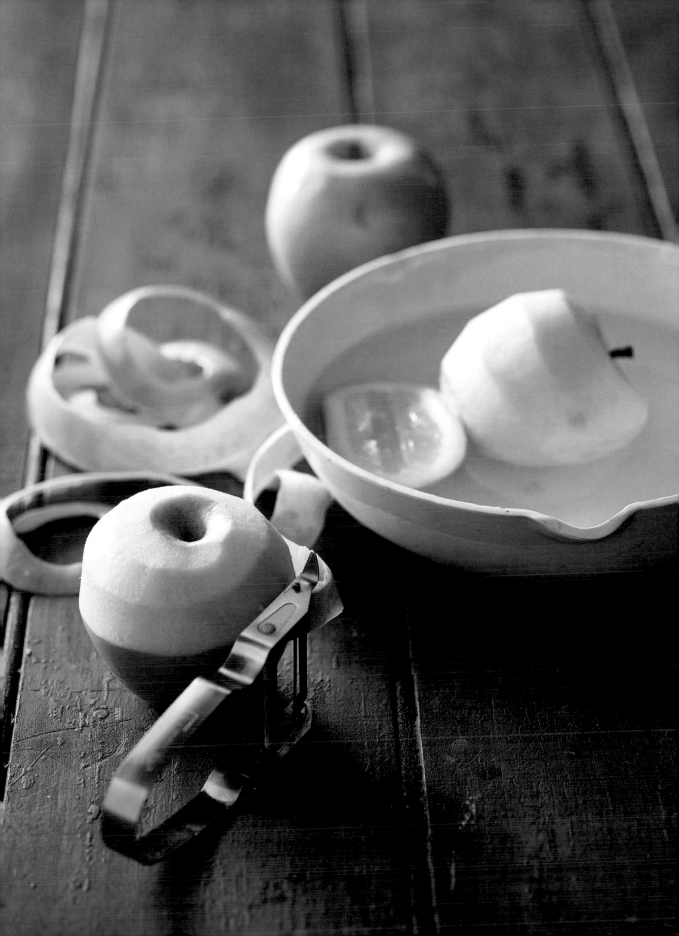

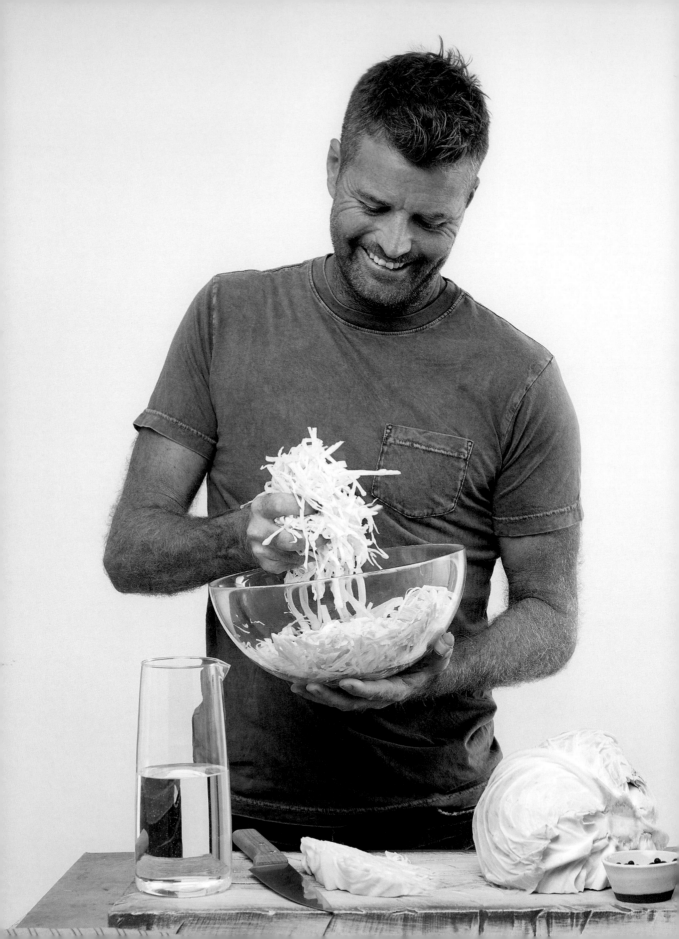

PART TWO GUT HEALTH RECIPES

100+ DELICIOUS RECIPES FOR ACHIEVING AND MAINTAINING OPTIMAL GUT HEALTH

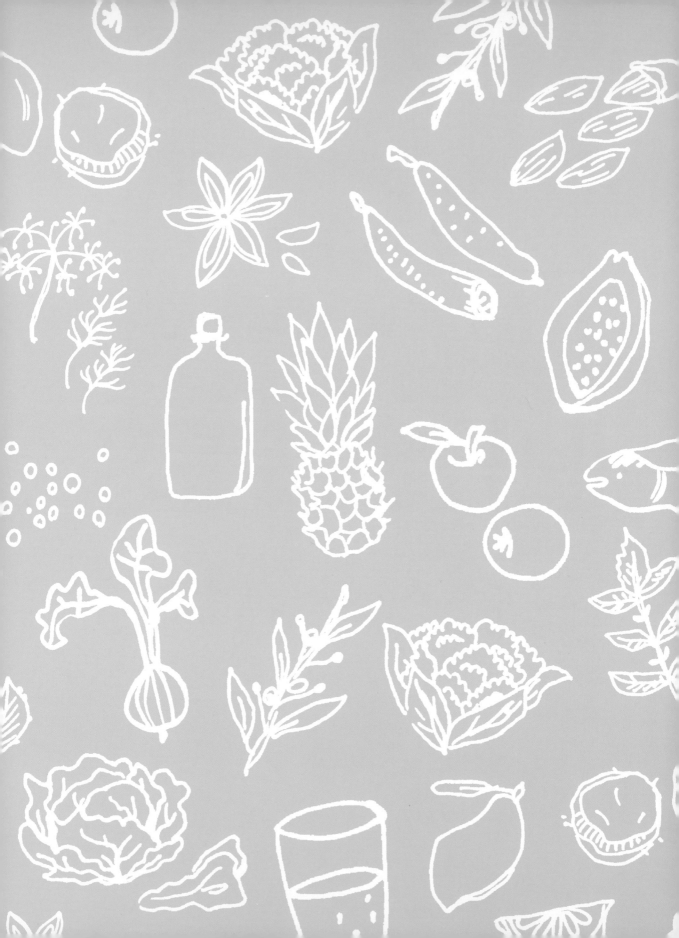

FERMENTS

COCONUT YOGURT (CANNED)

MAKES ABOUT 5½ CUPS

This super yummy coconut yogurt is a really simple way to get good dairy-free fats and healthy probiotics into your diet. We make this once or twice a week and use it in smoothies, sprinkle it on top of our paleo muesli, or eat it straight out of the jar. Feel free to add in some spices, cacao, berries, or other types of in-season fruit that you love or some activated nuts and seeds (unless you're doing AIP). If you want to get serious about yogurt-making, you might like to look for an electric yogurt maker or dehydrator that allows for at least twenty-four hours of fermenation time.

---

1 tablespoon powdered gelatin

3 x 13.5-ounce cans (5 cups) coconut milk

1 vanilla pod, split and seeds scraped
    (optional)

1–2 tablespoons honey, maple syrup, or
    coconut sugar

2 probiotic capsules or ¼ teaspoon
    vegetable starter culture*

1 tablespoon lemon juice (optional)

* See Glossary

MAKE AIP FRIENDLY

Omit: vanilla

Note: For those doing AIP, natural sweetener is allowed in this recipe as it is needed for the fermentation process. The bacteria fermenting the coconut milk consume the sugar, not you.

You'll need a 1½-quart preserving jar with a lid for this recipe. Wash the jar and all utensils thoroughly in very hot soapy water, then run them through a hot rinse cycle in the dishwasher to sterilize.

Put 3 tablespoons filtered water in a small bowl, sprinkle on the gelatin, and soak for 2 minutes.

Combine the coconut milk and vanilla seeds (if using) in a saucepan and gently heat, stirring with a spoon, over medium-low heat until just starting to simmer (200°F, if testing with a thermometer). Do not allow to boil. Immediately remove the pan from the heat. While still hot, mix in the gelatin mixture, then add the sweetener and mix well. Cover the pan with a lid and set aside to cool to lukewarm (100°F or less).

Pour ½ cup of the cooled coconut milk mixture into a sterilized bowl. Open the probiotic capsules (if using). Stir the probiotic powder or starter culture and lemon juice (if using) into the coconut milk in the bowl. Add the remaining coconut milk and mix well.

Pour the coconut milk mixture into the sterilized jar and seal the lid loosely. Ferment in a warm spot for 12 hours at 100–104°F. To maintain this temperature and allow the yogurt to culture, wrap your jar in a kitchen towel and place it on a plate in the oven with the door shut and the oven light on. The light's warmth will keep the temperature consistent. Alternatively, place the kitchen towel–wrapped jar in a cooler, fill a heatproof container with boiling water and place it beside the jar – do not allow them to touch – and close the lid. Replace the boiling water halfway through the fermenting process.

Once fermented, the yogurt tends to form air bubbles and looks as though it has separated. Stir well and refrigerate for at least 5 hours before eating. If it separates after chilling, give it a good whisk. Store in the fridge for up to 2 weeks.

TIP

Taste the yogurt after 12 hours. If you prefer a tangier taste, you can leave it to ferment for another couple of hours.

COCONUT YOGURT (FRESH)

MAKES ABOUT 2 CUPS

I have included two different types of coconut yogurt in this book – one is for when you have canned coconut milk, and this one is for when you have young coconuts and want to make something exciting with them.

---

4 young coconuts* (you'll need about 7 cups coconut flesh, woody bits removed, and 1 cup coconut water, plus extra coconut water if necessary)

juice of 1 lemon or lime

yacon syrup*, maple syrup, or honey, to taste

2 probiotic capsules or ¼ teaspoon vegetable starter culture*

* See Glossary

> AIP FRIENDLY

Note: For those doing AIP, natural sweetener is allowed in this recipe as it is needed for the fermentation process. The bacteria fermenting the coconut milk consume the sugar, not you.

You'll need a 1-quart preserving jar with a lid for this recipe. Wash the jar and all utensils thoroughly in very hot soapy water, then run them through a hot rinse cycle in the dishwasher to sterilize.

To make the coconut cream, combine the coconut flesh, coconut water, lemon or lime juice, and sweetener in a blender and process until smooth and creamy. Add a little more coconut water if you prefer a runnier texture, and mix well. Open the probiotic capsules (if using). Tip the starter culture or probiotic powder into the blender and pulse for 10 seconds. Pour into the prepared glass jar and seal loosely.

Ferment the yogurt in a warm spot for 12 hours at 100–104°F. To maintain this temperature and allow the yogurt to culture, wrap your jar in a kitchen towel and place it on a plate in the oven with the door shut and the oven light on. The warmth from the light will keep the temperature consistent. Alternatively, place the kitchen towel–wrapped jar in a cooler, fill a heatproof container with boiling water, and place it beside the jar – do not allow them to touch – and close the lid. Replace the boiling water halfway through the fermenting process.

Taste the yogurt after 12 hours. If you prefer a tangier flavor, leave it to ferment for another couple of hours. Once fermented, the yogurt tends to form air bubbles and looks as though it has separated. Stir well and refrigerate for at least 5 hours before eating. If it separates after chilling, give it a good whisk. Store the yogurt in the fridge for up to 2 weeks.

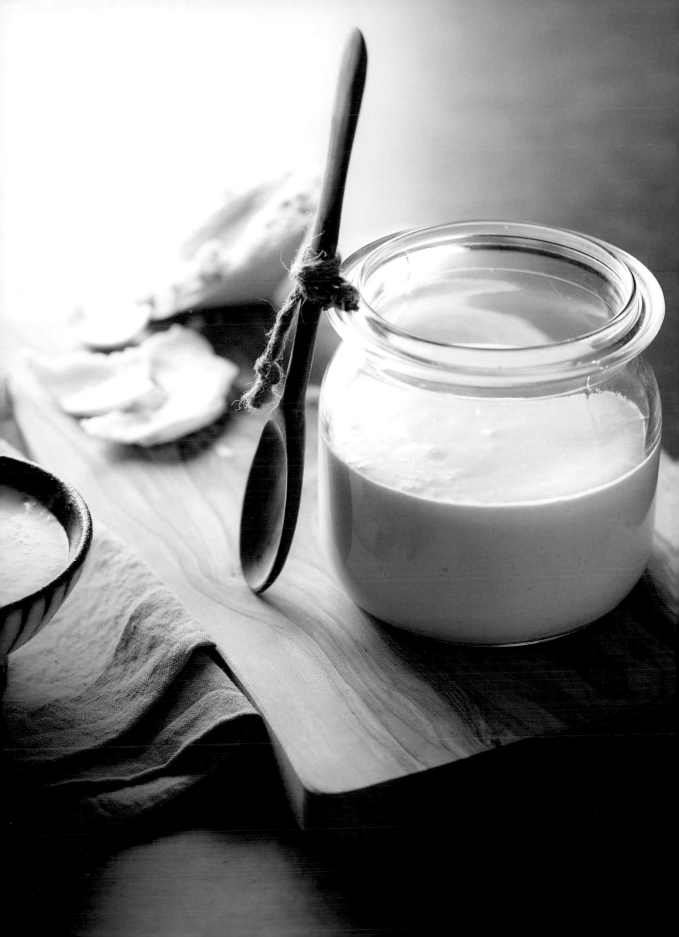

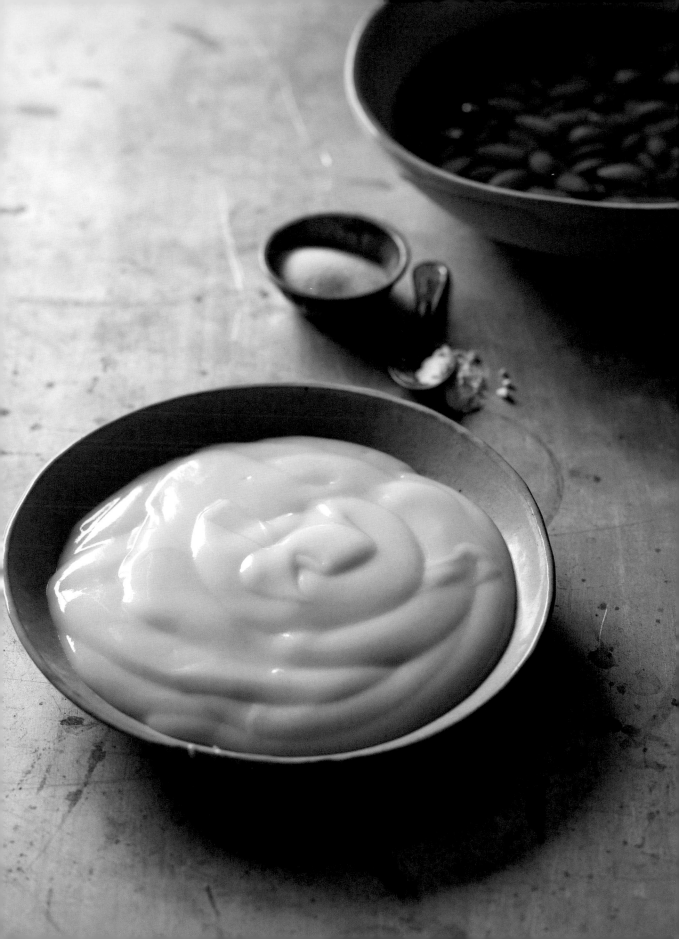

ALMOND MILK YOGURT

MAKES ABOUT 5½ CUPS

Some people have a reaction to nuts, while others cannot tolerate coconuts. I wanted to cover all bases with this book, so here I've included a yogurt for people who can't do coconuts or dairy, but still want that yogurt experience.

¼ cup tapioca flour*

1 quart (4 cups) Almond Milk (page 306)

1½ tablespoons powdered gelatin*

2 tablespoons honey or coconut sugar

2 probiotic capsules or ¼ teaspoon vegetable starter culture*

* See Glossary

TIP

Taste the yogurt after 12 hours. If you prefer a tangier taste, you can leave it to ferment for another couple of hours.

You'll need a 1½-quart preserving jar with a lid for this recipe. Wash the jar and all utensils thoroughly in very hot soapy water, then run them through a hot rinse cycle in the dishwasher to sterilize.

Mix the tapioca flour with ½ cup almond milk in a small bowl, and set aside.

Put 3 tablespoons filtered water in a small bowl, sprinkle the gelatin over, and soak for 2 minutes. Set aside.

Pour 1 cup filtered water into a saucepan, bring to a boil, and whisk in the remaining almond milk, the tapioca mixture, and the honey or sugar. Bring back to a boil and whisk constantly until the mixture coats the back of a spoon, 10–15 seconds.

Remove the pan from the heat, stir in the gelatin until dissolved, cover, and set aside to cool to 100°F or less.

Pour ½ cup of the cooled almond milk mixture into a sterilized bowl. Open the probiotic capsules (if using). Tip the probiotic powder or starter culture into the almond milk mixture in the bowl, and stir. Add the remaining cooled almond milk mixture, and mix well. Pour into the sterilized glass jar and seal loosely.

Ferment the yogurt in a warm spot for 10–12 hours at 100–104°F. To maintain this temperature and allow the yogurt to culture, wrap your jar in a kitchen towel and place on a plate in the oven with the door shut and the oven light on. The warmth from the light will keep the temperature consistent. (See page 86 for an alternative method using a cooler.)

Once fermented, the yogurt tends to form air bubbles and looks as though it has separated. Stir well and refrigerate for at least 5 hours before eating. If it separates after chilling, give it a good whisk. Store in the fridge for up to 2 weeks.

ACTIVATED CHARCOAL YOGURT

SERVES 4–6

Activated charcoal is a hot topic in health circles. It is touted as being able to do everything from whiten teeth to help with digestion and remove toxins from the body. My understanding is that a little activated charcoal isn't harmful, so I wanted to create an activated charcoal yogurt that will have your guests talking next time you serve it up. Activated charcoal powder can be obtained easily from health-food stores, pharmacies, and online.

4 cups Coconut Yogurt (page 86 or 88)
   or Almond Milk Yogurt (page 91)
1½–2 tablespoons activated charcoal
   powder

| MAKE AIP FRIENDLY |

Use: coconut yogurt

You will need a 1-quart preserving jar with a lid for this recipe. Wash the jar and all utensils thoroughly in very hot soapy water, then run them through a hot rinse cycle in the dishwasher to sterilize.

Combine the yogurt and charcoal in a bowl and mix well. Pour into the sterilized jar, seal with the lid, and store in the refrigerator for up to 2 weeks.

NOTE

Activated charcoal acts as a bit of a mop-up agent in the gut, binding to potential toxins. This can make it valuable when used as part of a detox program. It can also help relieve bloating and gas. Charcoal doesn't discriminate, though, so it will bind to nutrients, not just toxins. For this reason, it's best to have charcoal separate from main meals to prevent inhibiting the absorption of nutrients from your meal.

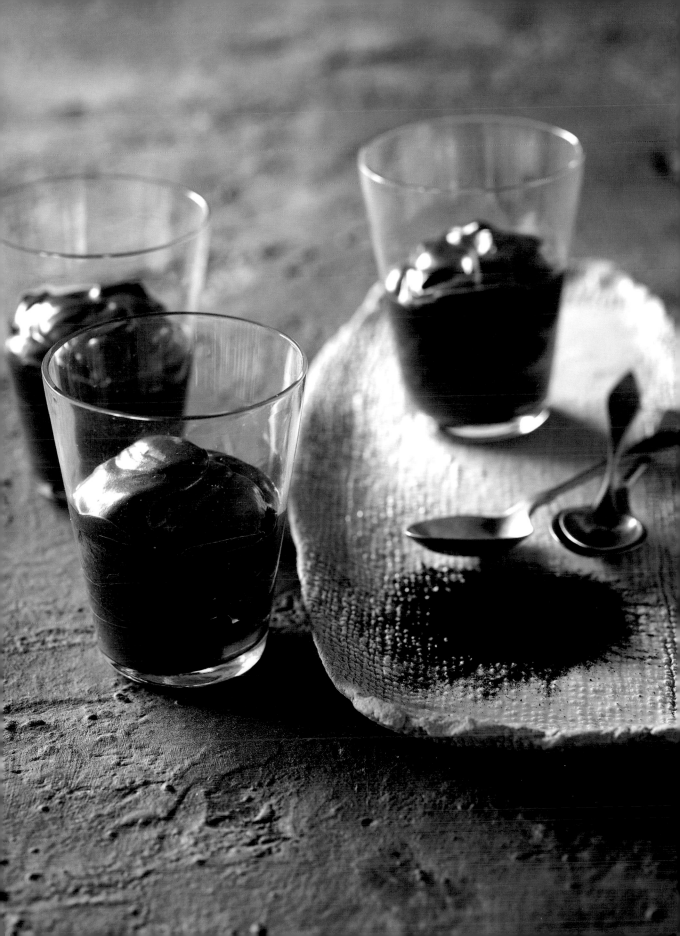

SAUERKRAUT

MAKES 1 x 1½-QUART JAR

If I had to choose only one dish to encourage you to eat daily, this would be it (closely followed by bone broth). Classic sauerkraut has been around for centuries, and is something that has fascinated me for years. I find it very rewarding spending the time shredding the cabbage and massaging it with salt, adding the spices and herbs, filling the glass jar, and pressing the cabbage mixture down. It is quite a meditative process, especially as you have to wait a couple of weeks to savor the fruits of your labor.

---

1 star anise
1 teaspoon whole cloves
1⅓ pounds cabbage (you can use green or red, or a mixture of the two)
1½ teaspoons sea salt (or 3 teaspoons if not using the vegetable starter culture – see opposite)

2 teaspoons caraway seeds
2 tablespoons juniper berries*
1 small handful dill fronds, roughly chopped
½ packet vegetable starter culture* (optional)

* See Glossary

MAKE AIP FRIENDLY

Omit: star anise, caraway seeds, and juniper berries
Substitute: parsley or thyme in place of omitted spices

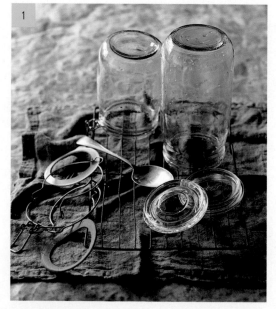

You will need a 1½-quart preserving jar with an airlock lid for this recipe. Wash the jar and all the utensils you will be using in very hot water, then run them through a hot rinse cycle in the dishwasher.

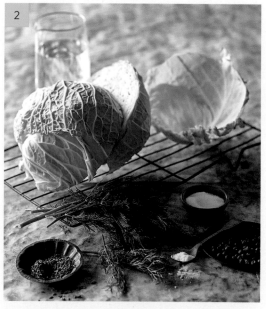

Place the star anise and cloves on a small piece of cheesecloth, tie into a bundle, and set aside. Remove the outer leaves of the cabbage, choosing one to wash well and set aside. Shred the cabbage head.

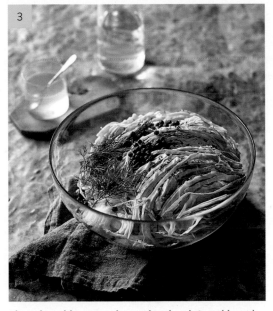

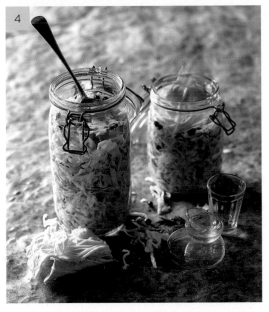

Place the cabbage in a large glass bowl. Sprinkle with the salt, caraway, juniper, and dill. Massage the cabbage for 10 minutes to release its juices. Dissolve the starter (if using) in water according to packet instructions. Add to the cabbage mix with the bag of spices. Mix well.

Fill the prepared jar with the cabbage mix, pressing down well with a large spoon or potato masher to remove any air pockets. Leave ¾ inch of room free at the top. The cabbage should be completely submerged in its juices; add more water if necessary.

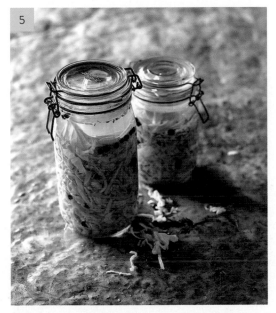

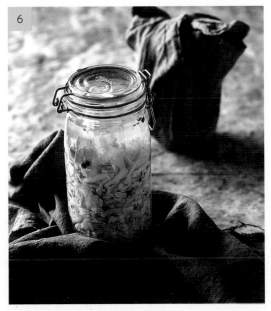

Take the clean cabbage leaf, fold it up, and place it on top of the cabbage mixture, then add a small glass weight (a shot glass is ideal) to keep everything submerged.

Close the lid. Wrap a kitchen towel around the jar to block out the light. Store in a dark place at 60–73°F for 8–15 days (add another 5 days if not using the starter culture). You can place the jar in a cooler to maintain a more consistent temperature. →

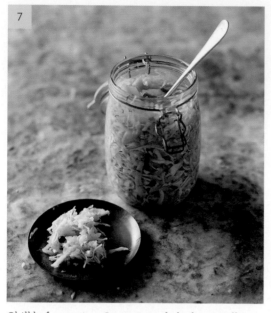

Chill before eating. Once opened, the kraut will last for up to 2 months in the fridge when kept submerged in the liquid. If unopened, it will keep for up to 9 months in the fridge. ■

NOTES

Different vegetables have different culturing times, and the warmer the climate, the shorter the time needed. The highest level of good bacteria usually occurs after 8–15 days of fermentation. It's up to you how long you leave it – from as little as 4 days to up to a couple of months. Some people prefer the tangier flavor that comes with extra fermenting time, while others prefer a milder flavor.

Remember never to heat kraut, as it is a live food, and heat destroys the beneficial bacteria.

Start off small with only a teaspoon, and work your way up to 1–2 tablespoons per meal each day.

TIPS

I use my Culture For Life starter jar as they are purpose-made for fermenting vegetables. If you do use one of these, there is no need to cover and weight the shredded cabbage with a folded cabbage leaf and shot glass, as the jar has an inbuilt weighting system. There is also no need to cover with a kitchen towel, as there is a silicone cover provided to block out the light.

Never throw out the sauerkraut brine when you've finished your kraut! Drink a shot of this every day to help the beneficial gut bacteria proliferate.

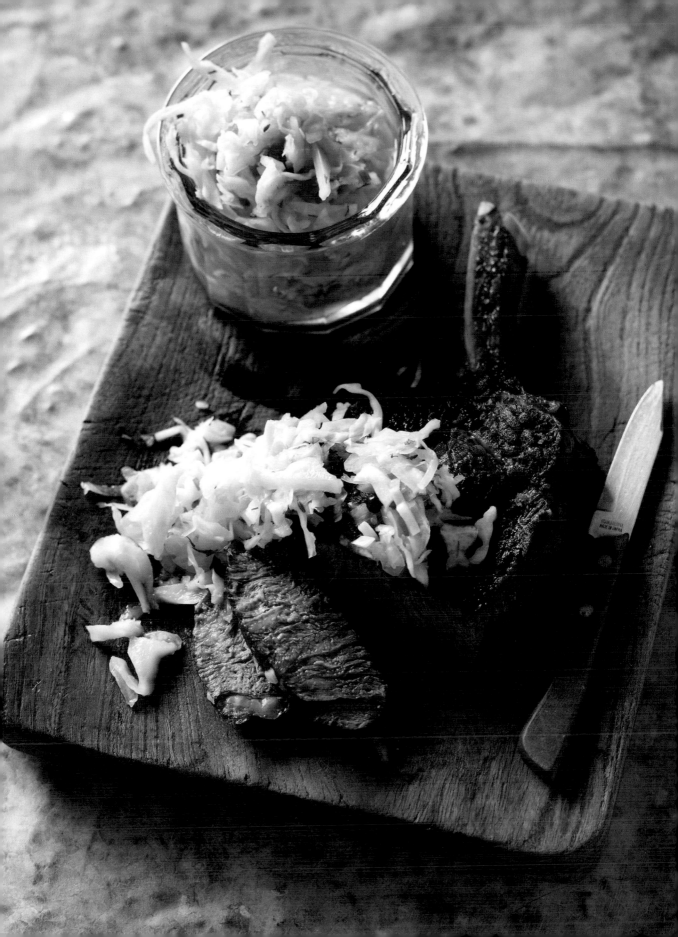

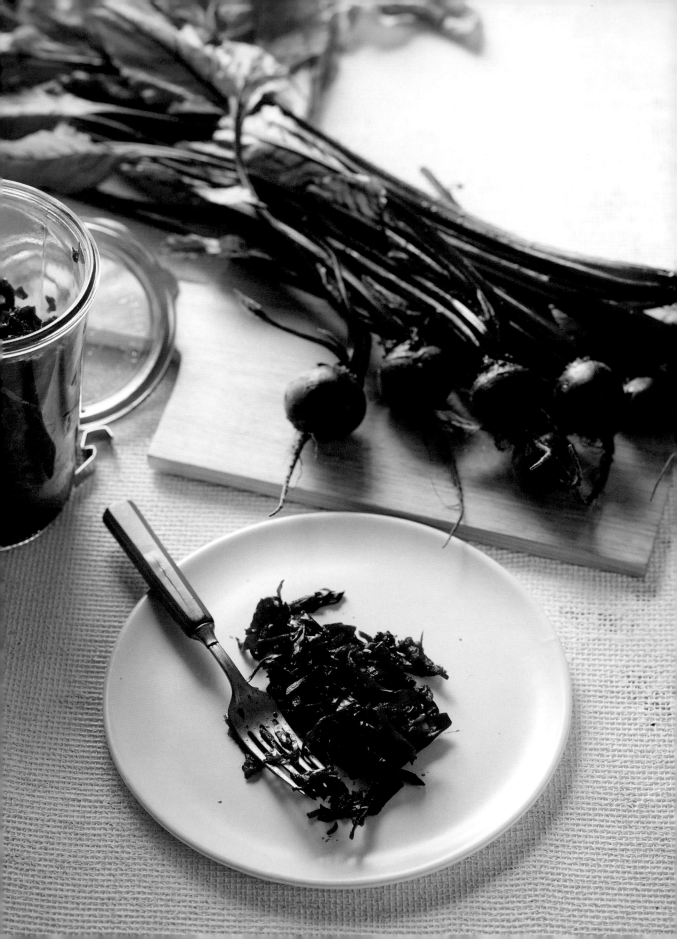

BEET KRAUT
WITH WATTLESEEDS

MAKES 1 x 1½-QUART JAR

Beet kraut goes with just about everything: roast beef, steak, roast pork with crackling, bacon and eggs, slow-cooked ribs – as well as seafood (salmon in particular). It is awesome on eggs or in a salad. Give this a go once you have mastered the classic kraut.

---

1 teaspoon black peppercorns
4 large beets, trimmed and sliced into very
  thin strips (you can use a food processor
  or mandoline for this)
¼ cabbage (you can use green or red,
  or a mixture of the two)
finely grated zest of 1 lemon
1 teaspoon ground and toasted wattleseeds*
  (optional)
1½ teaspoons sea salt (or 3 teaspoons
  if not using the vegetable starter
  culture – see below)
½ packet vegetable starter culture*
  (optional)

* See Glossary

MAKE AIP FRIENDLY

Omit: black peppercorns and wattleseeds
Substitute: parsley, mint, or your favorite
herb in place of wattleseeds

You'll need a 1½-quart preserving jar with an airlock lid for this recipe. Wash the jar and all utensils in very hot soapy water, then run them through a hot rinse cycle in the dishwasher to sterilize.

Place the peppercorns on a small piece of cheesecloth, tie into a bundle, and set aside. Put the beets in a large glass or stainless-steel bowl. Remove the outer leaves of the cabbage. Choose one of the outer leaves, wash it well, and set aside. Shred the cabbage in the food processor, or slice by hand or with a mandoline. Add the shredded cabbage, lemon zest and wattleseeds (if using) to the beets, then sprinkle with the salt. Mix well, cover, and set aside for 10 minutes (the cabbage will start to break down and release its liquid until it is quite wet) while you prepare the culture.

Dissolve the starter culture (if using) in filtered water according to the packet instructions (the amount of water will depend on the brand). Add to the beet mixture along with the cheesecloth bag containing the peppercorns, and mix well.

Fill the prepared jar with the beet mixture, pressing down well with a large spoon or potato masher to remove any air pockets. Leave ¾ inch of room free at the top. The vegetables should be completely submerged in the liquid; add more water if necessary.

Fold up the clean cabbage leaf and place it on top of the beet mixture, then add a small glass weight (a shot glass is ideal) to keep everything submerged. Close the lid, then wrap a kitchen towel around the jar to block out the light. Store in a dark place (e.g., a cooler) at 60–73°F for 8–15 days (add another 5 days if not using the culture). See Notes on page 96 for more information about vegetable culturing times.

Chill before eating. Once opened, it will last for up to 2 months in the fridge when kept submerged in the liquid. If unopened, it will keep for up to 9 months in the fridge.

FERMENTED INDIAN-SPICED CAULIFLOWER

MAKES 1 x 2-QUART JAR

Once you have mastered the classic kraut, it is time to take off your training wheels and open up a whole new world of fermented culinary masterpieces. Play around with different vegetables, spices, and herbs, and create your own gourmet delicacies. This kraut is one of my all-time favorites, and it's the one that my wife, Nic, always asks me to make.

---

1 large head of cauliflower (about 2 pounds), broken into small florets

7 ounces green cabbage, shredded (reserve one well-washed outer leaf)

2½ teaspoons sea salt (or 4 teaspoons if not using the vegetable starter culture – see below)

½ packet vegetable starter culture* (optional)

2½ teaspoons ground turmeric

2 teaspoons cumin seeds, toasted

½ teaspoon mustard seeds, toasted

½ teaspoon ground coriander

½ teaspoon finely grated ginger

20 fresh curry leaves

15 cardamom pods

* See Glossary

MAKE AIP FRIENDLY

Omit: cumin seeds, mustard seeds, ground coriander, and cardamom pods

You'll need a 2-quart preserving jar with an airlock lid for this recipe. Wash the jar and all utensils in very hot soapy water, then run them through a hot rinse cycle in the dishwasher to sterilize.

Combine the cauliflower and cabbage in a glass or stainless-steel bowl and sprinkle on the salt. Mix well, cover, and set aside.

Dissolve the starter culture (if using) in filtered water according to the packet instructions (the amount of water will depend on the brand you are using). Add to the cauliflower and cabbage along with the turmeric, cumin, and mustard seeds, ground coriander, grated ginger, curry leaves, and cardamom pods, and mix well.

Fill the prepared jar with the cauliflower mixture, pressing down with a large spoon to remove any air pockets and leaving ¾ inch of room free at the top. The vegetables should be completely submerged in the liquid; add more filtered water if necessary.

Take the reserved cabbage leaf, fold it up, and place it on top of the cauliflower mixture, then add a small glass weight (a shot glass is ideal) to keep everything submerged. Close the lid and wrap a kitchen towel around the jar to block out the light. Store in a dark place (e.g., a cooler) at 60–73°F for 8–15 days (add another 5 days if not using the starter culture). See Notes on page 96 for more information about vegetable culturing times.

Chill before eating. Once opened, the spiced cauliflower will last for up to 2 months in the fridge when kept submerged in the liquid. If unopened, it will keep for up to 9 months in the fridge.

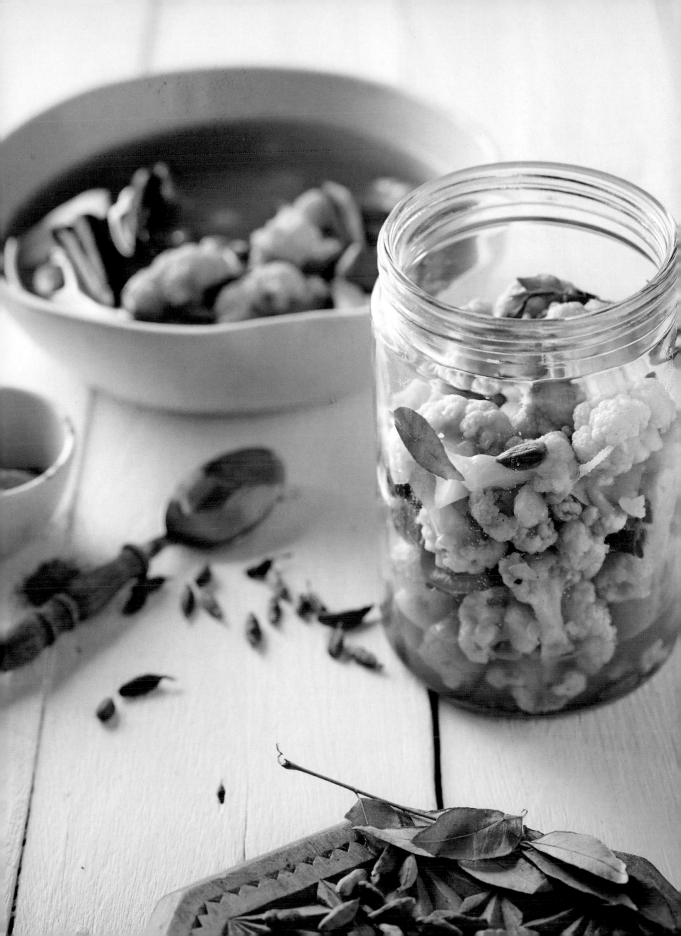

FERMENTED ESCABECHE

MAKES 1 x 1½-QUART JAR

Escabeche, a classic recipe from Europe, is basically an acidic dish of meat or seafood and vegetables. Here, I have used the base elements of a classic escabeche – onion, celery, and carrot – and fermented them to create the most amazing accompaniment to simple grilled fish, such as sardines, any type of crustacean, or grilled chicken thighs with the skin on.

---

1 teaspoon coriander seeds, lightly crushed

½ teaspoon cumin seeds, lightly crushed

1 teaspoon black peppercorns

1 onion, thinly sliced

1 fennel bulb, sliced

2 carrots, sliced

2 celery ribs, sliced

4 garlic cloves, sliced

2 fresh bay leaves

4 thyme sprigs

1½ teaspoons sea salt (or 3 teaspoons if not using the vegetable starter culture – see below)

½ packet vegetable starter culture* (optional)

1 well-washed small cabbage leaf

* See Glossary

MAKE AIP FRIENDLY

Omit: coriander seeds, cumin seeds, and black peppercorns

You'll need a 1½-quart preserving jar with an airlock lid for this recipe. Wash the jar and all utensils in very hot soapy water, then run them through a hot rinse cycle in the dishwasher to sterilize.

Combine the coriander and cumin seeds, peppercorns, onion, fennel, carrot, celery, garlic, bay leaves, and thyme in a glass or stainless-steel bowl. Add the salt, mix well, cover, and set aside.

Dissolve the starter culture (if using) in filtered water according to the packet instructions (the amount of water will depend on the brand you are using). Add to the vegetable mixture and mix well.

Fill the prepared jar with the vegetable mixture, pressing down well with a large spoon or potato masher to remove any air pockets. Leave ¾ inch of room free at the top. The vegetables should be completely submerged in the liquid; add more filtered water if necessary.

Take the clean cabbage leaf, fold it up, and place it on top of the vegetable mixture, then add a small glass weight (a shot glass is ideal) to keep everything submerged. Close the lid, then wrap a kitchen towel around the jar to block out the light. Store in a dark place (e.g., a cooler) at 60–73°F for 8–15 days (add another 5 days if not using the starter culture). See Notes on page 96 for more information about vegetable culturing times.

Chill before eating. Once opened, the escabeche will last for up to 2 months in the fridge when kept submerged in the liquid. Unopened, it will keep for up to 9 months in the fridge.

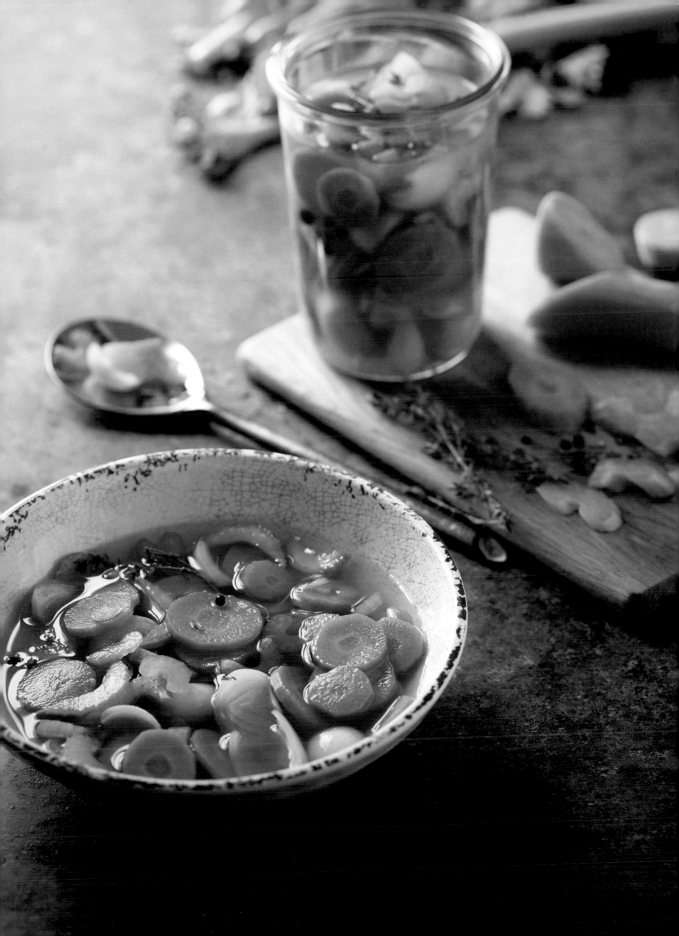

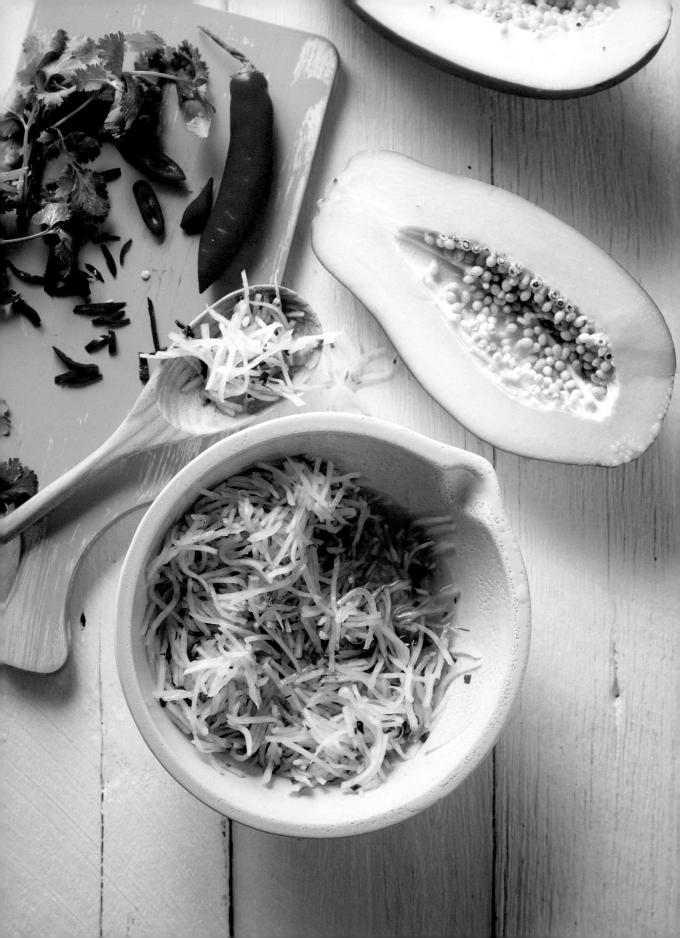

FERMENTED GREEN PAPAYA

MAKES 1 x 1½-QUART JAR

Hands down, this is my favorite fermented dish to serve alongside barbecued seafood or chicken. When papaya is green (unripe) it is at its healthiest for us to consume, as the sugars haven't yet concentrated – which is why the flesh is still rock hard. When like this, you have to grate or shred the papaya and add the flavors that you love – try ginger, chile, lemongrass, or garlic – and ferment for up to a week.

---

2 green papayas (about 1½ pounds each), peeled and seeded

3 teaspoons sea salt

1 long red chile, seeded and finely chopped

1½ tablespoons finely grated ginger

2 tablespoons finely chopped cilantro leaves

2 tablespoons lime juice

1 well-washed small cabbage leaf

MAKE AIP FRIENDLY

Omit: chile

You'll need a 1½-quart preserving jar with an airlock lid for this recipe. Wash the jar and all utensils in very hot soapy water, then run them through a hot rinse cycle in the dishwasher to sterilize.

Shred the papaya in a food processor with a grater attachment, or grate by hand, then put it in a large glass or stainless-steel bowl. Sprinkle with the salt, chile, ginger, cilantro, and lime juice. Mix well and massage with your hands for 5 minutes to release some liquid.

Fill the prepared jar with the papaya mixture, pressing down well with a large spoon or potato masher to remove any air pockets. Pour in the liquid from the bowl, leaving ¾ inch of room free at the top. The papaya should be completely submerged in the liquid; add some filtered water if necessary.

Take the clean cabbage leaf, fold it up, and place it on top of the papaya mixture, then add a small glass weight (a shot glass is ideal) to keep everything submerged. Close the lid, then wrap a kitchen towel around the jar to block out the light. Store in a dark place (e.g., a cooler) at 60–73°F for 8–15 days. See Notes on page 96 for more information about vegetable culturing times.

Chill before eating. Once opened, the cultured papaya will last for up to 2 months in the fridge when kept submerged in the liquid. Unopened, it will keep for up to 9 months in the fridge.

SUMMER KRAUT WITH PINEAPPLE AND MINT

MAKES 1 x 1½-QUART JAR

Kitsa Yanniotis of Kitsa's Kitchen is a legend in the fermenting world, and really knows her stuff when it comes to making the most amazing gut-healing concoctions. When I first tried this summer kraut with pineapple, it knocked my socks off. This is a great dish for introducing fermented foods to the kids. Start them on just a teaspoon of the juice, mashed up with some avocado or sprinkled over their salad, and then slowly work up to ¼ teaspoon, then up to a teaspoon or two per meal when they appreciate the taste.

1 pound red or green cabbage

2 ounces kale, central stems removed

½ fennel bulb (about 4 ounces), trimmed and chopped

½ red onion (about 4 ounces), chopped

2 red apples, cored and chopped but not peeled

1 small handful mint leaves

7 ounces pineapple, chopped (1 cup)

1½ teaspoons sea salt (or 3 teaspoons if not using the vegetable starter culture – see below)

1 packet vegetable starter culture* (optional)

* See Glossary

AIP FRIENDLY

You'll need a 1½-quart preserving jar with an airlock lid for this recipe. Wash the jar and all utensils in very hot soapy water, then run them through a hot rinse cycle in the dishwasher to sterilize.

Remove the outer leaves of the cabbage, choose one, wash it well, and set aside for later. Put the remaining cabbage in the bowl of a food processor, add the kale, fennel, onion, apple, and mint, and process to shred. Remove from the food processor and transfer to a large glass or stainless-steel bowl. (You can also use a mandoline or knife to chop, then mix by hand.) Stir the pineapple through, sprinkle with the salt, cover, and set aside.

Dissolve the starter culture in filtered water according to the packet instructions (the amount of water will depend on the brand). Add to the cabbage mixture and mix again.

Fill the prepared jar with the cabbage mixture, pressing down well to remove any air pockets. Leave ¾ inch of room free at the top. The cabbage mixture should be completely submerged in the liquid; add more filtered water if necessary.

Take the clean cabbage leaf, fold it up, and place it on top of the kraut mixture, then add a small glass weight (a shot glass is ideal) to keep everything submerged. Close the lid, then wrap a kitchen towel around the jar to block out the light. Store in a dark place (e.g., a cooler) at 60–73°F for 8–15 days (add another 5 days if not using the starter culture). See Notes on page 96 for more information about vegetable culturing times.

Chill before eating. Once opened, the kraut will last for up to 2 months in the fridge when kept submerged in the liquid. Unopened, it will keep for up to 9 months in the fridge.

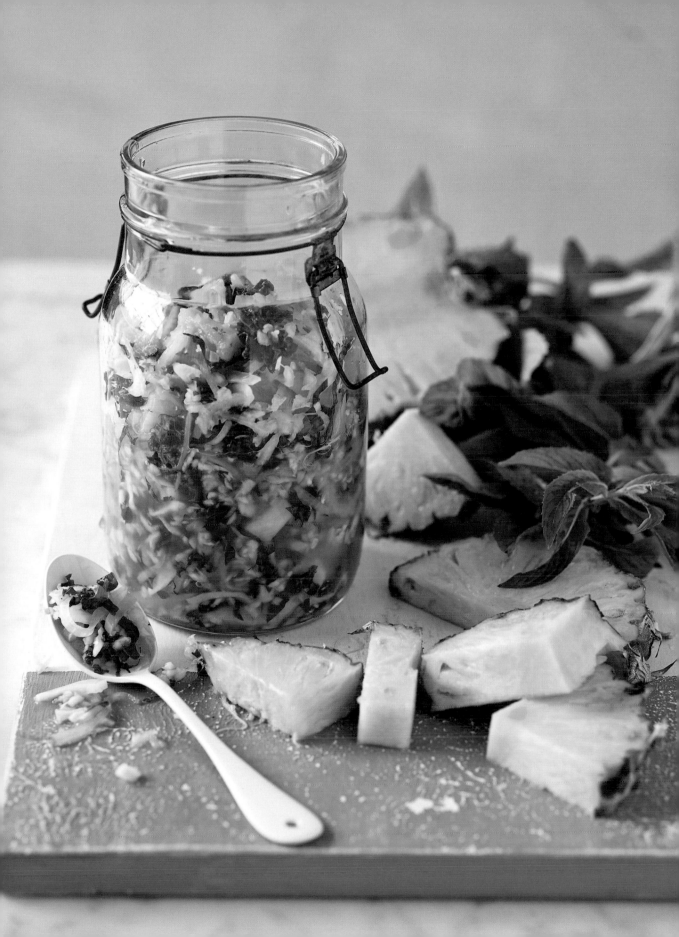

CLASSIC KIMCHI

MAKES 1 x 1½-QUART JAR

Kimchi is the national dish of Korea and Koreans eat close to 20 kilograms of it per person each year. They say their good health and vigor comes from having this fermented superfood every day. There are regional and seasonal variations, but at its heart kimchi is very similar to its European cousin, sauerkraut. I am a huge fan of kimchi and enjoy it on the side with many Asian dishes; it also works well with eggs for breakfast and with burgers when mixed with homemade mayonnaise.

½ napa cabbage (about 1¾ pounds)
1 yau choy (choy sum) or 1–2 bok choy, cut into 2-inch pieces
3 green onions, thinly sliced
1 bunch of cilantro, stalks and leaves, finely chopped
3 long red chiles, 2 seeded and finely chopped, 1 halved lengthwise and seeded
1½ teaspoons sea salt (or 3 teaspoons if not using the vegetable starter culture – see below)
3 garlic cloves, finely chopped
2-inch piece of ginger, cut into thin strips
1–2 tablespoons Korean chile powder (gochugaru) (see Note)
2–3 tablespoons fish sauce
½ packet vegetable starter culture* (optional)

* See Glossary

MAKE AIP FRIENDLY

Omit: chile and chile powder

You'll need a 1½-quart preserving jar with an airlock lid for this recipe. Wash the jar and all utensils in very hot soapy water, then run them through a hot rinse cycle in the dishwasher to sterilize.

Remove the outer leaves of the cabbage. Choose one, wash it well, and set aside. Cut the cabbage in half lengthwise, then cut crosswise into 2-inch pieces, discarding the root end.

Combine the cabbage, choy sum, green onions, cilantro, and chopped and halved chiles in a large glass or stainless-steel bowl, sprinkle with the salt, and mix well. Add the garlic, ginger, chile powder, and fish sauce. Mix well, cover, and set aside.

Dissolve the starter culture in filtered water according to the packet instructions (the amount of water will depend on the brand). Add to the vegetables and mix well. Fill the prepared jar with the vegetable mixture, pressing down well with a large spoon or potato masher to remove any air pockets. Leave ¾ inch of room free at the top. The vegetables should be completely submerged in the liquid; add more filtered water if necessary.

Fold the clean cabbage leaf, place it on top of the cabbage mixture, and add a small glass weight (a shot glass is ideal) to keep everything submerged. Close the lid, then wrap a kitchen towel around the jar to block out the light. Store in a dark place (e.g., a cooler) at 60–73°F for 8–15 days (add another 5 days if not using the starter culture). See Notes on page 96 for more information about vegetable culturing times.

Chill before eating. Once opened, the kimchi will last for up to 2 months in the fridge when kept submerged in the liquid. Unopened, it will keep for up to 9 months in the fridge.

NOTE
Korean chile powder has smoky, fruity, and sweet notes – and a hot kick. It is available from Asian grocers.

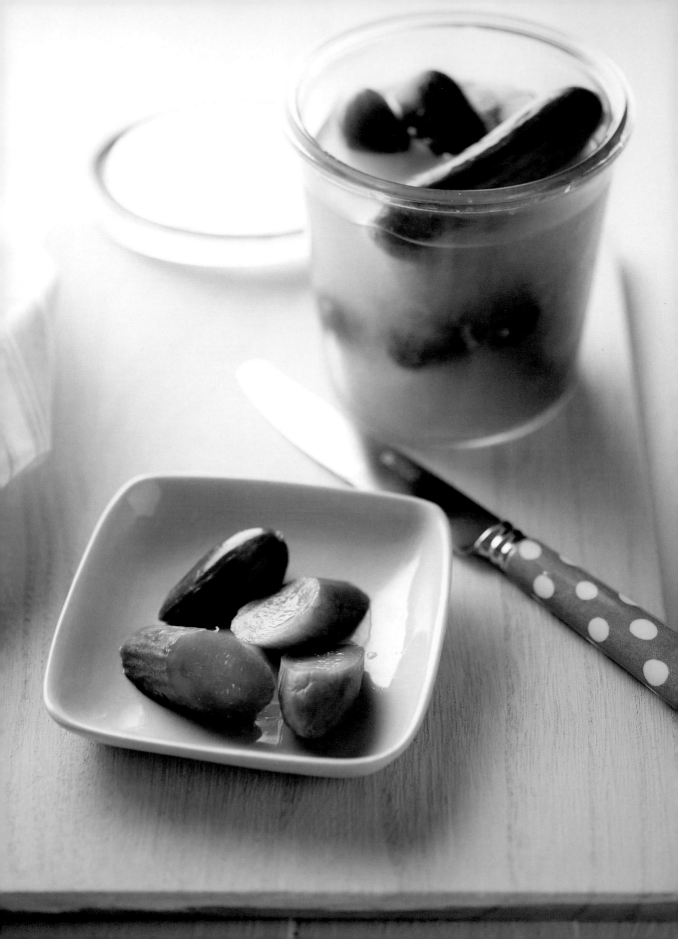

FERMENTED "PICKLES"

MAKES 1 x 1½-QUART JAR

Pickles and sweet pickle relish are hugely popular condiments used in hamburgers and fast food restaurants all over the world. Luckily, we can easily make our own fermented version (without the truckloads of sugar you'd find in sweet pickles) and have these wonderful probiotic-rich morsels on hand to elevate so many dishes. Try these fermented cucumbers with paleo burgers and meatloaf, pâtés and terrines, and add to tartar sauce to enjoy with a lovely piece of grilled fish.

1½ teaspoons Celtic sea salt (see Note)
   (or 3 teaspoons if not using the
   vegetable starter culture – see below)
10 baby or pickling cucumbers
1 teaspoon black peppercorns
1 garlic clove, peeled
2 fresh bay leaves
½ packet vegetable starter culture*
   (optional)
1 well-washed cabbage leaf

* See Glossary

> **MAKE AIP FRIENDLY**

Omit: black peppercorns

You'll need a 1½-quart preserving jar with an airlock lid for this recipe. Wash the jar and all utensils in very hot soapy water, then run them through a hot rinse cycle in the dishwasher to sterilize.

Mix the salt with ½ cup filtered water in a glass or stainless-steel bowl.

Combine the cucumbers, peppercorns, garlic, and bay leaves in the prepared jar, and set aside.

Dissolve the starter culture in filtered water according to the packet instructions (the amount of water will depend on the brand you are using). Add to the salt mixture and mix well.

Pour the cultured brine over the cucumbers, pressing down gently with a large spoon and leaving ¾ inch of room free at the top. The cucumbers should be completely submerged in the liquid; add more filtered water if necessary. Place the washed cabbage leaf and then a small glass weight (a shot glass is ideal) on top to keep everything submerged. Close the lid, then wrap a kitchen towel around the jar to block out the light. Store in a dark place (e.g., a cooler) at 60–73°F for 8–15 days (add another 5 days if not using the starter culture). See Notes on page 96 for more information about vegetable culturing times.

Chill before eating. Once opened, the cucumbers will last for up to 2 months in the fridge kept when submerged in the liquid. Unopened, they will keep for up to 9 months in the fridge.

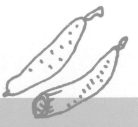

> **NOTE**
> *If you cannot source Celtic sea salt, use a good-quality pale grey sea salt.*

CURRIED "PICKLED" EGGS

MAKES 1 x 1½-QUART JAR

Yes, you can ferment eggs, and they are utterly delicious and very "moreish." They are perfect for packed lunches and as a snack for kids or adults to nibble on after school or work. This recipe is as simple as boiling some eggs until cooked to your liking, then fermenting them with your favorite spices, herbs, and flavorings – beet juice is a winner, as you get the most wonderful looking purple/pink eggs with a golden yolk inside, or try these turmeric-flavored golden delights.

---

10 eggs
1½ tablespoons sea salt
1 tablespoon ground turmeric
1½ tablespoons curry powder
1 tablespoon mustard seeds
4 fresh curry leaves
1 well-washed cabbage leaf

You'll need a 1½-quart preserving jar with an airlock lid for this recipe. Wash the jar and all utensils in very hot soapy water, then run them through a hot rinse cycle in the dishwasher to sterilize.

Put the eggs in a large saucepan and add enough cold water to completely cover them by at least 1 inch. Place the saucepan over medium-high heat and bring to a boil. As soon as the water begins to boil, reduce the heat to medium-low and simmer for 8 minutes. Remove the eggs from the heat. Place in cold water and allow to cool a little (this makes them easier to peel). Once they are cool enough to handle, peel off the shells and set the eggs aside to cool completely.

Meanwhile, mix the salt and 2½ cups filtered water in a glass jug or bowl, and stir until dissolved. Add the turmeric, curry powder, and mustard seeds and stir until well combined.

Pack the eggs into the prepared jar, adding the curry leaves as the jar is filled so the leaves are evenly distributed, then pour on the curry mixture. Leave ¾ inch of room free at the top. The eggs should be completely submerged in the liquid; add more filtered water if necessary.

Place the washed cabbage leaf and then a small glass weight (a shot glass is ideal) on top to keep the eggs submerged. Close the lid, then wrap a kitchen towel around the jar to block out the light. Store in a dark place (e.g., a cooler) at 60–73°F for 24 hours.

Transfer the jar to the refrigerator and allow the eggs to chill before serving. The pickled eggs will keep, submerged in the liquid, for up to 5 days in the fridge.

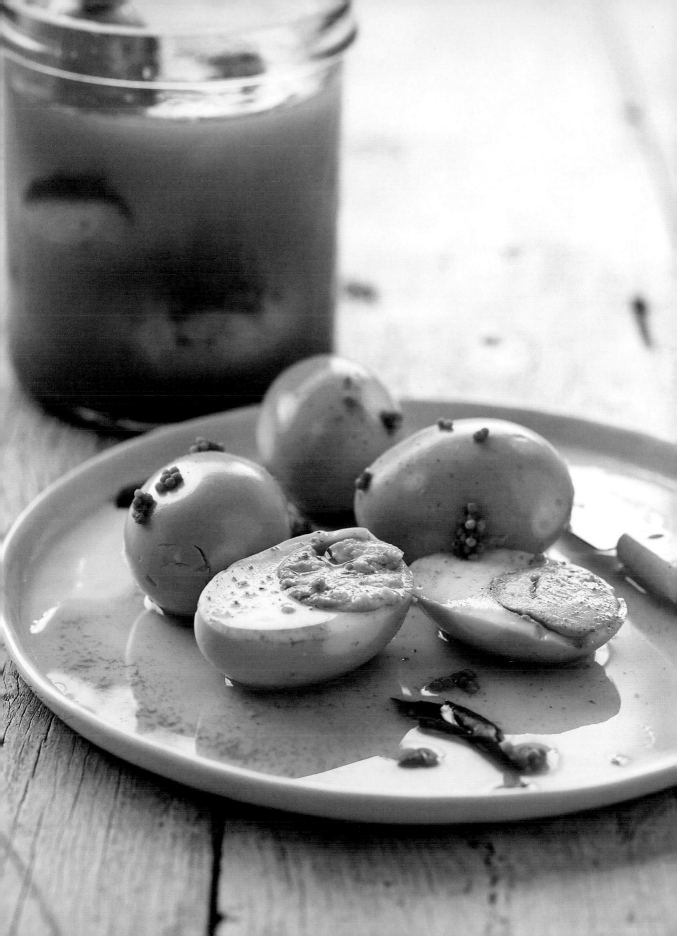

BROTHS AND SOUPS

CHICKEN BONE BROTH

BEEF BONE BROTH

FISH BONE BROTH

ASIAN MUSHROOM BROTH

CHIMICHURRI BONE BROTH

CHINESE LONG SOUP WITH FISH AND PRAWNS

AVGOLEMONO SOUP

BONE MARROW PHO

CHICKEN LIVER SOUP WITH CRISPY BACON AND WATERCRESS

CABBAGE AND BACON SOUP

TOM KHA GAI

MISO SOUP WITH CHICKEN MEATBALLS

ZUCCHINI SOUP WITH FRESH MINT

CHICKEN AND VEGETABLE SOUP

HEALING GARLIC SOUP

HAM HOCK SOUP

MIDDLE EASTERN MEATBALL SOUP

HUNTER SOUP (BIGOS)

CREAMY MUSHROOM SOUP

HEARTY OXTAIL SOUP

SPANISH SEAFOOD SOUP

CHILLED AVOCADO SOUP

SRI LANKAN CAULIFLOWER SOUP

STRACCIATELLA SOUP

THAI SQUASH SOUP WITH BRAISED BEEF CHEEK

ASPARAGUS SOUP WITH CRISPY BACON

CHICKEN BONE BROTH

MAKES 4 QUARTS

Everyone loves the humble chicken bone broth, and it is by far my favorite broth to make. Often when people start to include broths in their diet, they try beef first, find it too strong in flavor, and give up. Chicken broth is lighter, more subtle, and so yummy – in fact, as I write this, the bones from last night's roast chicken are simmering away in a pot on the stove. My daughters had a cup of broth this morning for breakfast with their eggs and veggies, and I enjoy it any time of the day.

See page 118 for pressure- and slow-cooker instructions.

5½ pounds bony chicken parts (such as necks, breastbones, and wings)
2–4 chicken feet (optional)
2 tablespoons apple cider vinegar
1 large onion, roughly chopped
2 carrots, roughly chopped
3 celery ribs, roughly chopped

1 leek, white part only, rinsed well and roughly chopped
1 garlic bulb, broken into cloves
1 tablespoon black peppercorns, lightly crushed
2 large handfuls flat-leaf parsley, leaves and stalks

> **MAKE** AIP FRIENDLY

Omit: black peppercorns

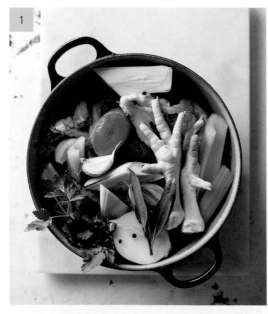

Place the chicken pieces in a stockpot or very large saucepan. Add 5 quarts cold water, the vinegar, onion, carrots, celery, leek, garlic, peppercorns, and parsley.

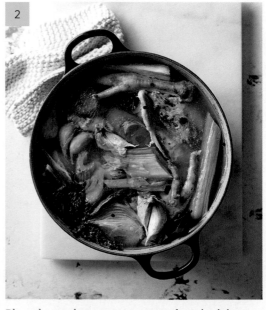

Place the stockpot or pan over medium-high heat and bring to a boil, skimming off the scum that forms on the surface. Reduce the heat to low and simmer for 6–12 hours. The longer you cook the broth, the more the flavor develops.

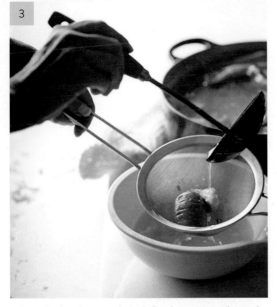

Allow the broth to cool slightly, then strain through a fine sieve into a large storage container. Cover and place in the fridge until the fat rises to the top and congeals.

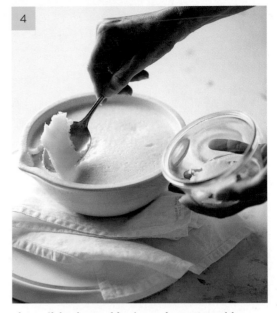

Skim off this layer of fat (it is a fantastic, stable cooking fat) and keep it in a glass storage container in the fridge for up to 2 weeks – use it for frying and sautéing.

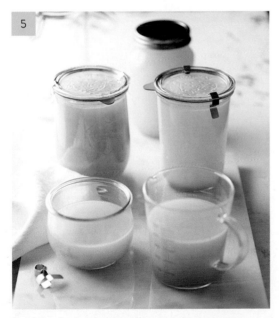

Transfer the broth to smaller airtight containers and store in the refrigerator for up to 4 days, or freeze for up to 3 months. ■

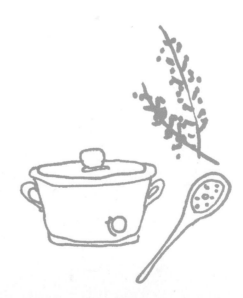

IN THE PRESSURE COOKER
MAKES ABOUT 2¾ QUARTS

Using exactly the same ingredients as on page 116, follow step 1 using your pressure cooker, but add only enough cold water to just cover the meat and vegetables. (Your cooker should be no more than two-thirds full, otherwise hot liquid may spray out.) Close the lid and lock it, then bring the cooker to high pressure and cook over medium-low heat for 2 hours. Let the pressure drop naturally before opening the lid. Follow steps 3 – 5.

IN THE SLOW COOKER
MAKES ABOUT 3 QUARTS

Using exactly the same ingredients as on page 116, follow step 1 using your slow cooker, but add only enough cold water to just cover the meat and vegetables. Cover with the lid and cook on low for 12 hours. Follow steps 3 – 5.

NOTES

It's important to fill the pressure cooker loosely to the marker indicated, or until no more than two-thirds full. If it is overfilled with tightly packed veggies and meat, it could explode or spray out hot liquid.

Letting the pressure drop naturally means turning the heat off and leaving the pressure cooker to sit on the stovetop. The food will keep on cooking, but the internal temperature will drop from 250°F to 212°F, which makes it possible to safely open the lid. This process will take about 15 minutes.

TIPS

Store the broth in glass jars or containers.

Always freeze a portion or two, so you have backup broth on hand.

When freezing broth in glass, to prevent the storage container from breaking:

- *Do not fill to the brim – leave ¾ inch at the top to allow the liquid to expand.*
- *Pop the lid on loosely until the liquid has frozen, then cap tightly.*

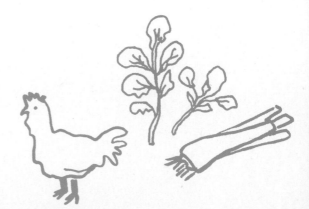

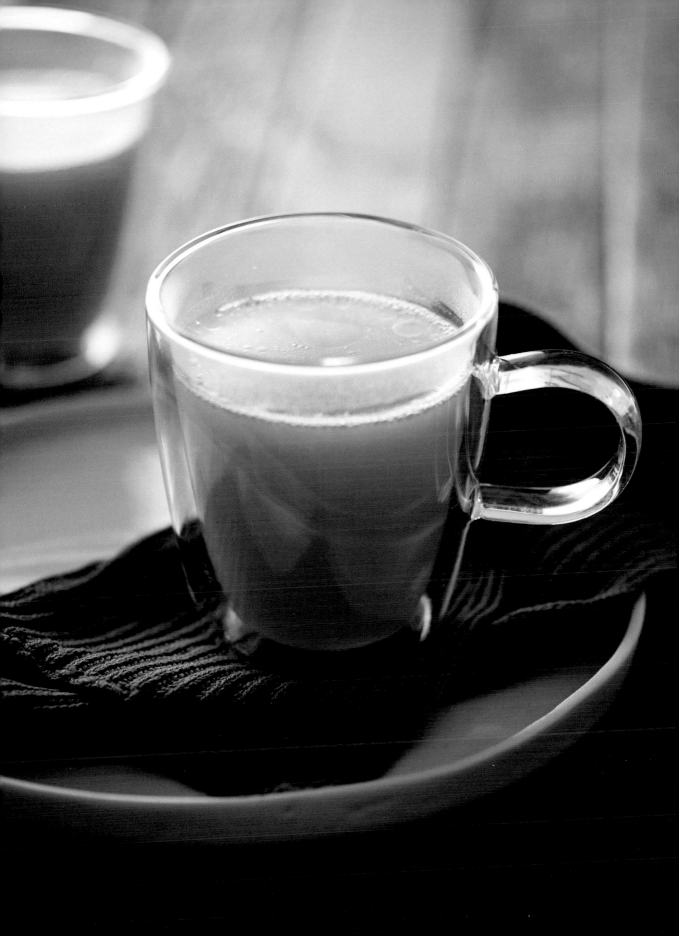

TIPS

Store the broth in glass jars or containers.

Freeze a portion or two so you always have broth on hand.

Keep the layer of fat that has solidified on top of your cooled broth. It is a fantastic, stable cooking fat that's perfect for frying and sautéing.

When freezing liquids in glass, do not fill to the brim; leave ¾ inch of room at the top to allow the broth to expand as it freezes. Loosely pop the lid on top until your broth is frozen, then cap tightly. This prevents the glass from breaking.

If you wish, add some grass-fed gelatin and collagen powder to further enrich your broth.

BEEF BONE BROTH

MAKES 4½ QUARTS

Helen has gone into great detail at the start of this book about why bone broths are important for optimal gut health, so here I'll talk about them from my point of view. The first thing you learn as a chef is how to make bone broths – the flavorsome building blocks for so many dishes. I urge you to cook at least one per week. Play around with different herbs and spices, or just keep it neutral and add flavor when you incorporate your broth into soups, braises, curries, tagines, casseroles, and sauces.

See page 122 for pressure- and slow-cooker instructions.

4½ pounds beef knuckle and marrow bones
3 tablespoons apple cider vinegar
3–3½ pounds meaty beef rib or neck bones
   (soup bones)
2 onions, roughly chopped
2 carrots, roughly chopped
2 leeks, white part only, rinsed well
   and roughly chopped
2 celery ribs, roughly chopped
6 thyme sprigs, tied together with
   kitchen string
1 teaspoon black peppercorns, crushed
1 garlic bulb, cut in half lengthwise
2 large handfuls flat-leaf parsley,
   leaves and stalks

MAKE AIP FRIENDLY

Omit: black peppercorns

1. Put the knuckle and marrow bones in a stockpot or very large saucepan. Add the vinegar and pour in 5 quarts cold water, or enough to cover.

2. Preheat the oven to 400°F.

3. Put the meaty bones, onions, carrots, leeks, and celery in a roasting pan and roast until well browned, 20–30 minutes.

4. Transfer the bones and vegetables to the stockpot or pan.

5. Pour the fat from the roasting pan into the stockpot or pan. Pour 1–2 ladlefuls of water into the roasting pan and, using a wooden spoon, loosen any brown bits and coagulated juices that are stuck to the pan. Pour the liquid back into the stockpot or pan.

6. Add additional water, if necessary, to just cover the bones; the liquid should come no higher than ¾ inch below the rim of the stockpot or pan, as the volume will expand slightly during cooking.

7. Bring the broth to a boil, skimming off the scum that rises to the top. Reduce the heat to low and add the thyme, peppercorns, garlic, and parsley. Simmer for 8–12 hours.

8. Strain the broth through a fine sieve into a large container. Cover and let cool in the fridge. Remove the congealed fat that rises to the top (store it in a glass container in the fridge for up to 2 weeks and use it for frying and sautéing). Transfer the broth to smaller airtight containers and store in the fridge for 3–4 days, or freeze for up to 3 months.

IN THE PRESSURE COOKER
MAKES ABOUT 2¾ QUARTS

2 pounds beef knuckle and marrow bones

1½ tablespoons apple cider vinegar

1⅔ pounds meaty beef rib or neck bones
   (soup bones)

1 onion, roughly chopped

1 carrot, roughly chopped

1 leek, white part only, rinsed well and
   roughly chopped

1 celery rib, roughly chopped

3 thyme sprigs, tied together with kitchen string

½ teaspoon black peppercorns, crushed

½ garlic bulb, cut in half lengthwise

1 large handful flat-leaf parsley, leaves and stalks

Follow step 1 using your pressure cooker, but add only enough cold water to just cover the bones. Follow steps 2 – 3 , then transfer the bones and vegetables to the pressure cooker. Follow step 5 . Add the thyme, peppercorns, garlic, and parsley, and pour in additional water, if necessary, to just cover the bones and vegetables; the pressure cooker should be no more than two-thirds full. (It's very important not to overfill the cooker, as this may cause hot liquid to spray out.) Close the lid and lock it, then bring the cooker to high pressure and cook over medium-low heat for 3 hours. Let the pressure drop naturally before opening the lid. Follow step 8 .

IN THE SLOW COOKER
MAKES ABOUT 3 QUARTS

2 pounds beef knuckle and marrow bones

1½ tablespoons apple cider vinegar

1⅔ pounds meaty beef rib or neck bones
   (soup bones)

1 onion, roughly chopped

1 carrot, roughly chopped

1 leek, white part only, rinsed well and
   roughly chopped

1 celery rib, roughly chopped

3 thyme sprigs, tied together with kitchen string

½ teaspoon black peppercorns, crushed

½ garlic bulb, cut in half lengthwise

1 large handful flat-leaf parsley, leaves and stalks

Follow step 1 using your slow cooker, but add only enough cold water to just cover the bones. Follow steps 2 – 3 , then transfer the bones and vegetables to the slow cooker. Follow step 5 . Add the thyme, peppercorns, garlic, and parsley, and pour in additional water, if necessary, to just cover the bones and vegetables. Cover with the lid and cook on low for 12–24 hours. Follow step 8 .

NOTES

It's important to fill the pressure cooker loosely to the marker indicated, or until no more than two-thirds full. If it is overfilled with tightly packed veggies and meat, it could explode or spray out hot liquid.

Letting the pressure drop naturally means turning the heat off and leaving the pressure cooker to sit on the stove top. The food will keep on cooking, but the internal temperature will drop from 250°F to 212°F, which makes it possible to safely open the lid. This process will take about 15 minutes.

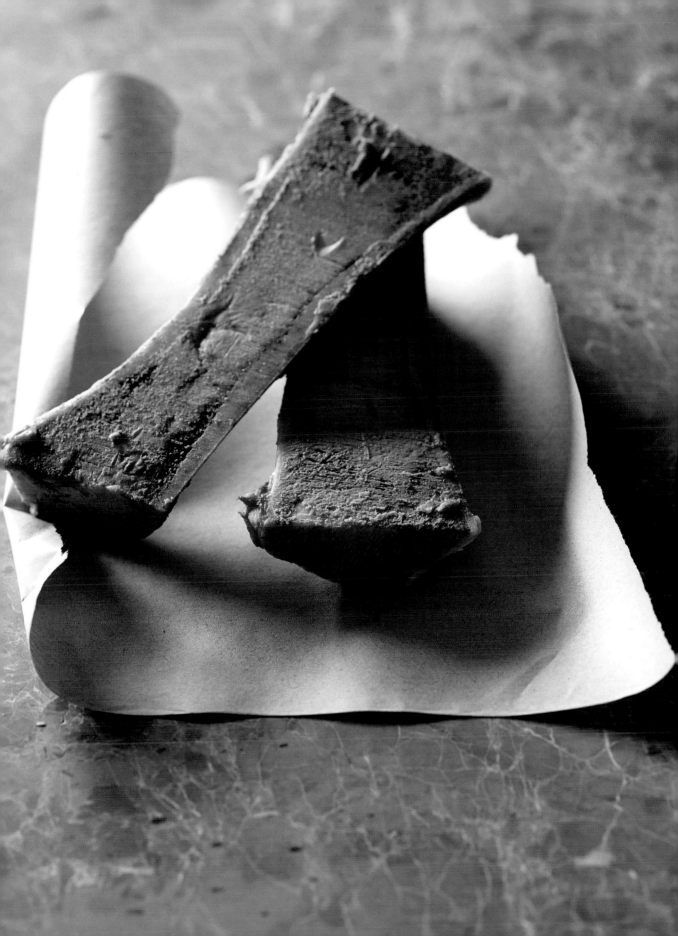

FISH BONE BROTH

MAKES ABOUT 3 QUARTS

Whenever you have a whole fish, make sure you keep the head and bones so that you can make a delicious broth. Fish bone broth can be used as an aromatic base to create the most amazing soups and curries. All you need to do is add seafood, vegetables, spices, and herbs – and, voilà, you have dinner in mere minutes.

3–4 non-oily fish carcasses and heads
(such as snapper, grouper, or kingfish)
2 celery ribs, roughly chopped
2 onions, roughly chopped
1 carrot, roughly chopped
2 tablespoons apple cider vinegar
1 handful thyme and flat-leaf
parsley sprigs
3 fresh or dried bay leaves

AIP FRIENDLY

1. Put the fish carcasses and heads in a stockpot or very large saucepan, add the veggies and apple cider vinegar, and cover with 3½ quarts cold water.

2. Bring to a boil, skimming off the scum and any impurities as they rise to the top. Tie the herbs together with kitchen string and add to the broth.

3. Reduce the heat to low, cover, and simmer for 3–4 hours.

4. Remove the fish carcasses and heads with tongs or a slotted spoon. Strain the broth into storage containers, cover, and chill in the refrigerator. Remove the congealed fat that rises to the top. (Store it in a glass container in the fridge for up to 2 weeks and use it for frying and sautéing.) The broth can be stored in the refrigerator for up to 4 days, or frozen for up to 3 months.

IN THE PRESSURE COOKER
MAKES ABOUT 2¾ QUARTS

Follow step 1 – 3 using your pressure cooker, but add only enough cold water to just cover the fish and vegetables, or until the cooker is two-thirds full. (It's very important not to overfill the cooker, as this may cause hot liquid to spray out.) Close the lid and lock it, then bring the cooker to high pressure and cook over medium-low heat for 1½ hours. Let the pressure drop naturally before opening the lid. Follow step 4.

IN THE SLOW COOKER
MAKES ABOUT 3 QUARTS

Place all the ingredients in your slow cooker, but add only enough water to just cover. Cover with the lid and cook on low for 8 hours, then follow step 4.

NOTES

It's important to fill the pressure cooker loosely to the marker indicated, or until no more than two-thirds full. If it is overfilled with tightly packed veggies and meat, it could explode or spray out hot liquid.

Letting the pressure drop naturally means turning the heat off and leaving the pressure cooker to sit on the stove top. The food will keep on cooking, but the internal temperature will drop from 250°F to 212°F, which makes it possible to safely open the lid. This process will take about 15 minutes.

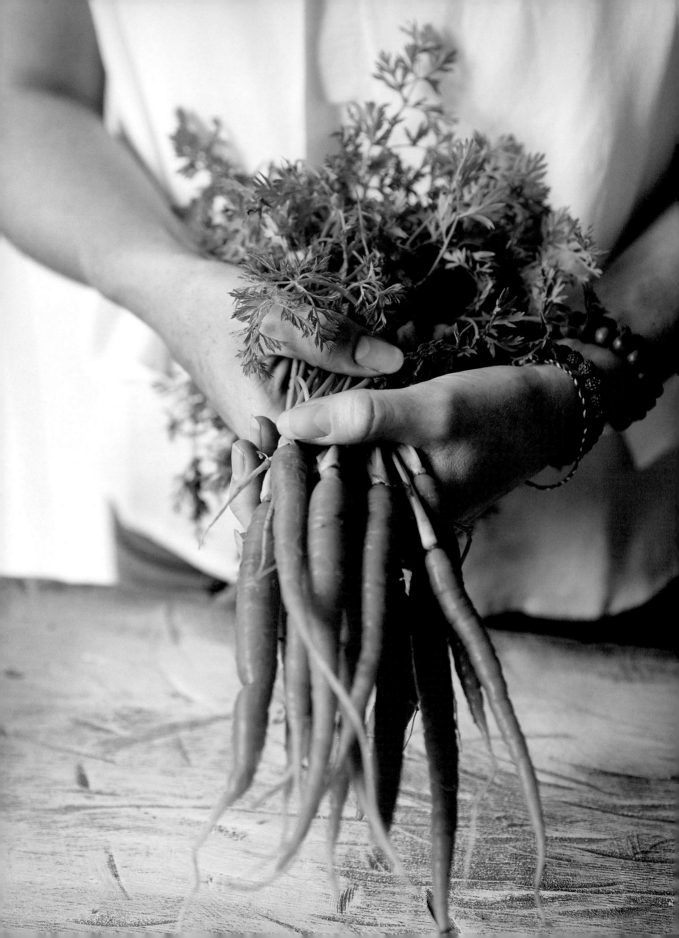

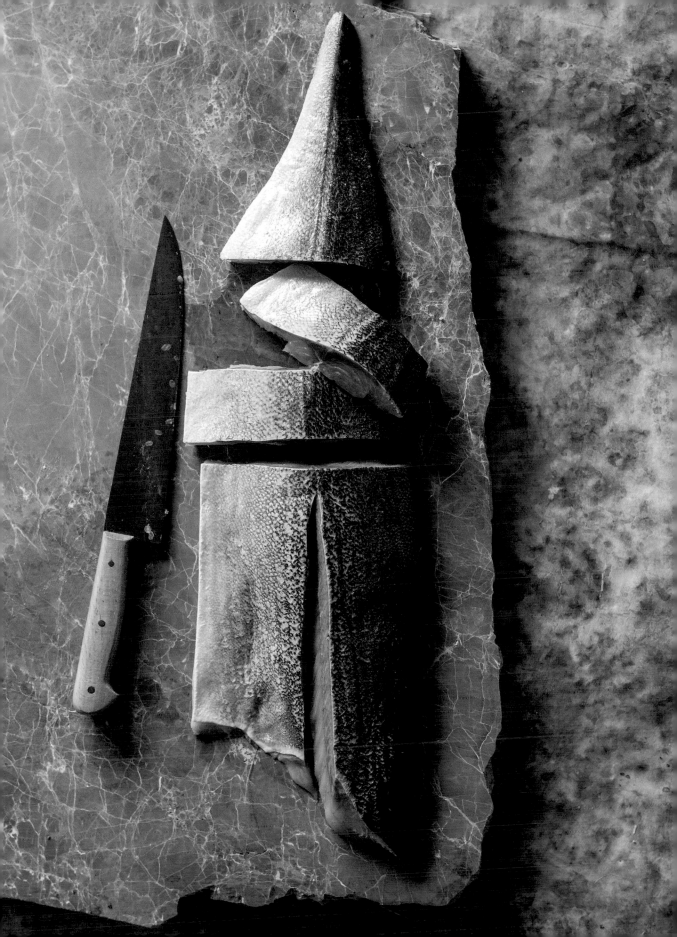

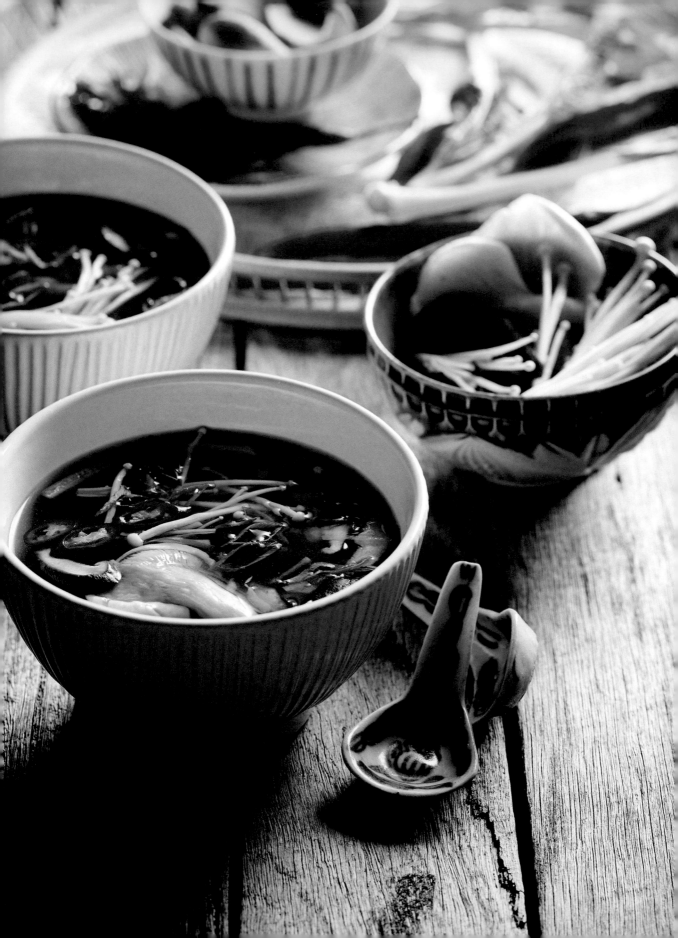

ASIAN MUSHROOM BROTH

SERVES 6

Seaweed is a great source of minerals – particularly iodine, calcium, iron, and magnesium. It also contains fucose (not to be confused with fructose!), which is a great prebiotic. This meat-free dish is absolutely delicious and is perfect for when you need a cleansing soup that will leave you feeling satisfied. Of course, if you want some more protein or fat, feel free to add bone marrow, scallops, prawns, mussels, crabmeat, or any fish or meat that you love.

---

2 tablespoons coconut oil

1 onion, chopped into 1¼-inch pieces

4 garlic cloves, thinly sliced

2-inch piece of ginger, cut into matchsticks

2 quarts (8 cups) vegetable stock or Chicken Bone Broth (page 116)

3 tablespoons tamari or coconut aminos*

1 tablespoon fish sauce

1 sheet of dried kombu seaweed*, rinsed

5 ounces shiitake mushrooms, sliced

5 ounces enoki mushrooms

4 ounces wood ear fungus*

5 ounces oyster mushrooms, torn

¼ napa cabbage, chopped into 1¼-inch pieces

1 ounce dried wakame seaweed*, soaked in 1 cup water for 10 minutes to expand

1 bunch Chinese broccoli (gai lan) (about 10 ounces), roughly chopped

2 green onions, sliced at an angle

1 long red chile, thinly sliced (optional)

* See Glossary

Heat the coconut oil in a large saucepan over medium heat. Add the onion and cook until softened, 5 minutes. Stir in the garlic and ginger and cook until fragrant, 1 minute. Pour in the stock or broth, tamari or coconut aminos, and fish sauce, add the kombu, and bring to a simmer.

Add the mushrooms and cabbage to the broth and continue to simmer until the mushrooms are tender and the broth is infused nicely with the kombu, 20 minutes. Remove the kombu and discard.

Drain the excess water from the wakame. Add the wakame and Chinese broccoli to the broth and simmer until the broccoli is tender, 3–4 minutes. Remove from the heat. Ladle the broth and vegetables into serving bowls and top with the green onions and sliced chile (if using).

MAKE AIP FRIENDLY

Omit: tamari and chile

Substitute: coconut aminos in place of tamari

CHIMICHURRI BONE BROTH

SERVES 4

Bone broth is well known for its health-giving properties, and we encourage everyone to incorporate it into his or her diet. This age-old recipe is dirt cheap – about 20–30 cents per serving – and sustainable, using all parts of the animal, which are good things in anyone's book. If you're having your daily broth, then you might like to jazz it up a little from time to time with different spices or herbs. Here is something we do when we have leftover chimichurri. Adding the chimichurri to the broth takes it to another level, and as a bonus you get all those wonderful herbs into your system, too.

CHIMICHURRI (makes ¾ cup)

3 garlic cloves, peeled

sea salt

1 jalapeño or long red chile, seeded and finely chopped

1 very large handful flat-leaf parsley leaves

1 very large handful cilantro leaves

3 tablespoons apple cider vinegar

½ teaspoon ground cumin

3 tablespoons extra-virgin olive oil or melted coconut oil

freshly ground black pepper

1 quart (4 cups) Chicken, Beef or Fish Bone Broth (pages 116, 121, and 124)

MAKE AIP FRIENDLY

Omit: chile, cumin, and black pepper

To make the chimichurri, combine the garlic and a little salt in a mortar and crush with the pestle. Add the chile, parsley, and cilantro, and pound to a paste. Stir in the vinegar, cumin, and olive or coconut oil, then taste and season with salt and pepper. (You could also make the chimichurri in a food processor.)

Pour the broth into a saucepan and bring to a simmer. Remove from the heat and stir in ½ cup chimichurri. Taste and season again with salt and pepper, if necessary. Ladle the broth into soup bowls or mugs, and serve.

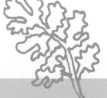

TIP

Store the remaining chimichurri in an airtight glass container in the fridge for up to 3 days. You can use it as a sauce, condiment, or marinade, or thin it with a little water or apple cider vinegar to make a salad dressing.

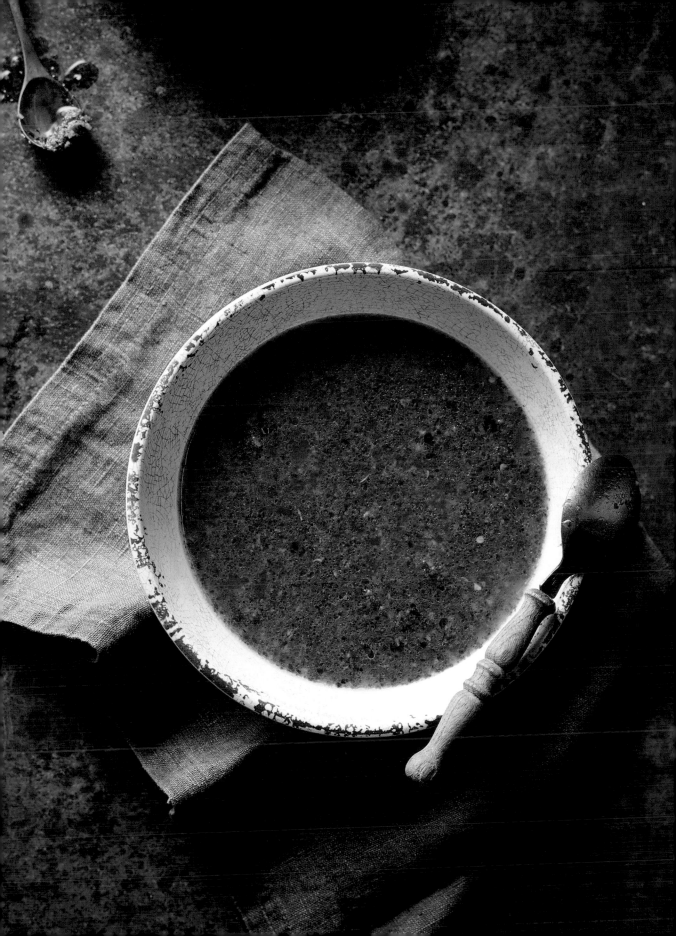

CHINESE LONG SOUP
WITH FISH AND SHRIMP

SERVES 4

A lot of people believe being paleo is all about consuming meat, meat, and more meat, which couldn't be further from the truth. Paleo is really about including in your diet gut-healthy broths, small to moderate amounts of well-sourced protein from land or sea, and an abundance of vegetables, as well as some good fats and fermented foods. This dish is the perfect paleo meal, and one which I encourage you to try. Enjoy with some fermented vegetables on the side.

---

10 ounces kelp noodles or other
    vegetable noodles
2 teaspoons tamari or coconut aminos*
½ teaspoon sesame oil
1 teaspoon finely grated ginger
1 quart (4 cups) Chicken or Fish Bone
    Broth (pages 116 and 124)
1 baby bok choy, quartered and roughly
    chopped
6 shiitake mushrooms, sliced
3 ounces wood ear fungus*, roughly
    chopped (optional)
7 ounces broccoli, broken into florets
7 ounces white-fleshed fish fillet (such as
    mackerel, whiting, or snapper), skin on
    or removed, cut into 1¼-inch pieces
12 large raw shrimp, shelled and deveined
    with tails intact
1 carrot, cut into matchsticks
sea salt and freshly ground black pepper
1 green onion, cut into matchsticks

* See Glossary

Rinse the kelp noodles in cold running water. Set aside.

Combine the tamari or coconut aminos, sesame oil, ginger, and broth in a large saucepan, and bring to a simmer over medium heat. Add the kelp noodles, bok choy, shiitake mushrooms, wood ear fungus, and broccoli and cook for 2 minutes.

Next, add the fish, shrimp, and carrot to the pan, cover with the lid, and simmer until the fish and shrimp are just cooked through, about 2½ minutes. Season with salt and pepper if needed. Carefully ladle the soup into warm serving bowls, and serve with the green onion sprinkled on top.

MAKE AIP FRIENDLY

Omit: tamari and black pepper
Substitute: coconut aminos in place of tamari

TIP
*Add some red pepper flakes or sliced fresh chile
if you like it a little spicy.*

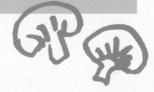

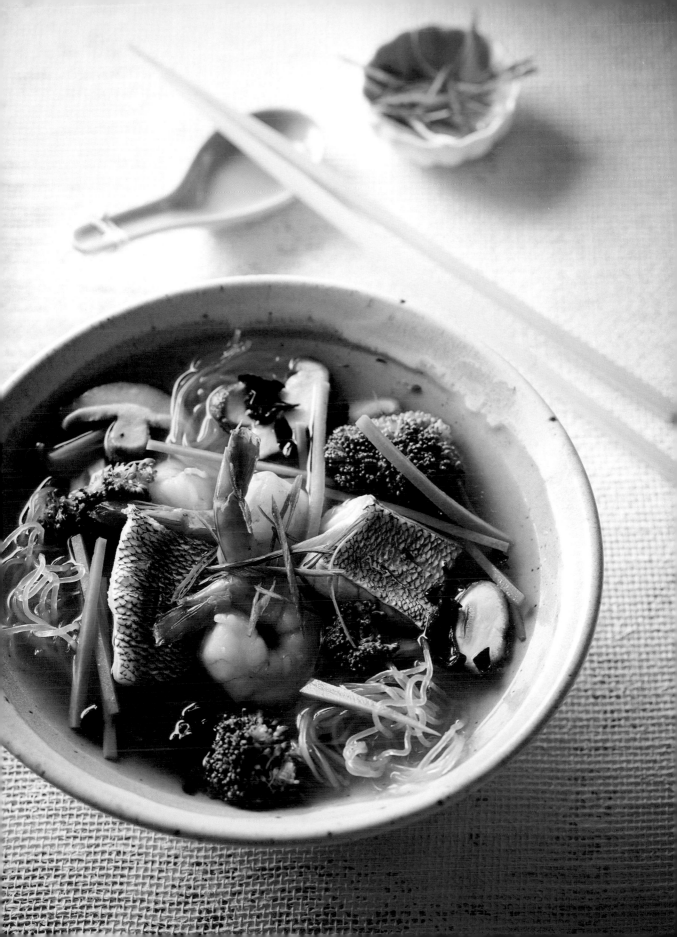

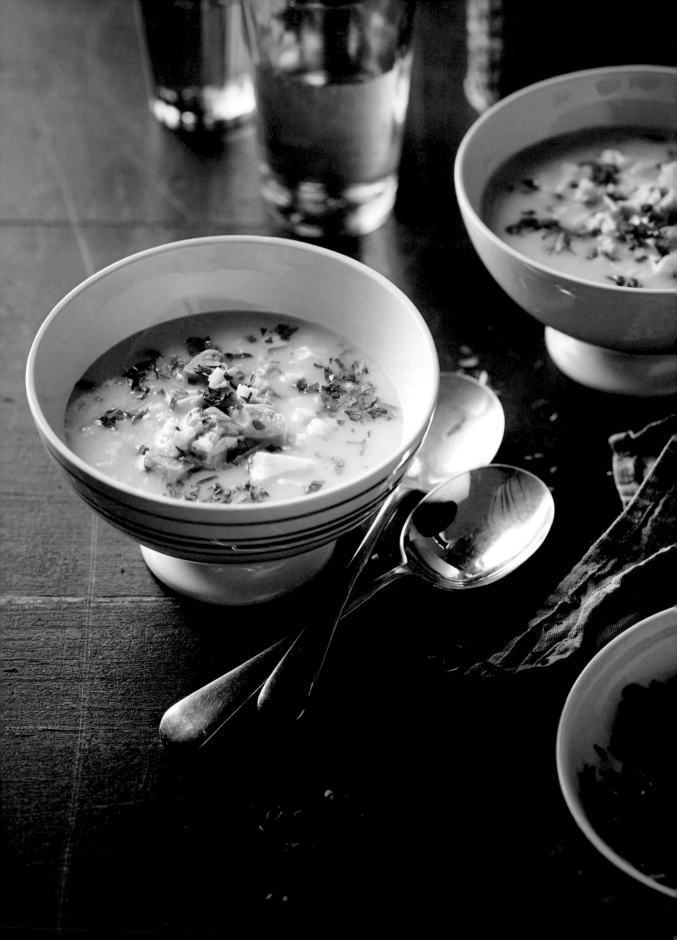

AVGOLEMONO SOUP

SERVES 4

I have to love a soup that contains all my favorite things: yummy chicken bone broth, eggs, lemon, herbs, and chicken. This classic Greek dish is a winner in the cooler months and can be on the table in a short period of time. If you like, you can add in extra vegetables in the form of broccoli or zucchini rice, parsnip noodles, Swiss chard, or asparagus.

½ head of cauliflower (about 1⅓ pounds)
2 tablespoons coconut oil
2 large onions, finely chopped
2 garlic cloves, finely chopped
1½ quarts (6 cups) Chicken Bone Broth
   (page 116)
3 boneless, skinless chicken thighs,
   cut into small cubes
3 eggs
¼ cup lemon juice, plus extra
   to taste
sea salt and freshly ground black pepper
2 tablespoons chopped flat-leaf parsley
   leaves, to serve

MAKE AIP FRIENDLY

Omit: eggs and black pepper

Put the cauliflower in the bowl of a food processor and pulse into tiny, fine pieces that look like rice. Set aside.

Heat the coconut oil in a large saucepan over medium heat. Add the onions and sauté until soft and translucent, 5–6 minutes. Add the garlic and sauté until fragrant, 1 minute. Pour in the broth and bring to a boil, then reduce the heat to low.

Add the cubed chicken and the cauliflower rice to the broth and simmer, stirring occasionally, until the chicken is cooked through, 10 minutes.

Put the eggs in a large bowl and whisk in the lemon juice. Slowly pour in 2 cups of the hot soup (the liquid only) in a steady stream, whisking constantly until combined. Then, slowly pour the warm egg mixture into the soup, still whisking vigorously, until creamy and cloudy looking. Taste and season with salt, pepper, and more lemon juice to your liking. Serve immediately with the parsley sprinkled on top.

BONE MARROW PHO

SERVES 6

I recently served this in one of my restaurants as part of a tasting menu – and it was a huge hit! I can always tell that a dish is going to be great when my chefs unanimously give it a thumbs up. This might look a little tricky, but in all honesty it is really quite simple and is perfect for a wonderful family meal or dinner party. If the kids or your guests are a bit squeamish about bone marrow, simply remove the marrow from the bones, finely chop it up, and add to the dish. Serve with a side of fermented veg, like kimchi, for extra gut health benefits.

5½ pounds beef bones, cut into 3-inch lengths (ask your butcher to do this)
2 tablespoons coconut oil
6 x 4-ounce boneless beef short ribs
1 pound oxtail, cut into 2-inch lengths (ask your butcher to do this)
2 onions, chopped
6 garlic cloves, chopped
3 ounces ginger, thinly sliced
2 pieces of cassia bark* or 2 cinnamon sticks
1 tablespoon coriander seeds
1 tablespoon fennel seeds
6 star anise
6 cardamom pods
8 cloves
3 tablespoons fish sauce
1 tablespoon coconut sugar (optional)
sea salt and freshly ground black pepper
2 pounds bone marrow, cut lengthwise, then into 2-inch pieces (ask your butcher to do this)
2 baby bok choy, quartered
8 oyster mushrooms, torn
12 ounces daikon, spiralized into thin noodles

TO SERVE

1 large handful *each* mint, cilantro, Thai basil, and Vietnamese mint leaves
1 handful sliced green onion
2 long red chiles, sliced (optional)
lime wedges

* See Glossary

Preheat the oven to 400°F.

Put the beef bones in a large roasting pan and roast for 30 minutes. Remove from the oven and set aside.

Heat the coconut oil in a stockpot over high heat. Add the short ribs and oxtail in batches and seal on each side for 2 minutes. Remove from the stockpot and set aside.

Add the onions, garlic, and ginger to the stockpot and cook until they get a bit of color, 5 minutes. Pour in 5 quarts water, add the roasted beef bones, the short ribs, oxtail, and spices, and bring to a boil, frequently skimming any scum from the surface. Reduce the heat to low, cover, and simmer until the short ribs are tender, 3½ hours. Remove the short ribs from the broth, put in a bowl, and refrigerate until needed.

Continue to simmer the broth, skimming occasionally, until well flavored, 1½–2 hours. Stir in the fish sauce and coconut sugar (if using), season to taste, and remove from the heat. Let cool slightly, then strain into a large bowl and skim all the fat that rises to the top. (Reserve the fat for cooking.) Remove the meat from the oxtail and set aside.

Preheat the oven to 400°F. Put the bone marrow cut-side up on a baking sheet, season with salt and pepper, and roast until cooked through, 12 minutes.

Return the broth to the stockpot, add the short ribs, oxtail meat, bok choy, oyster mushrooms, and daikon noodles, and bring to a boil. Simmer until the meat is heated through and the bok choy is wilted, 4 minutes. Fill warm serving bowls with the vegetables, oxtail meat, and short ribs, then top with the hot broth and roasted bone marrow. Sprinkle on the herbs and green onions and serve with the chile (if using) and lime wedges.

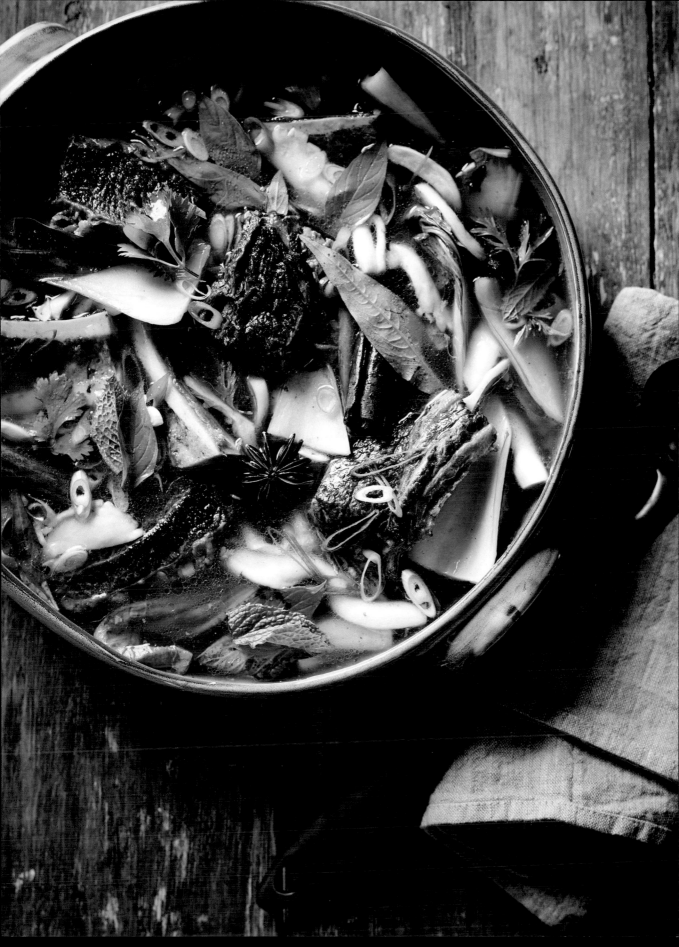

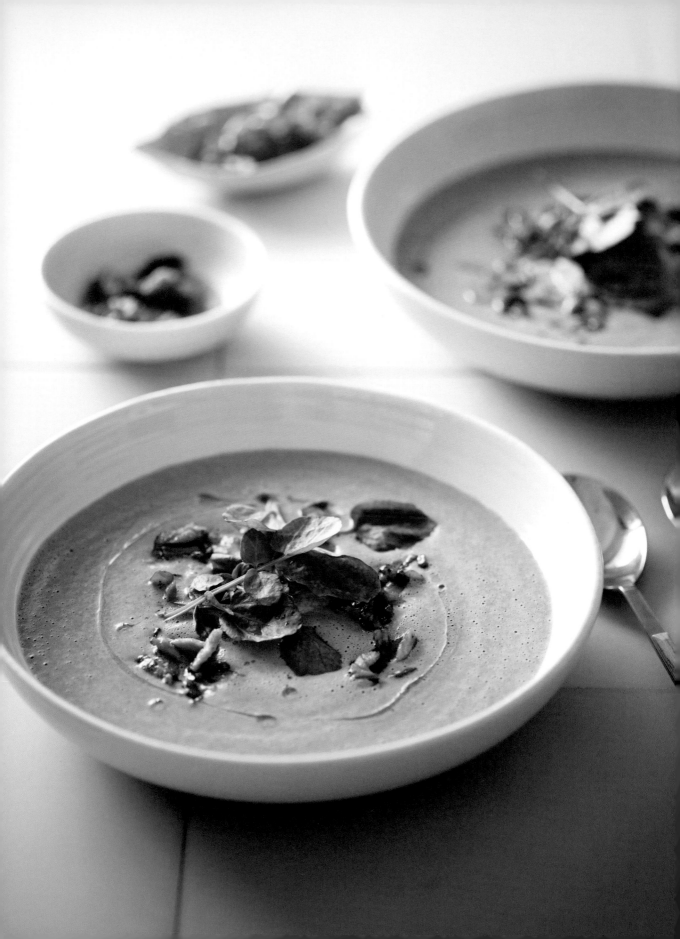

CHICKEN LIVER SOUP WITH CRISPY BACON AND WATERCRESS

SERVES 4

We should be eating a lot more organic offal, especially liver, as, in my humble opinion, it is the world's greatest superfood. This nourishing chicken broth flavored with bacon, mushrooms, thyme, and liver is a luxurious and medicinal meal fit for a queen or king.

---

2 tablespoons coconut oil or good-quality animal fat*

1 large onion, chopped

4 garlic cloves, chopped

1 pound chicken livers, sinew removed (or use duck, lamb, or beef liver)

8 ounces mushrooms (such as white or brown button), chopped

4 thyme sprigs, leaves picked and chopped

3⅓ cups Chicken Bone Broth (page 116), plus extra if needed

3 slices bacon

sea salt and freshly ground black pepper

1 handful watercress

drizzle of extra-virgin olive oil

* See Glossary

MAKE AIP FRIENDLY

Omit: black pepper

Melt the oil or fat in a saucepan over medium heat. Add the onion and cook, stirring occasionally, until softened and starting to caramelize, 8 minutes. Stir in the garlic and cook until fragrant, 1 minute. Next, add the livers and cook until browned but still pink on the inside, 3 minutes. Remove the livers from the pan and set aside. Add the mushrooms and thyme to the pan, pour in the broth, and bring to a boil. Reduce the heat to low and simmer for 10 minutes, stirring occasionally.

Meanwhile, preheat the oven to 400°F.

Arrange the bacon on a baking sheet and cook in the oven for 4–5 minutes. Flip the bacon and cook until golden brown and crispy, 4–5 minutes more. When cool enough to handle, chop the bacon into small pieces.

Return the chicken livers to the pan and cook for 3 minutes. Season with salt and pepper. Blend the soup with a handheld blender until smooth. Add more broth if desired. Ladle the soup into warm serving bowls, sprinkle with the bacon crisps, and top with the watercress. Finish with a drizzle of olive oil.

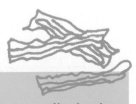

TIP

If you use half the amount of broth in this recipe, this soup becomes a wonderful pâté. Simply place in ramekins and chill in the fridge until set. Serve with veggie sticks and seeded crackers.

CABBAGE AND BACON SOUP

SERVES 4–6

Now, please don't be put off by the name of this soup. Cabbage soup may not sound like something worth celebrating, but you will be surprised at how comforting, warming, and absolutely addictive this is. It is just like a big, warm hug for your body, and the fact that it contains bacon may get it across the line with the rest of the family. Maybe we should rename this "OMG Bacon Soup"!

2½ tablespoons coconut oil or good-quality animal fat*

1 onion, chopped

2 garlic cloves, chopped

8 ounces Swiss chard, leafy green part and stems separated, all trimmed and chopped

8 ounces green cabbage, shredded

7 ounces bacon

½ teaspoon ground turmeric

1½ quarts (6 cups) Chicken Bone Broth (page 116)

sea salt and freshly ground black pepper

1 large handful flat-leaf parsley leaves

* See Glossary

MAKE AIP FRIENDLY

Omit: black pepper

Melt 2 tablespoons of the oil or fat in a large saucepan over medium heat. Add the onion and cook until softened, 5 minutes. Stir in the garlic, Swiss chard stems, and cabbage and cook until softened, 5 minutes.

Meanwhile, melt the remaining oil or fat in a frying pan over medium-high heat. Add the bacon and cook, turning once, until lightly golden (about 4 minutes on each side). Remove from the pan, reserving any fat in the pan.

Chop the bacon into ¾-inch pieces and stir into the cooked cabbage mixture, then add the turmeric, broth and any bacon fat from the pan. Bring to a boil, reduce the heat to low, and gently simmer, stirring occasionally, for 30 minutes. Stir in the chopped Swiss chard leaves and cook until wilted, 5 minutes more. Season with salt and pepper. To finish, stir in the parsley leaves and serve.

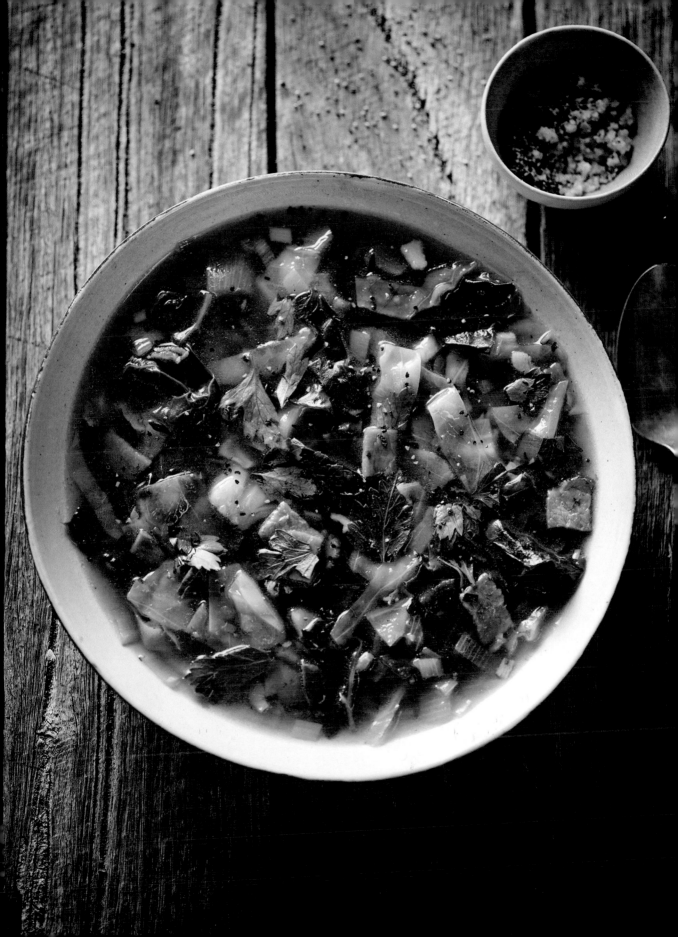

TOM KHA GAI

SERVES 4

Tom kha gai is a classic dish in Lao and Thai cuisine, and it's easy to see why. This hot and sour soup has coconut milk or cream as its base, and the addition of chicken, vegetables, and medicinal aromatics (like galangal, chile, garlic, kaffir lime leaves, lemongrass, and cilantro) make it satisfying for even the biggest eater. It really is a most delicious concoction that the whole family will love.

---

2 x 13.5-ounce cans coconut milk
2 cups Chicken Bone Broth
   (page 116)
2 lemongrass stems, white part only,
   bruised and cut into 3-inch lengths
12 slices of fresh galangal* or ginger
   (about 1½ ounces)
1 long red chile, seeded and sliced,
   plus extra chile if desired
5 fresh kaffir lime leaves, lightly bruised
   (or use dried)
10 oyster mushrooms, torn
14 ounces boneless, skinless chicken
   breasts or thighs, cut into strips
2 tablespoons lime juice
2½ tablespoons fish sauce (or to taste)
7 ounces kelp noodles or other
   vegetable noodles
1½ bunches of yau choy (choy sum) or
   other Asian greens (about 13 ounces),
   roughly chopped
1 large handful cilantro leaves, torn
1 lime, cut into wedges, to serve

* See Glossary

MAKE AIP FRIENDLY

Omit: chile

Combine the coconut milk, broth, lemongrass, galangal or ginger, chile, and kaffir lime leaves in a large saucepan over medium heat, bring to a simmer, and cook for 5 minutes.

Add the mushrooms and chicken to the pan and simmer until the chicken is just cooked through, 4–6 minutes. Stir in the lime juice and fish sauce, add the kelp noodles and yau choy, and cook until the yau choy is wilted, 2 minutes. Taste and add a little more fish sauce if required.

Ladle the soup into warm bowls, add the cilantro, and serve with the lime wedges on the side.

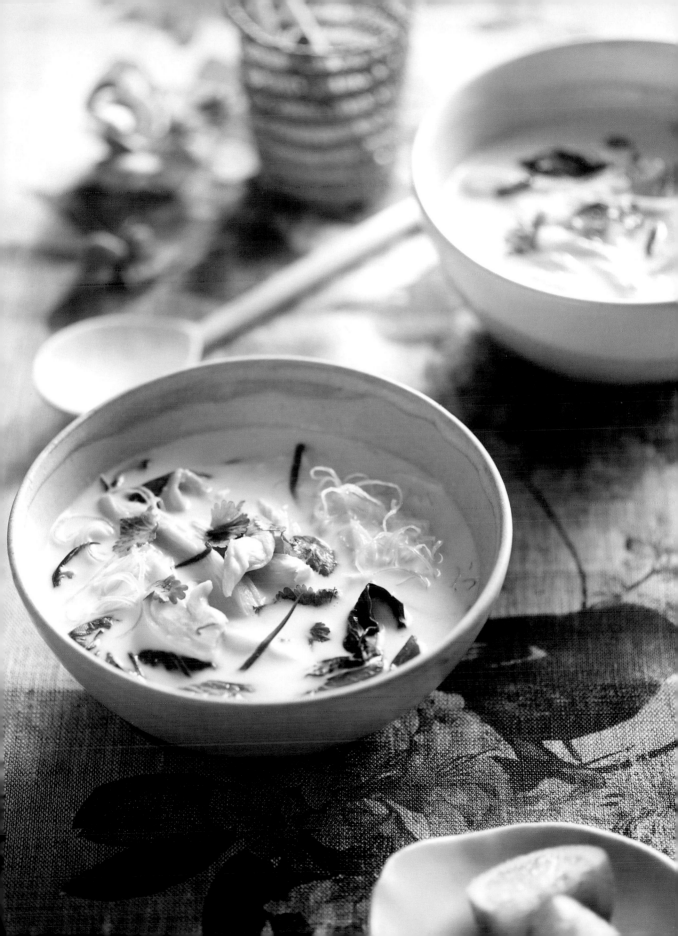

MISO SOUP WITH CHICKEN MEATBALLS

SERVES 4

Here, I have taken the classic miso soup and swapped out the bland pieces of tofu (yes, tofu is about as exciting as watching golf on the TV) and replaced it with something that will please the whole family – meatballs! I use chicken, but any ground protein, such as pork, shrimp, or beef, will work well. You can even gently poach a fillet of fish if you prefer. You can also leave out the miso paste, if you like, so it becomes a simple chicken broth base.

MEATBALLS
1 pound ground chicken
1 tablespoon finely grated ginger
2 red Asian shallots, finely chopped
2 garlic cloves, finely chopped
1 tablespoon tamari or coconut aminos*
¼ teaspoon fine sea salt
¼ teaspoon freshly ground black pepper

SOUP
1 quart (4 cups) Chicken Bone Broth
   (page 116)
3 teaspoons dried wakame seaweed*
7 ounces cauliflower, roughly chopped
3 green onions, thinly sliced
10 okra pods, sliced (optional)
½ cup miso paste
1 tablespoon toasted sesame seeds
   (optional)
sesame oil

* See Glossary

MAKE AIP FRIENDLY

Omit: tamari, black pepper, and sesame seeds
Substitute: coconut aminos in place of tamari

To make the meatballs, combine all the ingredients in a bowl and mix well. Shape the meat mixture into 18–20 balls, depending on how big or small you like your meatballs (a small ice-cream scoop is perfect for this).

To make the soup, bring the broth to a boil in a large saucepan over medium heat. Add the wakame and meatballs and simmer until the wakame has expanded, 8 minutes. Add the vegetables and cook for a couple of minutes. Add the miso – the best way to do this is to push it through a strainer into the pan (this evenly distributes it in the broth). Simmer until the miso has dissolved, stirring gently if required, 1–2 minutes.

Spoon the soup into warm serving bowls and finish with the sesame seeds (if using) and a drop or two of sesame oil.

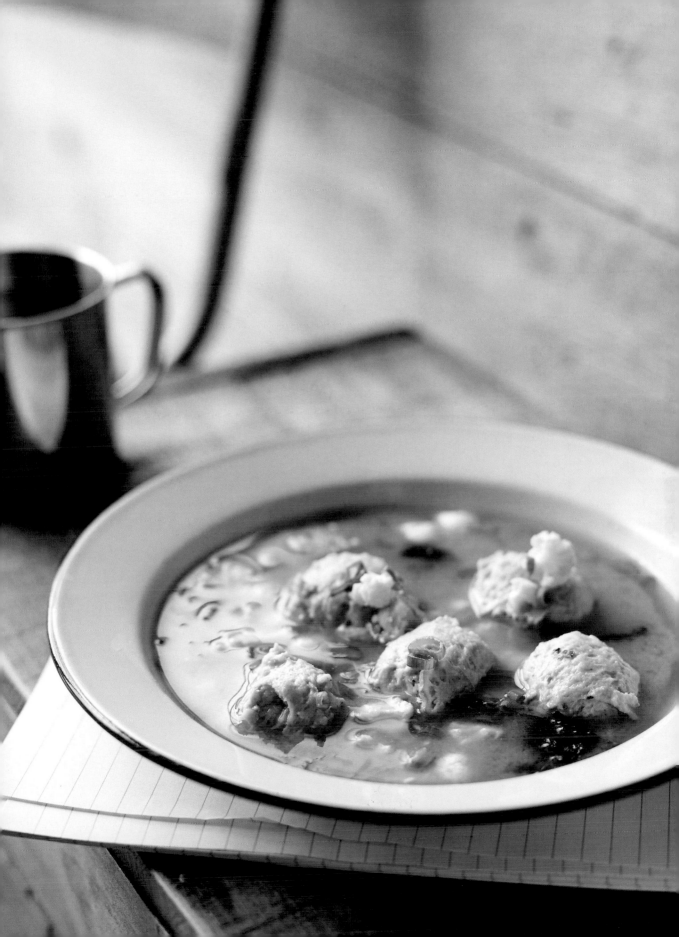

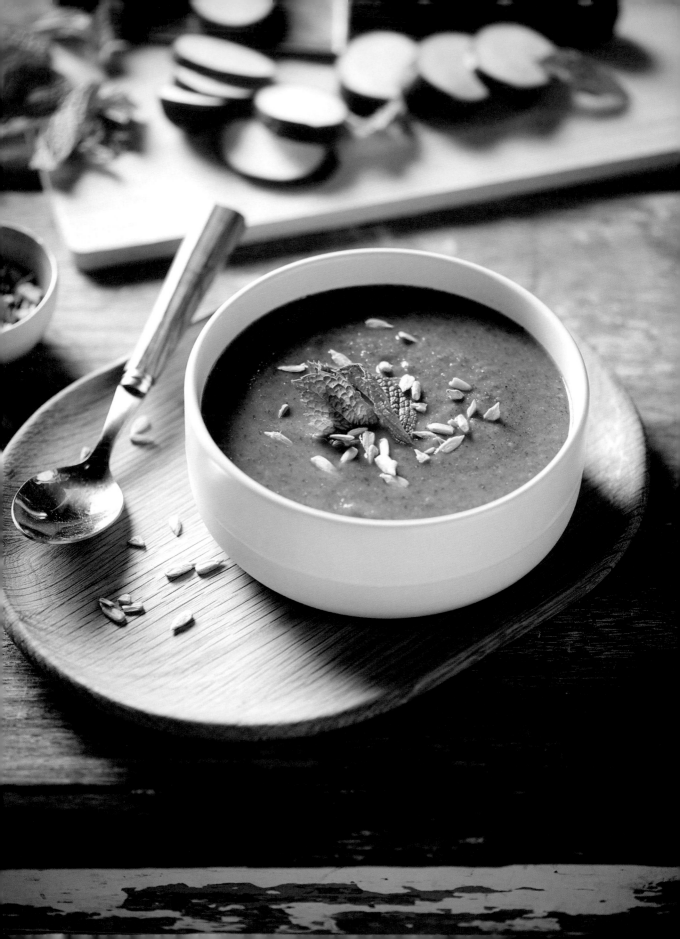

ZUCCHINI SOUP WITH FRESH MINT

SERVES 6

I suggest making this amazing and nourishing soup for your family in summer, when zucchini are overtaking your garden or you see them on sale at your local farmers' market or supermarket. The addition of mint is a masterstroke; if you want to make it even more delicious, add some red pepper flakes and any type of seafood.

---

1 tablespoon coconut oil
1 onion, chopped
3 garlic cloves, chopped
6 large zucchini, chopped
12 ounces cauliflower florets
5½ cups Chicken Bone Broth (page 116),
    plus extra hot broth if needed
2 handfuls baby spinach leaves
sea salt and freshly ground white pepper
mint leaves, to serve
hulled sunflower seeds, to serve

MAKE AIP FRIENDLY

Omit: white pepper and sunflower seeds

Melt the coconut oil in a large saucepan over medium heat, add the onion and garlic, and sauté for a few minutes until the onion is translucent, 4–5 minutes.

Add the zucchini to the pan and cook until softened, 5 minutes. Add the cauliflower and broth and bring to a boil. Reduce the heat to low, cover, and simmer until the cauliflower is tender, 20 minutes.

Stir the spinach into the soup, then purée with a handheld blender until smooth. Add more hot broth if the soup is too thick. Season with salt and white pepper. Serve hot or cold, topped with some mint leaves and sunflower seeds.

CHICKEN AND VEGETABLE SOUP

SERVES 6-8

If you want to cook a meal that will get the double thumbs up from the whole family, then look no further than the humble but always pleasing chicken soup. Different cultures all over the globe have been slowly simmering aromatic pots of chicken, fowl, or game with vegetable goodness for millennia. This is a very basic version. Feel free to add in or take out whatever you like … you really can't go wrong.

2 tablespoons coconut oil or
    good-quality animal fat*
1 onion, chopped
3 garlic cloves, finely chopped
1 large carrot, chopped
1 celery rib, halved lengthwise and
    cut into ½-inch-thick slices
3 thyme sprigs, leaves picked
1 fresh bay leaf
7 cups Chicken Bone Broth (page 116),
    plus extra if needed
1 tablespoon finely grated ginger
1 zucchini, cut into ¾-inch cubes
10 ounces kabocha or butternut squash,
    cut into ¾-inch cubes
1 pound boneless, skinless chicken thighs,
    cut into pieces
10 ounces kale or Swiss chard, shredded
sea salt and freshly ground black pepper
1 handful flat-leaf parsley leaves,
    finely chopped

* See Glossary

MAKE AIP FRIENDLY

Omit: black pepper

Melt the oil or fat in a stockpot or very large saucepan over medium heat. Add the onion, garlic, carrot, celery, thyme, and bay leaf, and cook, stirring occasionally, until the vegetables are soft but not brown, 6 minutes. Pour in the chicken broth and bring to a boil, then reduce the heat to low, cover, and simmer for 20 minutes.

Add the ginger, zucchini, and squash to the stockpot or pan and continue to cook until the squash is tender, 15 minutes. Gently add the chicken and simmer until the chicken is cooked through, 10 minutes or so. Add the kale or Swiss chard and cook until wilted, 5 minutes. Season with salt and pepper and sprinkle with the parsley before serving.

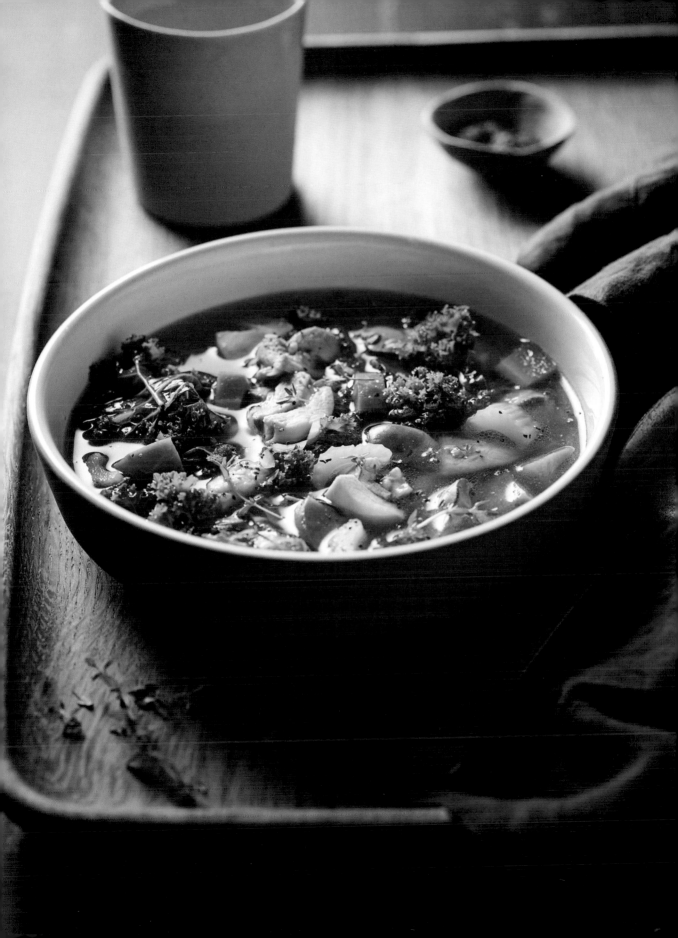

HEALING GARLIC SOUP

SERVES 4–6

I can't possibly count the number of times I have been asked, "What is great to eat when you have a cold or flu?" Apart from drinking water with some lemon juice in it, I thoroughly recommend this warming and nourishing soup that is chock-full of goodness: garlic, onion, leek, chicken stock, and good-quality fats.

---

3 tablespoons coconut oil or
    good-quality animal fat*
32 garlic cloves, roughly chopped
1 onion, chopped
1 leek, white part only, rinsed well
    and chopped
1½ quarts (6 cups) Chicken Bone Broth
    (page 116)
1 parsnip, chopped
2 pinches of freshly grated nutmeg
sea salt and freshly ground black pepper
4 egg yolks
3 tablespoons extra-virgin olive oil
1 cup almonds (activated if possible*),
    toasted and chopped
2 tablespoons chopped flat-leaf
    parsley leaves
drizzle of Turmeric Oil (page 314)

* See Glossary

MAKE AIP FRIENDLY

Omit: nutmeg, black pepper, egg yolks,
and almonds

Melt the coconut oil or fat in a large saucepan over medium heat. Add the garlic, onion, and leek and sauté, stirring occasionally, until softened and fragrant, 5 minutes. Pour in the broth, add the parsnip, and simmer until the vegetables are tender, 30 minutes.

Puree the soup with a handheld blender and season with the nutmeg, salt, and pepper. Reheat the soup over low heat.

Combine the egg yolks and olive oil in a bowl and whisk. Add a ladle of the hot soup to the egg mixture and whisk to incorporate. Pour the warm egg mixture into the soup and stir gently to heat through, 1 minute. Do not allow the soup to boil, or the egg yolks will curdle. Ladle the soup into warm serving bowls. Sprinkle with the almonds and parsley, and drizzle on a little turmeric oil.

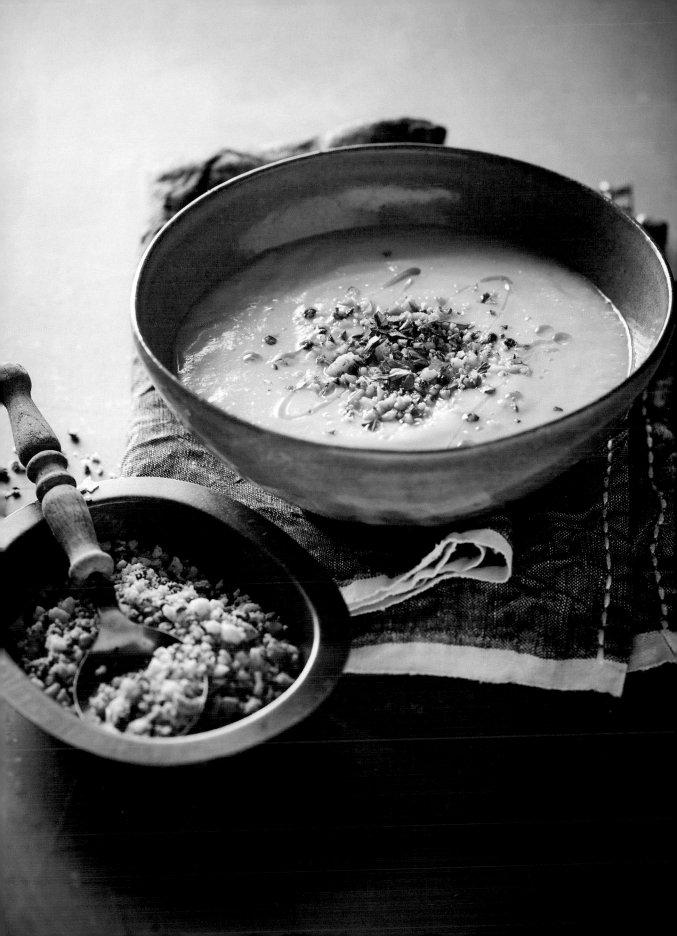

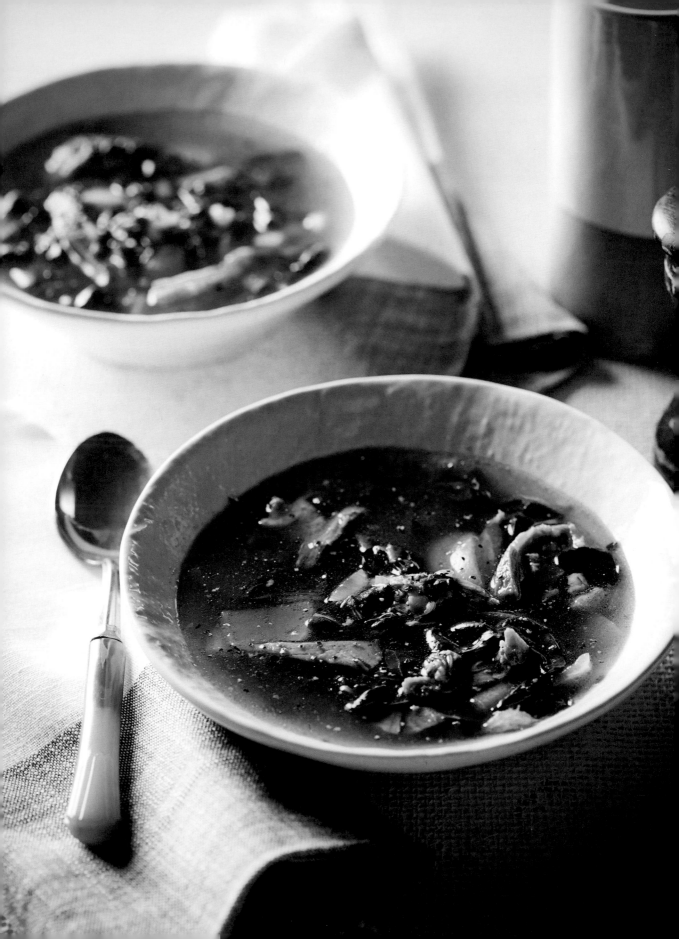

HAM HOCK SOUP

SERVES 6–8

Slowly simmering smoky ham hock fills the kitchen with the most amazing and hard-to-resist aroma. I am sure many of us remember coming home during the cooler months to find a yummy bowl of pea and ham soup being prepared. Here, I have swapped the split peas for Swiss chard, as Swiss chard is a lot gentler on the gut. You still have the same amazing flavor, but without the bloating effect afterwards. If you need a little more substance, then add in some sweet potato, squash, or bone marrow.

---

1 tablespoon coconut oil or
   good-quality animal fat*
2 onions, chopped
1 large smoked ham hock
   (about 2–2½ pounds)
3 garlic cloves, sliced
2 celery ribs, sliced
2 carrots, cut into ¼-inch slices
1 turnip, cut into ½-inch cubes
3 quarts Chicken Bone Broth (page 116)
   or water
1 teaspoon ground turmeric
½ teaspoon ground cumin
2 zucchini, cut into ½-inch cubes
14 ounces butternut squash, cut into
   ¾-inch pieces
2 large handfuls roughly chopped
   Swiss chard leaves (about ¼ bunch
   with stems removed)
juice of 1 lemon, or to taste
sea salt and freshly ground black pepper

* See Glossary

Heat the oil or fat in a large stockpot over medium heat. Add the onions and cook, stirring often, until softened, 3–5 minutes. Add the ham hock, garlic, celery, carrots, and turnip, pour in the broth or water, stir in the turmeric and cumin, and bring to a boil. The ham hock must be completely submerged, so add a little more broth or water if necessary. Reduce the heat to low, cover, and simmer until the meat is just starting to fall off the bone, 1½–2 hours.

Add the zucchini and squash to the soup and cook until the zucchini and squash are soft and the meat is falling off the bone, 30 minutes more.

Remove the ham hock from the soup and set aside. When cool enough to handle, remove the meat from the bone, discarding the skin, bone, and fat. Shred or chop the meat and return it to the soup. Stir in the Swiss chard and continue to cook until wilted, 5 minutes. Pour in the lemon juice, and season with salt and pepper. Ladle the soup into warm bowls, and serve.

MAKE AIP FRIENDLY

Omit: cumin and black pepper

MIDDLE EASTERN MEATBALL SOUP

SERVES 4–6

With ground meat in the freezer, you can create countless different meals. We have a chest freezer on the farm and like to order in ten two-pound lots of ground beef, chicken, pork, and lamb, so we are well and truly stocked up at all times. I would much rather eat ground meat than have beef tenderloin or a lamb chop; not only is it more economical, it is way more tasty. Here is a delicious soup that pairs meatballs with the health benefits and wonderful flavors of medicinal spices.

MEATBALLS

1 pound ground lamb

2 garlic cloves, finely chopped

2 tablespoons finely chopped flat-leaf
    parsley leaves

1½ teaspoons ground cumin

1 teaspoon dried mint

1 teaspoon finely chopped oregano

2 teaspoons sweet paprika

sea salt and freshly ground black pepper

3 tablespoons coconut oil or
    good-quality animal fat*

2 onions, chopped

4 garlic cloves, chopped

pinch of saffron threads

1 teaspoon ground cumin

1 teaspoon sweet paprika

1 teaspoon ground turmeric

½ teaspoon ground cinnamon

½ teaspoon ground ginger

3 tomatoes, chopped

5 cups Beef Bone Broth
    (page 121) or lamb bone broth

14 ounces cauliflower, chopped into
    small pieces

1 handful mint leaves

1 lemon, cut into wedges (optional)

* See Glossary

Combine all the meatball ingredients in a bowl. With wet hands, shape the mixture into walnut-sized balls.

Heat 2 tablespoons of the oil or fat in a large frying pan over medium heat. Add the meatballs in batches and seal until brown all over (about 2 minutes). Remove from the heat and drain on paper towels.

Melt the remaining oil or fat in a large saucepan over medium-high heat. Add the onion and sauté, stirring occasionally, until the onion is translucent, 4–5 minutes. Add the garlic and spices and sauté until fragrant, 30 seconds. Stir in the tomatoes and cook until they start to break down, 3–4 minutes. Pour in the broth and add the meatballs and cauliflower. Bring to a boil, reduce the heat to medium-low, and simmer until the meatballs are cooked through and the cauliflower is tender, 20 minutes. Adjust the seasoning, if necessary, stir in the mint, and serve with the lemon wedges (if using).

MAKE AIP FRIENDLY

Omit: cumin, paprika, tomatoes, and black pepper

Substitute: ½ cup stock in place of tomatoes

TIP

Try asking your butcher to add some offal to your ground lamb – to make up 5–20 percent of the ground meat.

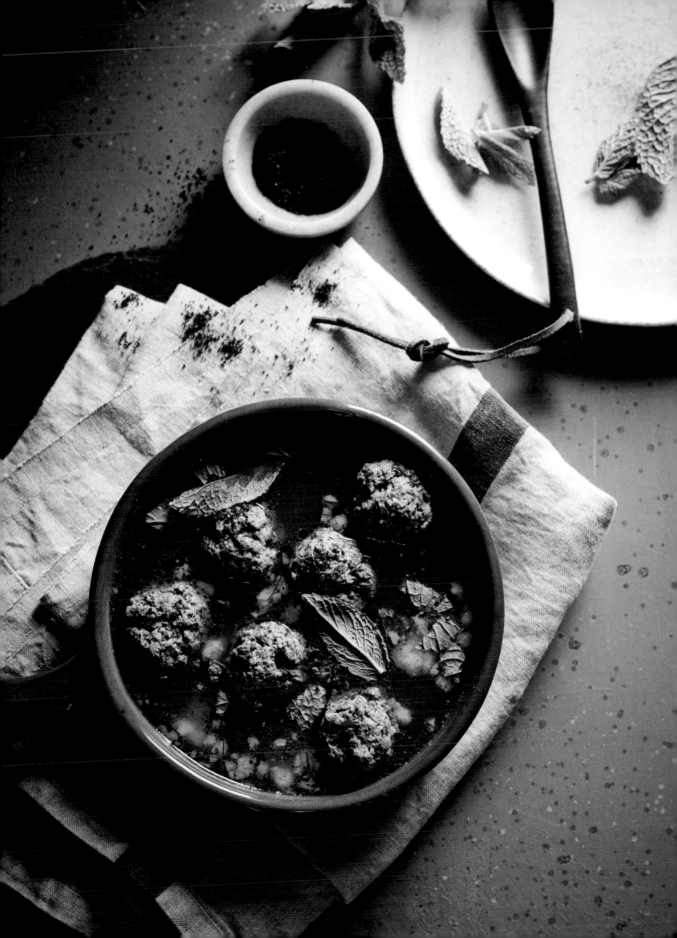

HUNTER SOUP (BIGOS)

SERVES 6–8

Bigos is a national treasure of Poland. This hearty hunter's soup, with its full-bodied and irresistible combination of offal, sausages, and smoky meats, fits perfectly in any dining room around the world. The sauerkraut rounds it all out and gives a pleasant sour note – but make sure to add the sauerkraut only once the soup has cooled to eating temperature, so as not to kill its beneficial bacteria.

2 tablespoons coconut oil or good-quality animal fat*

1⅓ pounds beef chuck or boneless short-rib meat, cut into 1-inch pieces

2 beef, chicken, or pork sausages (about 7 ounces), cut into ¾-inch slices

7 ounces beef heart, cut into ½-inch cubes

5 ounces bacon, chopped

1 large onion, chopped

2 large carrots, cut into ¾-inch cubes

2 celery ribs, cut into ¾-inch cubes

4 garlic cloves, chopped

3 tomatoes, chopped

2 fresh bay leaves

4 thyme sprigs, leaves picked

1 teaspoon sweet paprika

2 quarts Beef or Chicken Bone Broth (pages 121 and 116)

1 zucchini, cut into ¾-inch cubes

7 ounces butternut squash, cut into ¾-inch dice

7 ounces broccoli, cut into small florets

7 ounces mushrooms (such as white or brown button or portobello), thickly sliced

sea salt and freshly ground black pepper

1½ cups Sauerkraut (page 94)

* See Glossary

MAKE AIP FRIENDLY

Omit: tomatoes, paprika, and black pepper
Substitute: ½ cup stock in place of tomatoes

Heat the oil or fat in a large saucepan over medium-high heat. Add the beef, sausages, and heart and cook in batches until brown on all sides, 3–4 minutes. Remove from the pan and set aside.

Add the bacon to the pan and cook until starting to crisp, 5 minutes. Stir in the onion, carrots, and celery, and continue to cook until the vegetables start to soften, 5 minutes. Add the garlic and return the beef, sausages, and heart to the pan. Add the tomatoes, bay leaves, thyme, and paprika, stir to combine, then pour in the broth. Bring to a boil, reduce the heat to low, cover, and simmer gently until the beef is almost tender, 2 hours.

Add the zucchini, squash, broccoli, and mushrooms to the soup and cook until the squash and zucchini are tender, 20 minutes. Remove from the heat and season with salt and pepper.

Ladle the soup into warm bowls and serve with the sauerkraut on the side to mix through the soup (once the soup has cooled to eating temperature) or eat separately.

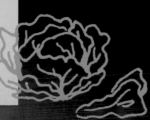

TIPS

I recommend doubling or tripling this recipe, as it will go down well as a treat with the family, and they will be asking for more over the coming days.

You can freeze the leftovers to have on hand for a rainy night.

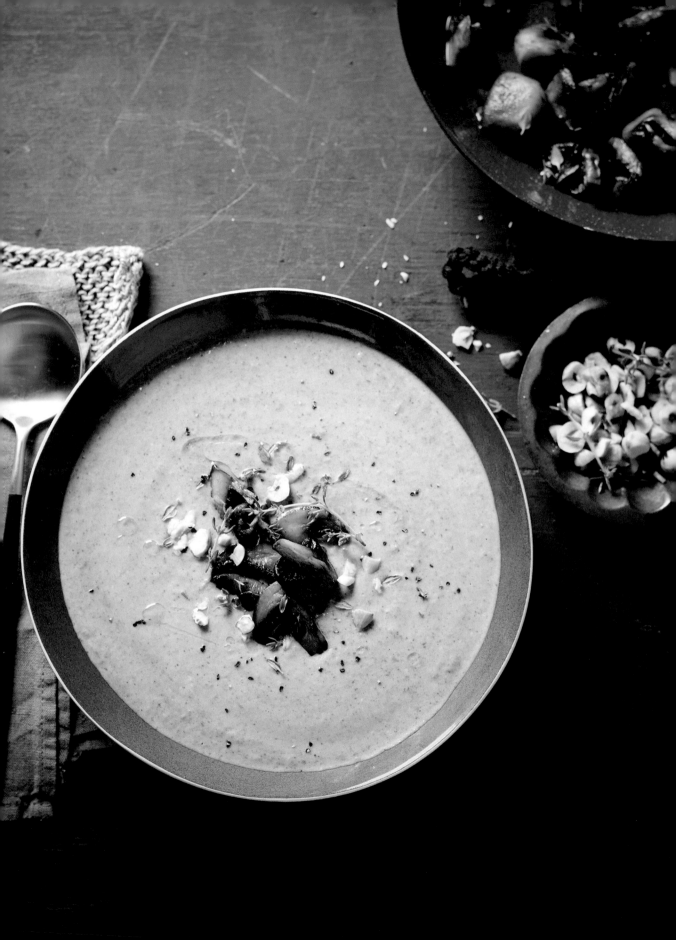

CREAMY MUSHROOM SOUP

SERVES 4

When the weather starts to turn from summer to autumn I get excited, as it means that wild mushroom season is about to be upon us again. Mushrooms are an excellent source of antioxidants, such as polyphenols, selenium, and ergothioneine (which some researchers call a "master antioxidant"). So, when you are feeling like a broth of nourishing goodness, fire up this little legend.

2½ tablespoons coconut oil or
   good-quality animal fat*
2 pounds mushrooms (such as portobello,
   white or brown button, or wild), sliced
sea salt
1 large onion, chopped
4 garlic cloves, chopped
1½ teaspoons thyme leaves
1 quart (4 cups) Chicken Bone Broth
   (page 116) or vegetable stock
½ cup coconut cream
freshly ground black pepper
½ cup hazelnuts (activated if possible*),
   toasted and chopped
1 tablespoon truffle oil, hazelnut oil,
   or extra-virgin olive oil

* See Glossary

MAKE AIP FRIENDLY

Omit: black pepper and hazelnuts

Melt 2 tablespoons of the coconut oil or fat in a large saucepan over medium-high heat. Add the mushrooms and a little salt and sauté until softened and starting to color (about 5 minutes). Remove about 2 heaping tablespoons of mushrooms from the pan and set aside. Reduce the heat to medium and continue to cook the mushrooms in the pan until the juices start to evaporate, 5 minutes or so. Add the onion, garlic, and 1 teaspoon of thyme leaves, and cook, stirring occasionally, until the onion has softened, 5 minutes.

Pour the broth or stock into the pan and bring to a boil. Turn the heat down to low, cover, and simmer for 15 minutes. Add the coconut cream and cook until heated through, 2 minutes. Season with salt and pepper and, using a handheld or stand blender, purée the soup until smooth.

Melt the remaining coconut oil or fat in a frying pan. Add the reserved mushrooms and sauté until the mushrooms are heated through. Add the remaining thyme and toss through the mushrooms. Season to taste with a little salt.

Ladle the mushroom soup into warm serving bowls. Top with some of the reserved sautéed mushrooms, sprinkle with the hazelnuts, and finish with some pepper and a drizzle of truffle, hazelnut, or olive oil.

HEARTY OXTAIL SOUP

SERVES 6

Every chef and home cook I know loves to use gelatinous, luscious, and "moreish" oxtail in his or her cooking. There is something very comforting and rewarding about turning an under-utilized cut of meat into one of the best things you will cook all week. Here is a very simple recipe that the whole family will love. I recommend serving it with some fermented veg on the side.

4½ pounds oxtail, chopped into 2½-inch pieces
sea salt and freshly ground black pepper
3 tablespoons coconut oil or good-quality animal fat*
1 large onion, roughly chopped
1 leek, white part only, rinsed well and roughly chopped
2 celery ribs, chopped into ½-inch pieces
3 large carrots, chopped into ½-inch pieces
½ teaspoon ground turmeric
½ teaspoon ground cumin
¼ teaspoon sweet paprika
a few thyme sprigs, leaves picked
2 fresh bay leaves
4 Roma tomatoes, roughly chopped
1 quart (4 cups) Beef or Chicken Bone Broth (pages 121 and 116)
1–2 tablespoons chopped flat-leaf parsley leaves

* See Glossary

MAKE AIP FRIENDLY

Omit: black pepper, cumin, paprika, and tomatoes
Substitute: ½ cup stock in place of tomatoes

Season the oxtail with salt and pepper.

Melt the oil or fat in a large saucepan or stockpot over high heat. Add the oxtail pieces in batches and cook for 3 minutes on each side to brown. Remove from the pan and set aside.

Reduce the heat to medium. Add the onion to the pan and cook until softened, 5 minutes. Add the leek, celery, and carrots, and cook until the vegetables start to color slightly, 5 minutes. Return the oxtail to the pan, then add the turmeric, cumin, paprika, thyme, bay leaves, and tomato. Pour in the broth, cover with a lid, and simmer until the meat is falling off the bone, 2½ hours.

Remove the oxtail from the soup. Using tongs (or your fingers when the meat is cool enough to handle), pull the meat away from the bone and chop into small pieces. Return the meat to the soup and gently stir through. Season to taste with salt and pepper. Ladle the soup into warm serving bowls and sprinkle with the parsley to finish.

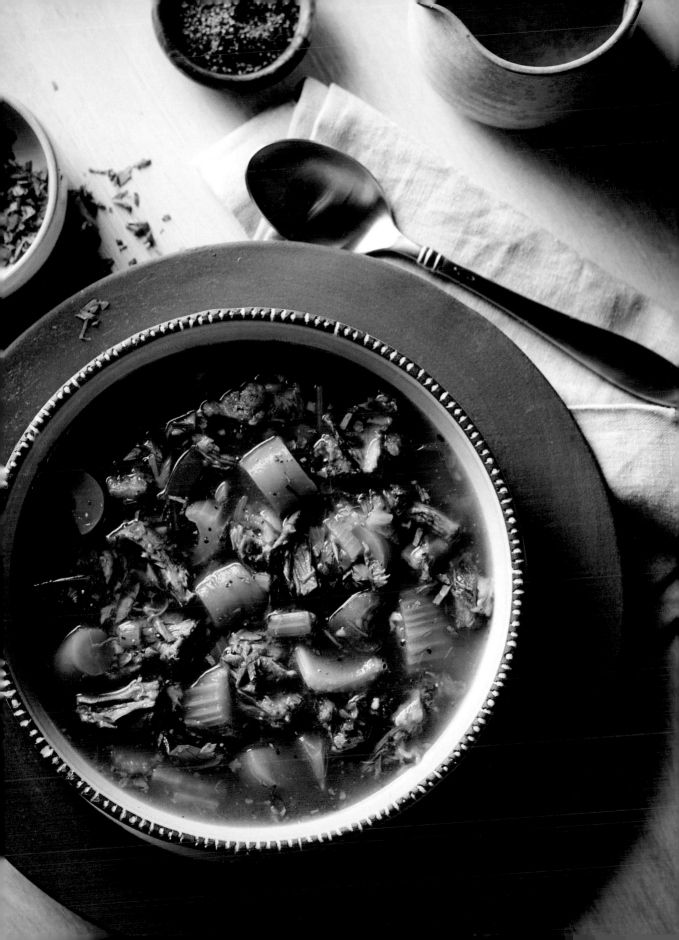

SPANISH SEAFOOD SOUP

SERVES 6-8

The Spanish really know how to take the taste of seafood to another level, while still retaining its authentic flavor. The way they combine pork and seafood and enhance them with the addition of saffron makes for a memorable meal. This delicious, easy, and relatively quick recipe is sensational for a weeknight meal – and it's good enough to impress guests for a special occasion. Pop some cauliflower rice into the soup to make it more of a meal, or add any other vegetables you like. Don't forget to serve with fermented veg on the side.

1½ quarts (6 cups) Fish or Chicken Bone Broth (pages 124 and 116)

2 pinches of saffron threads

2 tablespoons coconut oil or good-quality animal fat*

2 cured chorizo sausages, cut into ½-inch pieces

1 red bell pepper, chopped

1 long red chile, halved lengthwise and seeded

1⅓ pounds tomatoes, chopped

1 onion, chopped

4 garlic cloves, sliced

1 tablespoon tomato paste

2 teaspoons smoked paprika

½ cup organic dry white wine (such as Chardonnay) (optional)

¼ bunch kale (about 4 ounces), central stems discarded, leaves roughly chopped (optional)

10 ounces raw shrimp, peeled and deveined

1 pound mussels, scrubbed and debearded

1 pound white-fleshed fish (such as snapper or Spanish mackerel), skin on or removed, cut into large chunks

sea salt and freshly ground black pepper

1 handful flat-leaf parsley leaves

drizzle of extra-virgin olive oil

1½ tablespoons lemon juice, plus extra if needed

* See Glossary

Pour the broth into a saucepan, place over medium heat, and bring to a simmer. Remove from the heat, stir in the saffron threads, and set aside to infuse for 5–10 minutes.

Heat the coconut oil or fat in a stockpot over medium heat. Add the chorizo and fry, turning once, until golden and crispy. Add the bell pepper, chile, tomatoes, onion, garlic, tomato paste, and smoked paprika and cook, stirring occasionally, until the vegetables are soft (about 5 minutes). Pour in the wine (if using) and bring to a boil.

Add the warm broth to the pan and bring to a boil. Reduce the heat to low and simmer for 10 minutes, then add the kale (if using), shrimp, mussels, and fish, and cover with a lid. Cook until the mussels are open and the shrimp are just cooked, 2–3 minutes. Season with salt and pepper. Transfer the soup to warm serving bowls, scatter with the parsley leaves, and drizzle with the olive oil and lemon juice.

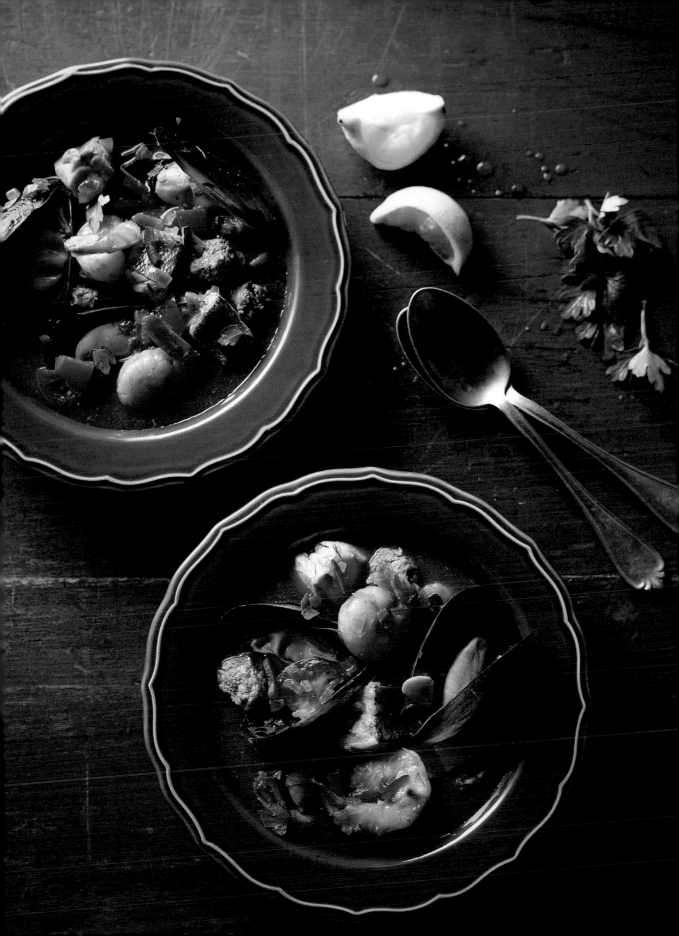

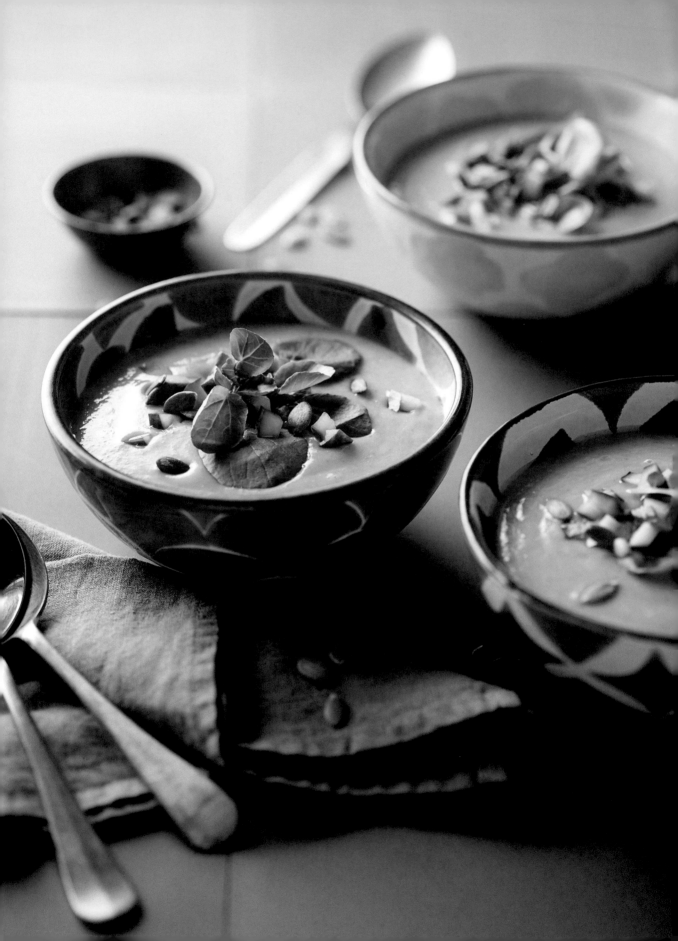

CHILLED AVOCADO SOUP

SERVES 4

We have just planted four different varieties of avocado tree on our property, and cannot wait for the harvest in coming years. I know we are going to have avocados coming out of our ears! We have a chest freezer in preparation for this, so we can blend and store the avocados to last us throughout the year. This recipe can be whipped up in a matter of minutes, and is a wonderful source of good fats. To make it a more substantial meal, just add some cooked crabmeat, prawns, chicken, or bacon.

---

2 cups Chicken Bone Broth
   (page 116), plus extra if needed
1 x 13.5-ounce can coconut milk
1½ teaspoons grated ginger
½ teaspoon ground cumin
2 avocados, pitted and peeled
1 large handful cilantro leaves, chopped
1½ tablespoons lime juice
sea salt and freshly ground black pepper
1 handful watercress, to serve
pumpkin seeds (activated if possible*),
   to serve
1 Persian cucumber, diced, to serve

* See Glossary

Combine the broth, coconut milk, ginger, and cumin in a large saucepan, and bring to a boil over medium heat. Reduce the heat to medium-low and simmer for 5 minutes. Remove from the heat and let cool.

Once cool, pour the soup into a blender. Add the avocado flesh, cilantro, and lime juice and blend until smooth and creamy. Add more broth or water to thin if necessary. Season to taste with salt and pepper. Place in the fridge to chill, or serve at room temperature, if desired.

Ladle the avocado soup into serving bowls, sprinkle with some watercress, and scatter on the pumpkin seeds and diced cucumber.

MAKE AIP FRIENDLY

Omit: cumin, black pepper, and pumpkin seeds

SRI LANKAN CAULIFLOWER SOUP

SERVES 4

Cauliflower has become one of my all-time favorite vegetables, thanks to its incredible versatility. From eating it raw to roasting, stir-frying, steaming, fermenting, pickling, and chargrilling – you name it, you can do it with cauliflower. As for the types of cuisine it works well in, here is a Sri Lankan–inspired soup that will have everyone asking for more.

---

3 tablespoons coconut oil
1 large head of cauliflower
    (about 2½ pounds), cut into florets
sea salt
1 sprig fresh curry leaves (about 10 leaves)
2 onions, chopped
3 garlic cloves, finely chopped
2 teaspoons ground cumin
2 teaspoons garam masala
1–2 pinches of cayenne pepper, or to taste
1½ quarts (6 cups) Chicken Bone Broth
    (page 116) or vegetable stock
1½ teaspoons apple cider vinegar
freshly ground black pepper
1 small handful cilantro leaves, to serve
toasted cumin seeds, to serve
Turmeric Oil (page 314), to serve

MAKE AIP FRIENDLY

Omit: cumin (ground and seeds), garam masala, cayenne, and black pepper

Substitute: 1½ teaspoons ground turmeric in place of the omitted spices

Preheat the oven to 350°F.

Melt 1 tablespoon of coconut oil on a large baking sheet in the oven. Remove the sheet from the oven, add the cauliflower florets, and toss them in the hot coconut oil. Sprinkle with a little salt, and roast until the cauliflower is golden, 20 minutes. Remove from the oven and set aside.

Heat the remaining coconut oil in a large saucepan over medium-high heat. Add the curry leaves and cook for 1 minute, or until the leaves start to crisp a little. Add the onions and cook until softened, 5 minutes. Stir in the garlic, cumin, garam masala, cayenne pepper, and three-quarters of the roasted cauliflower (reserve the remaining roasted cauliflower for serving) and cook for a few minutes until fragrant.

Add the broth or stock to the pan and bring to a boil. Reduce the heat to low, cover, and simmer until the cauliflower is very tender, 30 minutes. Remove from the heat and discard the curry leaves. Blend the soup until smooth. Stir in the vinegar, taste, and add salt and pepper if necessary.

Ladle the soup into warm bowls and top with the cilantro leaves, a sprinkle of cumin seeds, and some of the reserved cauliflower florets. Finish with a drizzle of turmeric oil.

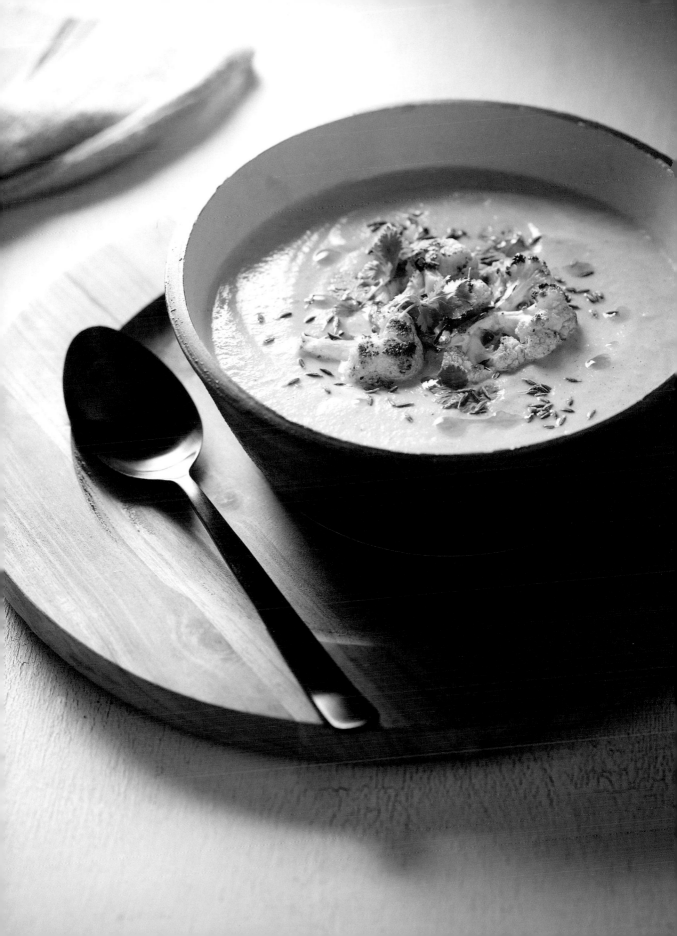

STRACCIATELLA SOUP

SERVES 4

The first time I ever made this soup I was so blown away by its simplicity and flavor that I couldn't believe I'd not encountered it earlier in my life. The delicious chicken bone broth enriched with organic eggs and vibrant greens and herbs is a marriage made in gut-healing heaven. Add some leftover roast chicken or gently poach some chicken wings in your stracciatella soup, and you have a wonderful meal that the whole family will love and crave. Serve with some fermented veggies on the side.

---

1 quart (4 cups) Chicken Bone Broth (page 116)

4 ounces cavolo nero (Tuscan kale)

12 thin slices pancetta, bacon, or lardo, cut into 1-inch lengths (see Note)

3 eggs

2 teaspoons lemon juice

¼ cup chopped flat-leaf parsley leaves

sea salt and freshly ground black pepper

extra-virgin olive oil, to drizzle

MAKE AIP FRIENDLY

Omit: eggs and black pepper

Pour the broth into a saucepan and bring to a boil. Add the cavolo nero and blanch for 30 seconds. Remove from the pan, transfer to a chopping board, and roughly chop. If using pancetta or bacon, add to the broth and simmer for 1 minute. (If using lardo, this is added at the end.)

Combine the eggs, lemon juice, and parsley in a bowl, and beat with a fork. Pour into the broth and stir for 1 minute. Return the cavolo nero to the pan and season with salt and pepper. Spoon into warm bowls, top with the pancetta, bacon, or lardo, and drizzle with some olive oil.

> **NOTE**
> *Lardo is pork fat that is cured with rosemary, spices, and herbs. It is available at specialty markets.*

TIP

You can use baby spinach, Swiss chard, kale, or broccoli florets instead of the cavolo nero.

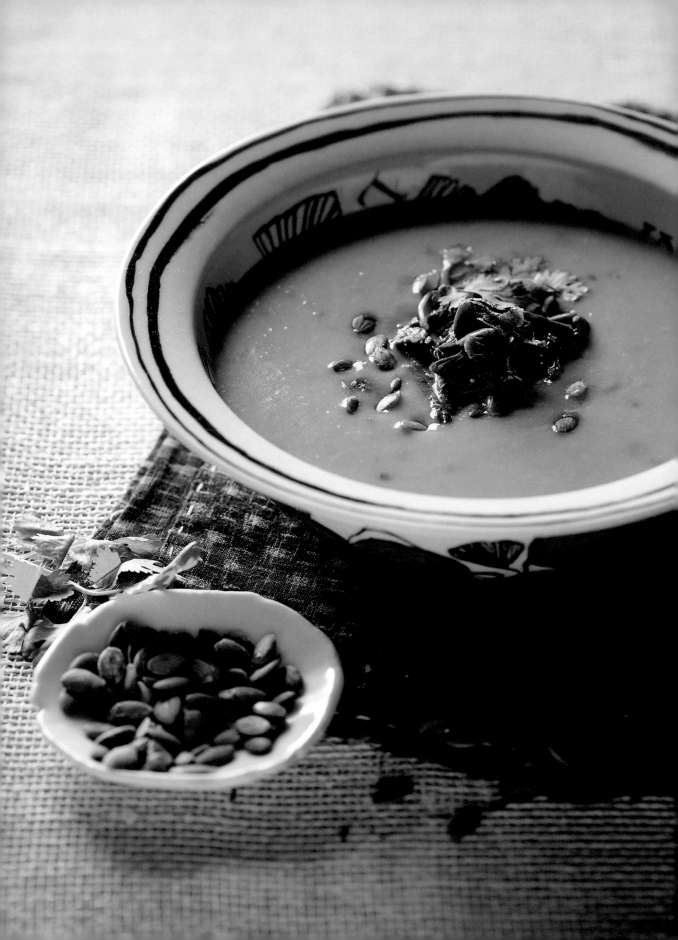

THAI SQUASH SOUP
WITH BRAISED BEEF CHEEK

SERVES 4

You'll probably know by now that I'm a fan of making life easier by cooking in bulk. Cooking and freezing in big batches means you will always have some good-quality meals on hand. This recipe came together when I had a big batch of Thai squash soup and some leftover braised beef in the freezer. I combined the two to create a super leftover meal. The end result is one of my favorite creations. Serve with some seeded bread.

BEEF CHEEK BROTH

1 tablespoon coconut oil or good-quality animal fat*

2 beef cheeks (about 1 pound each)

sea salt and freshly ground black pepper

½ onion, chopped

3 garlic cloves, chopped

1½ quarts (6 cups) Chicken or Beef Bone Broth (pages 116 and 121), vegetable stock, or water

SOUP

2 tablespoons coconut oil

1 large onion, chopped

2 garlic cloves, chopped

2 lemongrass stems, bruised and cut into 2-inch lengths

1 long red chile, seeded and finely chopped

2 tablespoons finely chopped cilantro roots and stalks

2-inch piece of ginger, finely grated

4 kaffir lime leaves, torn

1¾ pounds butternut squash, cut into ¾-inch pieces

zest of ½ lime

2 tablespoons fish sauce

1 tablespoon lime juice

½ cup coconut cream

pumpkin seeds (activated if possible*), toasted, to serve

cilantro leaves, to serve

* See Glossary

To make the beef cheek broth, melt the oil or fat in a large saucepan over medium-high heat. Season the beef cheeks generously with salt and pepper, and seal the meat for 3 minutes on each side until browned. Add the onion and garlic and cook until softened, 5 minutes, then pour in the broth, stock, or water, making sure the meat is fully submerged. Bring to a simmer, cover with a lid, and reduce the heat to low. Cook until the beef is tender, 2½ hours. Shred the beef cheeks and keep warm.

Meanwhile, to make the soup, melt the oil in a large saucepan over medium heat. Add the onion and garlic and cook until softened, 5 minutes. Stir in the lemongrass, chile, cilantro roots and stalks, ginger, and kaffir lime leaves, and sauté until fragrant, 3 minutes. Add the squash, lime zest, and 1 quart beef cheek broth, and bring to a boil. Cover, reduce the heat to low, and simmer until the squash is tender, 20 minutes. Remove the lemongrass and lime leaves. Blend the soup with a handheld blender until smooth. Mix in the fish sauce, lime juice, and coconut cream and reheat over low heat.

Ladle the soup into warm serving bowls, add some shredded beef cheek, and finish with the pumpkin seeds and cilantro leaves.

MAKE AIP FRIENDLY

Omit: black pepper, pumpkin seeds, and chile

ASPARAGUS SOUP WITH CRISPY BACON

SERVES 4

When asparagus is abundant, cheap, and in season, I love to incorporate it into as many meals as possible – stir-fries, curries, breakfasts, salads, seafood, and meat dishes – and I can never go past turning it into a delicious soup. This wonderful recipe works on so many levels, as bacon and asparagus truly go hand in hand. To round this off perfectly and make it more of a meal, simply add some pan-fried scallops, wild-caught salmon, or a poached egg.

---

2 tablespoons coconut oil or good-quality animal fat*

1 onion, chopped

3 garlic cloves, chopped

1 pound asparagus (about 4 bunches), woody ends trimmed

7 ounces cauliflower, chopped into florets

3 cups Chicken Bone Broth (page 116)

2 tablespoons chopped flat-leaf parsley leaves

sea salt and freshly ground black pepper

3 slices bacon

extra-virgin olive oil, to serve

* See Glossary

MAKE AIP FRIENDLY

Omit: black pepper

Melt the oil or fat in a large saucepan over medium heat. Add the onion and cook, stirring occasionally, until translucent, 5 minutes. Stir in the garlic and cook until softened, 1 minute. Add the asparagus and cauliflower and stir for 1 minute, then pour in the broth. Bring to a boil, reduce the heat to low, and simmer for 2 minutes. Remove four asparagus spears and reserve. Continue to cook the soup until the vegetables are very tender, 20 minutes. Add the parsley, and blend with a handheld blender until smooth. Season with salt and pepper.

Meanwhile, preheat the oven to 400°F.

Arrange the bacon on a baking sheet and roast for 4 minutes. Flip the bacon and roast for a further 4 minutes, or until golden and crisp. Cut into bite-sized pieces and set aside, keeping warm.

Ladle the soup into warm bowls, and top with some crispy bacon. Cut the reserved asparagus spears in half lengthwise, then cut into 2-inch lengths and add a few pieces to each bowl. Drizzle with olive oil, and serve.

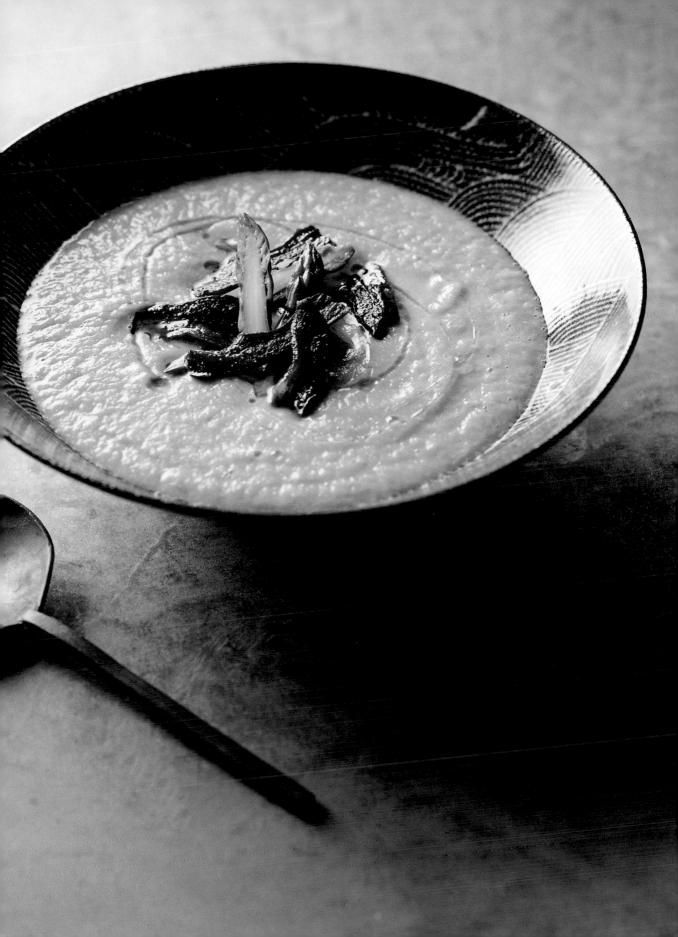

LIGHT MEALS AND SNACKS

WARM FLAXSEED PORRIDGE

STEWED APPLE WITH LICORICE ROOT
AND FLAXSEED MEAL

BACON CHIPS WITH GUACAMOLE

BEET HUMMUS WITH VEGGIE STICKS

VIETNAMESE NORI ROLLS

DEVILED EGGS WITH SMOKED TROUT SALAD AND NAM JIM

LEMONGRASS AND LIME CHICKEN WINGS

PIG'S HEAD PÂTÉ

TURMERIC CABBAGE ROLLS WITH LARB

BEEF TARTARE WITH SOFT-BOILED EGGS

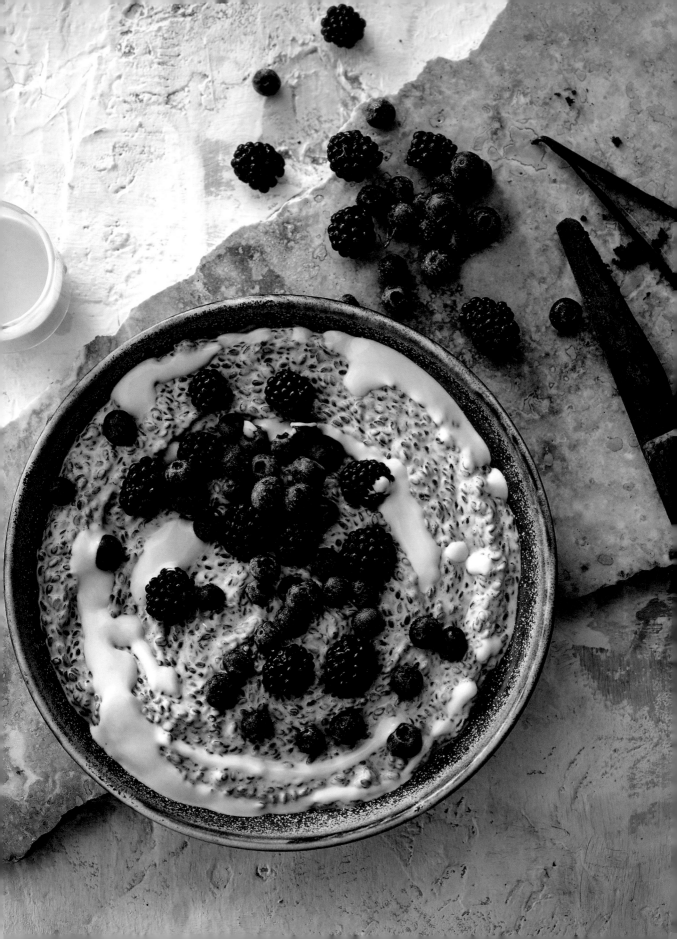

WARM FLAXSEED PORRIDGE

SERVES 2-3

Flaxseeds are a great source of anti-inflammatory omega-3 fatty acids and lignans. They also have a demulcent (slippery or jelling) property, which is both very soothing to the gut and helpful for keeping you regular. This is a delicious and nourishing way to start your day.

1⅓ cups flaxseeds
2½ cups coconut milk or Almond Milk
   (page 306), plus extra to serve
1 tablespoon honey (optional)
1 vanilla pod, split and seeds scraped
¼ teaspoon ground cinnamon
blueberries and blackberries, to serve

In a saucepan, combine the flaxseeds with the milk, honey (if using), and vanilla seeds. Mix well, and bring to a simmer over medium heat. Reduce the heat to low, cover, and simmer, stirring occasionally to prevent the porridge from sticking to the bottom of the pan, until the porridge is light and fluffy, 3 minutes.

Let cool a little before stirring in the cinnamon.

Spoon the porridge into two bowls and scatter with the berries. Serve with some extra almond milk on the side.

STEWED APPLE WITH LICORICE ROOT AND FLAXSEED MEAL

SERVES 2

Another tasty breakfast jam-packed with gut health benefits. The soluble fiber and plant-based nutrients support a healthy gut, and licorice root adds extra soothing and anti-inflammatory effects. The skin of the apples can be harder to digest, but stewing the peel before discarding it releases the pectin (a great source of soluble fiber). Make a big batch of this and store in the fridge and/or freezer so you always have some on hand for a quick gut-soothing breakfast.

---

2 Granny Smith apples
1 cinnamon stick
1 vanilla pod, split and seeds scraped
½ teaspoon licorice root powder*
1–2 teaspoons flaxseed meal

* See Glossary

MAKE AIP FRIENDLY

Omit: vanilla and flaxseed meal

Peel and core the apples, reserving the skin. Chop the apple into ¾-inch pieces.

In a saucepan, combine the apple, reserved apple peel, cinnamon, vanilla pod and seeds, and licorice. Add ½ cup filtered water, cover with a lid, and bring to a simmer. Cook, stirring occasionally so the apple doesn't stick to the bottom of the pan, until the apple is tender, 10–12 minutes. Let cool.

Remove the cinnamon stick, apple peel, and vanilla pod from the pan and discard (or reserve to use as a garnish, but not to eat).

Spoon the stewed apple into serving bowls and sprinkle with some flaxseed meal. Serve.

> **TIP**
>
> *Always make your own flaxseed meal by grinding fresh, whole flaxseeds in a coffee grinder or good-quality blender. The omega 3 oils in flaxseeds oxidize very quickly once exposed to air, light, and heat, so the oils in store-bought flaxseed meal will be less potent by the time you bring it home. Make enough at home to last you 3 or 4 days only, and store in a dark, airtight container (a dark glass jar is ideal) in the fridge.*

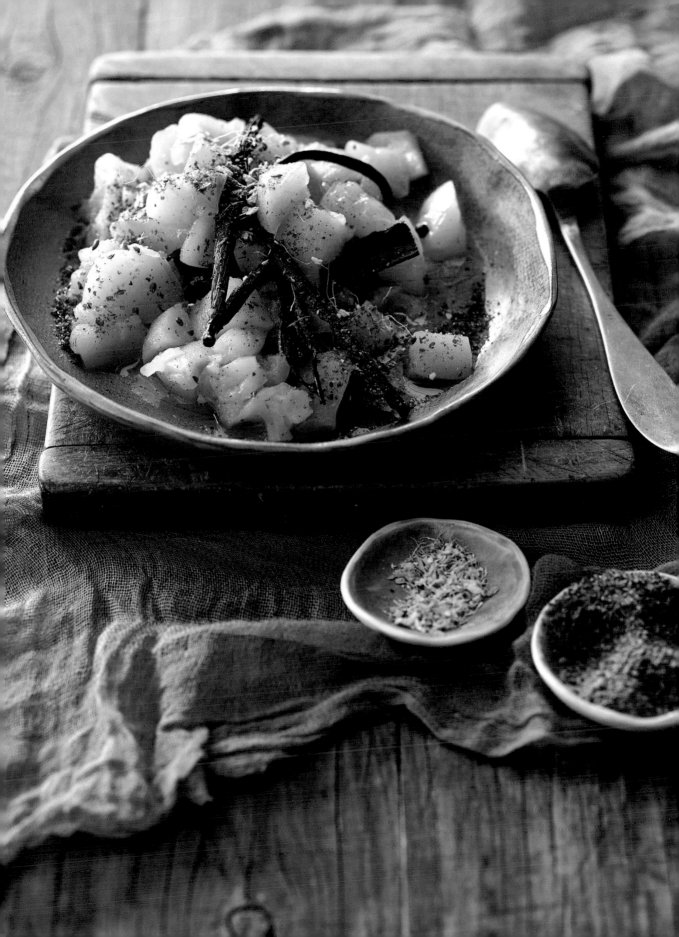

BACON CHIPS WITH GUACAMOLE

SERVES 4

I love it when I show people the types of food that a paleo lifestyle encourages, as they're usually gobsmacked by the variety. Take this recipe, for example. Not too long ago, low-fat foods were believed to be the healthiest way to go and fat was demonized as the leading cause of poor health. Now, thankfully, fat is back, and the science behind it makes perfect sense. So, break out the guacamole and, instead of corn chips, serve with these delicious bacon chips and maybe some chopped raw veg, too.

---

1 pound bacon

GUACAMOLE

2 avocados, diced
1 long red chile, halved lengthwise,
    seeded and finely chopped,
    plus extra to serve (optional)
juice of 1 lime, plus extra to taste (or use
    the equivalent amount of kraut juice)
2 tablespoons finely diced red onion
1 tablespoon chopped cilantro leaves
1 tablespoon extra-virgin olive oil
sea salt and freshly ground black pepper

MAKE AIP FRIENDLY

Omit: black pepper and chile

Preheat the oven to 400°F. Grease and line a large baking sheet with parchment paper.

Arrange the bacon in a single layer on the prepared sheet, making sure that the strips are not touching. Bake, turning the sheet once for even cooking, until the bacon is golden and crisp, 12–15 minutes. Keep a close eye on the bacon to prevent it from burning. Let cool completely, then cut into bite-sized pieces. Set aside until needed.

To make the guacamole, combine the avocados, chile, lime juice, onion, cilantro, and olive oil in a small bowl, and gently mix. Season with salt and pepper and sprinkle a little extra chile over the top (if desired).

Serve the guacamole straightaway with the bacon chips.

TIP

To make this a super snack, add some fermented veg to the guacamole, and enjoy every single mouthful.

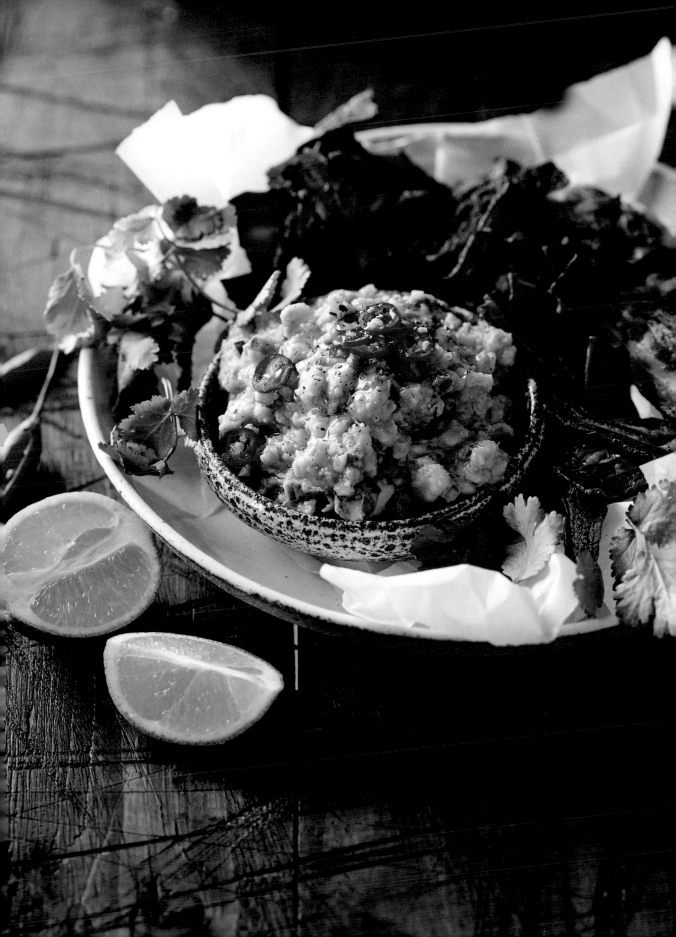

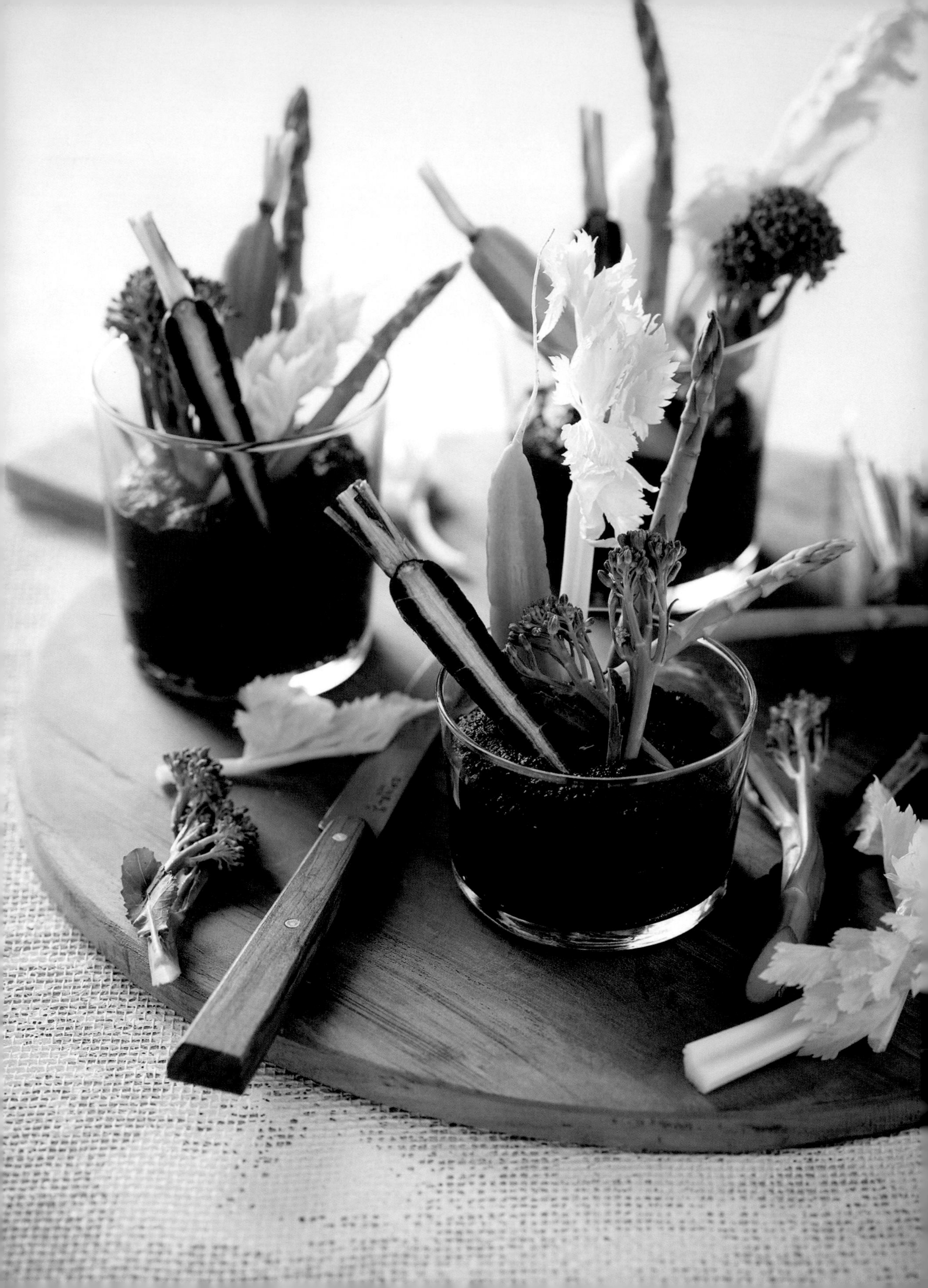

BEET HUMMUS
WITH VEGGIE STICKS

SERVES 6

I am often asked what to eat for a healthy snack. My response is always the same: real food! I'll often leave the house with some cucumber, carrot, or celery to eat when I want a snack. Here is a tricked-up, pretty version of just that. This delicious dip is a take on the classic hummus, but one that, in my eyes, is a lot better for your digestive system. Add some fermented kraut juice to the beet hummus for a probiotic kick.

---

1 pound beets (about 2 large or 4 small)
3 tablespoons unhulled tahini*
1 garlic clove, chopped
2 tablespoons extra-virgin olive oil
2 tablespoons lemon juice
1 tablespoon apple cider vinegar
2 teaspoons ground cumin
½ teaspoon sea salt
vegetables (such as purple and orange
   carrots, celery tips, cucumber,
   asparagus, broccolini), cut into batons

* See Glossary

Preheat the oven to 350°F.

Wrap the beets in foil and roast in the oven until tender, 1½–2 hours. Set aside to cool. When cool enough to handle, peel and roughly chop.

Put the beets in the bowl of a food processor. Add the tahini, garlic, olive oil, lemon juice, vinegar, cumin, and salt, and process until smooth. Let cool completely before serving.

Spoon some hummus into small jars, glasses, or bowls. Stick the veggie batons in the hummus, and serve.

VIETNAMESE NORI ROLLS

SERVES 4

Who doesn't love a Vietnamese rice paper roll? Here is my reinvented version – there are no bland fillers, just the most flavorsome food. I've replaced the rice paper wrappers with toasted nori seaweed, which is quicker to use and much tastier. Serve with some fermented veg or pop some inside, and feel free to use cooked chicken in place of the prawns.

DIPPING SAUCE

2 tablespoons *each* honey and fish sauce
2½ tablespoons lime juice
1 garlic clove, finely chopped
1 long red chile, halved lengthwise,
    seeded and finely chopped

CASHEW SATAY SAUCE

½ cup cashew nuts (activated if possible*)
¼ cup almond butter
1 tablespoon finely grated ginger
½ long red chile, halved lengthwise,
    seeded and finely chopped
1 tablespoon tamari or coconut aminos*
1 teaspoon *each* sesame oil and honey
sea salt

4 nori seaweed* sheets
1 handful mint leaves
6 cooked king prawns, shelled and
    deveined, cut in half lengthwise
1 carrot, cut into matchsticks
1 cucumber, seeded and cut into
    matchsticks
5 ounces daikon, finely shredded
1 handful cilantro leaves
1½ tablespoon mixed white and
    black sesame seeds, toasted

* See Glossary

MAKE AIP FRIENDLY

Omit: sesame seeds and chile
Substitute: puréed avocado in place of cashew sauce

To make the dipping sauce, whisk together the honey, 1½ tablespoons water, fish sauce, and lime juice until well combined. Add the garlic and chile, and allow to stand for 30 minutes before serving.

To make the cashew satay sauce, combine the cashews and almond butter in the bowl of a food processor and pulse to grind the nuts. Add the ginger and chile and pulse to combine. Pour in the tamari or coconut aminos, sesame oil, and honey, and blend well. Gradually pour in ¼ cup water and pulse until the sauce is smooth. If the sauce is a little too thick, simply add more water. Season with salt, and set aside until needed.

Place a nori sheet on a clean work surface with the long side facing you. Arrange 5 mint leaves along the bottom of the nori, about 1¼ inches away from the edge. Add 3 prawn pieces, smear some cashew satay sauce over the prawns, then top with one-quarter of the carrot, cucumber, daikon, cilantro, and a sprinkle of sesame seeds. Tightly roll up to enclose the filling, brush the long edge of the nori with a little water, then roll to fully enclose and press to seal. Repeat with the remaining nori sheets and filling.

Using a very sharp knife, cut the nori rolls into bite-sized pieces. Serve with the dipping sauce and enjoy.

NOTE
Leftover cashew satay sauce can be stored in an airtight container in the fridge for up to 2 weeks.

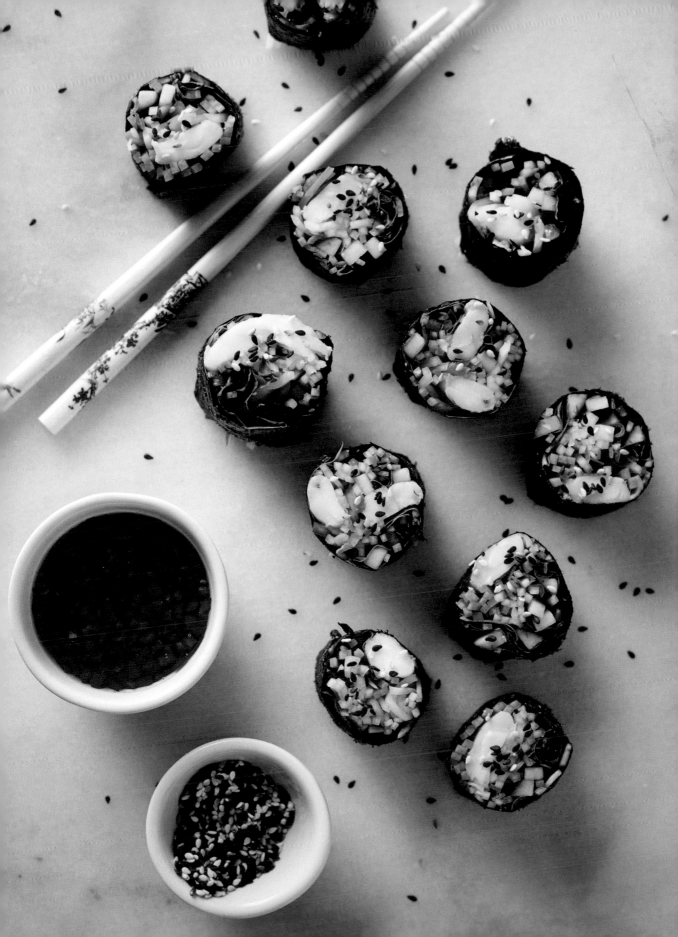

DEVILED EGGS WITH
SMOKED TROUT SALAD AND NAM JIM

SERVES 4–6

Deviled eggs are making a comeback in culinary circles, with versions containing everything from smoked eel to pulled pork and truffles. Here, I've created what I think is one of the nicest flavor explosions you can have: a mixture of salty, sweet, sour, and spicy. Try this at your next special occasion and watch the expressions on your guests' faces as they experience just how good healthy food can be.

---

6 hard-cooked eggs, peeled

1 hot-smoked rainbow trout
(about 8 ounces), bones and
skin removed, flesh flaked

2 red Asian shallots, thinly sliced

1 long red chile, halved lengthwise,
seeded and thinly sliced

1 handful Vietnamese mint leaves, torn

1 handful Thai basil leaves, torn

1 handful mint leaves, torn

3 kaffir lime leaves, thinly sliced

1 large handful cilantro leaves

½ cup Nam Jim Dressing (page 312),
plus extra if needed

12 betel leaves (optional) (see Note)

2 ounces trout or salmon roe

¼ cup Crispy Shallots (page 307)

Slice the eggs in half lengthwise. Carefully remove half of the egg yolks, put them in a bowl, and mash with a fork. Remove the remaining egg yolks from the egg whites and save for another dish, such as a salad, or eat as a delicious snack.

Add the trout, shallots, and chile to the mashed egg yolk and gently mix. Add the Vietnamese mint, Thai basil, mint, kaffir lime leaves, and cilantro, and gently dress with the nam jim dressing. Add more dressing if needed.

Lay each egg cut-side up on a betel leaf (if using), then fill the cavity with about 2 tablespoons of trout salad. Top with some trout or salmon roe and a sprinkle of crispy shallots.

NOTE

Slightly spicy and peppery betel leaves originate from Southeast Asia, and are popular in Vietnamese and Thai dishes. Mainly eaten raw, the fresh leaves can be found in good produce markets and Asian grocers. If betel leaves are not available, the deviled eggs are just as good on their own.

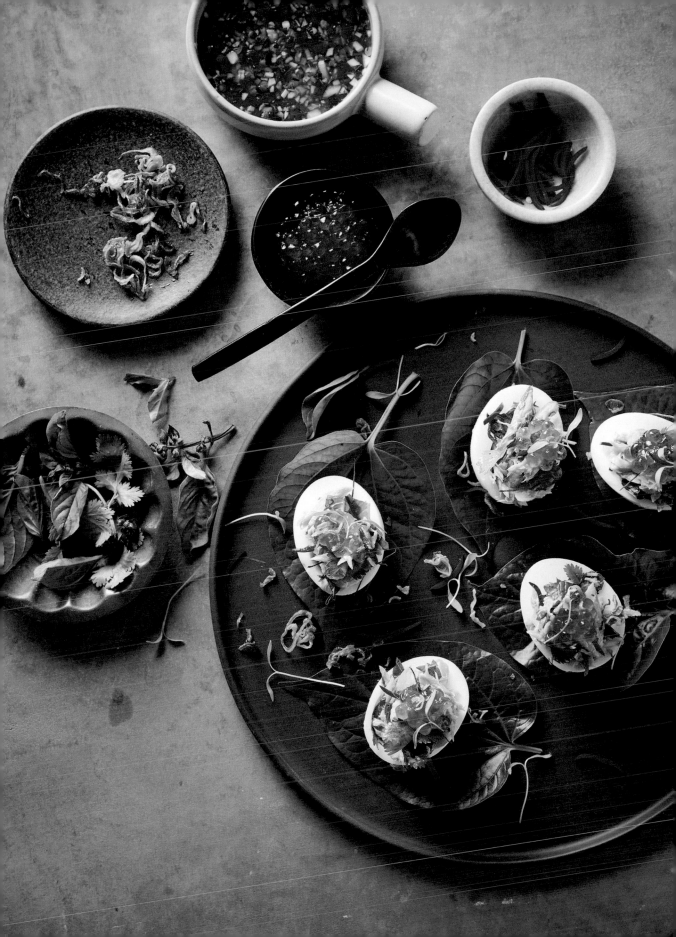

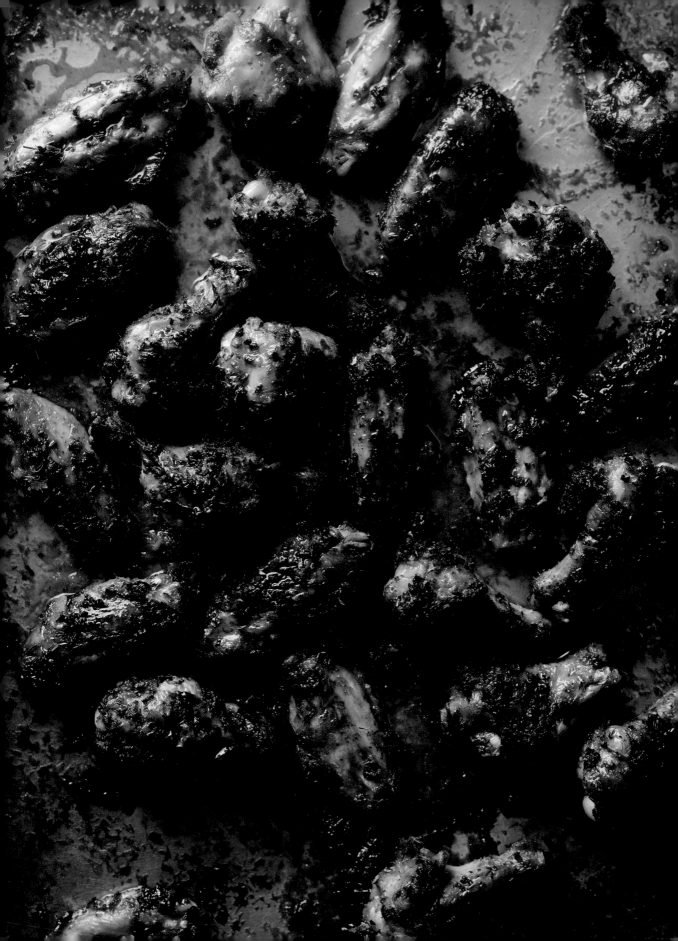

LEMONGRASS AND LIME CHICKEN WINGS

SERVES 4–6

Chicken wings are a favorite food memory from my childhood. Recently I was talking to an organic chicken producer, who told me chicken wings are not selling as well as they used to. I think it's time to bring them back and make them one of the most popular choices. This simple Thai-inspired number will have you licking your lips in glee. Serve with a refreshing salad and some fermented veg on the side.

3 lemongrass stems, white part only, roughly chopped

4 kaffir lime leaves, roughly chopped

3 shallots, roughly chopped

3 garlic cloves, roughly chopped

1 long red chile, halved lengthwise, seeded and chopped (leave the seeds in if you like it extra spicy)

1 tablespoon chopped cilantro stalks

2 tablespoons honey

2½ tablespoons fish sauce

2 tablespoons tamari

juice of 2 limes

20 chicken wings (or a combination of wings and drumettes)

2 tablespoons coconut oil or good-quality animal fat*

sea salt

* See Glossary

Combine the lemongrass, kaffir lime, shallots, garlic, chile, and cilantro in the bowl of a food processor, and process until finely chopped. Add the honey, fish sauce, tamari, and lime juice, and process until well combined.

Put the chicken wings and/or drumettes in a large bowl, and tip the lemongrass mixture over the top. Using your hands, massage the mixture into the chicken. Cover with plastic wrap and marinate in the fridge for 2 hours, or overnight for a stronger flavor.

Preheat the oven to 400°F. Grease a baking sheet with the oil or fat.

Spread the marinated chicken out evenly on the prepared sheet. Roast for 15 minutes, rotate the sheet and toss the chicken, then roast for another until the chicken is nicely colored and cooked all the way through, 15 minutes more. Season with a little salt if needed. Place the chicken on a large platter and serve while still hot.

MAKE AIP FRIENDLY

Omit: chile, honey, and tamari

Substitute: ¼ cup freshly squeezed orange juice in place of honey, and coconut aminos instead of tamari

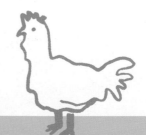

NOTE

Chicken wings are awesome in stocks, soups, curries, braises and, of course, when flavored with a delicious rub or marinade and cooked on the barbecue or in the oven.

PIG'S HEAD PÂTÉ

SERVES 10

Recently, I flew to the United Kingdom to cook with and interview Dr. Natasha Campbell-McBride, pioneer of Gut and Psychology Syndrome (GAPS), at her wonderful farm. Natasha is a revolutionary neurosurgeon and neurologist who has spent the last decade or two researching the link between the health of our guts and our emotional well-being and overall health. This is one of the terrific recipes she prepared with me. I will never forget the flavor and simplicity of this dish – it is one of the top ten meals I have ever eaten. Natasha included pig's heart in her version, too.

½ pig's head (about 6 pounds), cut in half
    (ask your butcher to do this)
1⅔ pounds pig's or lamb's liver
6 garlic cloves, peeled
2 tablespoons sea salt
1 tablespoon freshly ground black pepper

TO SERVE
thyme sprigs
seeded crackers
sliced carrots
celery sticks

MAKE AIP FRIENDLY

Omit: black pepper and seeded crackers

Put the pig's head and liver in a stockpot or very large saucepan. Add the garlic, salt, and pepper, and fill with just enough water to completely cover the head and liver. Cover with a lid and cook on low heat until the meat from the head is falling off the bone, 8–10 hours. (This step can also be done in a slow cooker on low for 10 hours.) Remove from the heat and let cool. Scoop out the garlic and set aside. Carefully strain the stock into a jug.

Remove and discard all the skin, soft tissue, and bone from the head, leaving only the meat.

Combine the garlic, meat, liver, and 1 cup stock (store the remaining stock in airtight containers in the fridge or freezer and use in other recipes – you'll have 3–3½ quarts left over) in the bowl of a food processor and process until smooth. Season to taste with salt and pepper. Pour the pâté into ramekins (it should fill 5) and refrigerate for 4 hours to set. Scatter with some thyme, and serve with the seeded crackers and veggie slices and sticks. The pâté will keep in the fridge for 5 days.

TIPS

Feel free to use pork belly instead of the pig's head.

If you find the flavor of liver too strong, you can cook the liver separately until it is just pink, and then blend it together with the other ingredients in the food processor later.

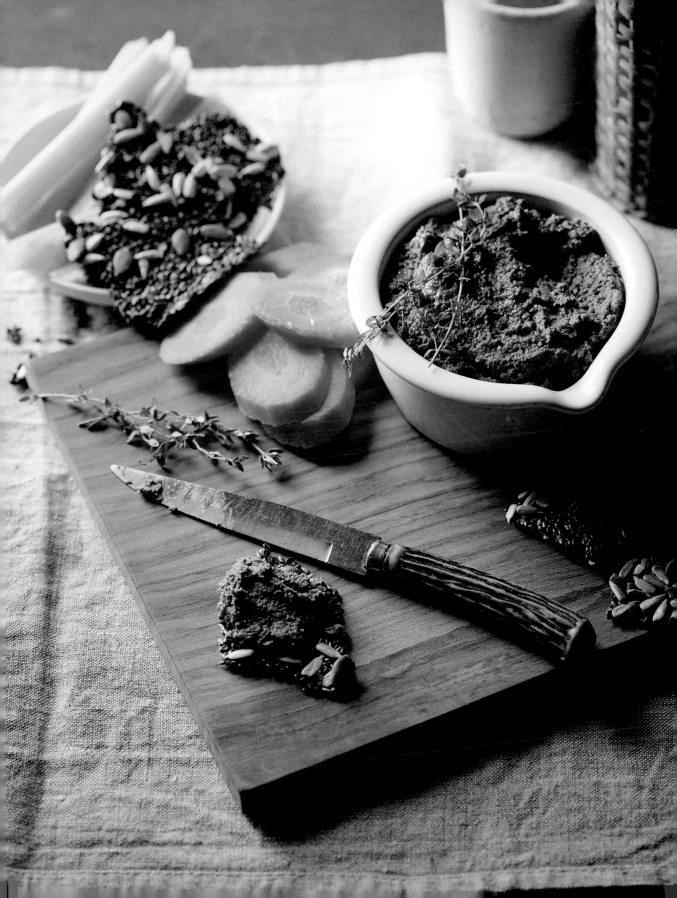

TURMERIC CABBAGE ROLLS WITH LARB

MAKES 16

Travel through Thailand or Laos, and on most menus you will notice a dish called "larb" – which, loosely translated, is a chopped meat salad that can be eaten raw or cooked. It is generally served with raw vegetables such as cabbage, cucumber, and beans. Here, I have chosen to cook the meat to appeal more to a Western palate. Add some liver or other offal to the mix if you are game (we always add liver and marrow), and simply pop in a bowl on the table with your raw vegetables, or wrap up in cabbage leaves. Serve with some fermented veg on the side, too.

1 tablespoon ground turmeric
2 teaspoons sea salt
8 large green cabbage leaves

LIME AND FISH SAUCE DRESSING

½ cup lime juice
3 tablespoons fish sauce
1 long green or red chile, halved lengthwise,
   seeded and finely chopped
1 green onion, thinly sliced,
   plus extra to serve

2 tablespoons coconut oil or good-quality
   animal fat*
1 pound ground chicken
3 red Asian shallots, finely diced
1 large handful mint leaves, torn
1 large handful cilantro leaves, torn,
   plus extra to serve
1 small handful Thai basil leaves, torn,
   plus extra to serve
3 tablespoons white sesame seeds, toasted
1 carrot, cut into thin matchsticks
1 Persian cucumber, seeded and cut into
   thin matchsticks
1 handful bean sprouts
1 lime, cut into wedges

* See Glossary

Bring 1½ quarts (6 cups) water to boil in a saucepan. Add the turmeric and salt and cook the cabbage leaves in batches until tender, 2–3 minutes. Drain on paper towels. Set aside to cool completely.

Meanwhile, to make the dressing, combine the lime juice, fish sauce, chile, and green onion in a bowl, and mix well.

Heat a wok or large frying pan over medium-high heat. Add the oil or fat and the ground chicken and cook, stirring frequently, until cooked and crumbly, 2–3 minutes. Pour in half the dressing, add the shallots, and toss to combine. Remove from the heat and let cool for 1 minute. Toss the mint, cilantro, Thai basil, and sesame seeds through the chicken.

Cut the thickest part of the vein (about 1¼–1½ inches) from each cabbage leaf, then cut each leaf in half. Place a leaf on a flat surface and spoon 2 heaping tablespoons of the chicken-and-herb mixture along the base. Arrange some carrot, cucumber, and bean sprouts on top. Roll up the cabbage leaf, folding in the sides, to enclose the filling. Repeat with the remaining cabbage leaves and filling.

Arrange the cabbage rolls on a platter, sprinkle on the extra herbs and green onion, and serve with the lime wedges and the remaining dressing on the side.

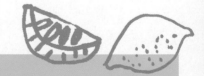

MAKE AIP FRIENDLY

Omit: sesame seeds, bean sprouts, and chile

TIP
You can use romaine or iceberg lettuce leaves, or fermented cabbage leaves, instead of fresh cabbage.

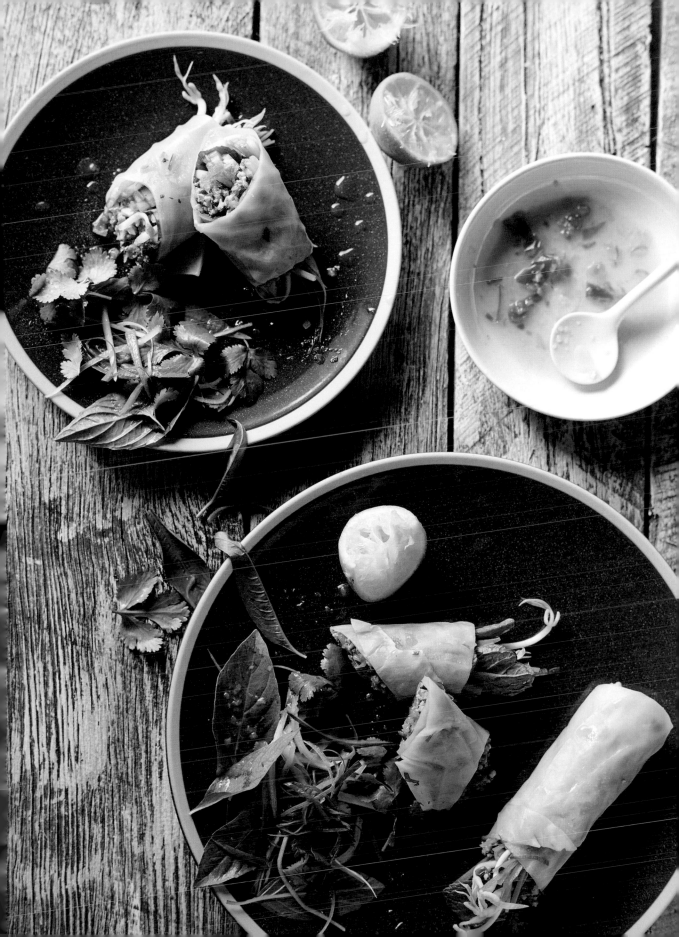

BEEF TARTARE WITH SOFT-BOILED EGGS

SERVES 4

Raw beef is one of my favorite foods to eat during the summer months. Whether it be tartare, sashimi, carpaccio, kibbeh, or sliced and marinated in a Thai-style salad, there is not much that comes close. A lot of research shows that a raw meat and seafood diet is good for our health. And, if you think about it, this is how our Paleolithic ancestors ate their meat. Most cultures around the world have preparations for raw meat and seafood, perhaps with a dipping sauce or a marinade. Here is a classic tartare.

MUSTARD VINAIGRETTE

2 tablespoons Fermented Mustard
  (page 309)
1 teaspoon honey
2 tablespoons apple cider vinegar
¼ cup extra-virgin olive oil
sea salt

4 eggs

TARTARE

2 teaspoons Dijon mustard
4 salted anchovy fillets, rinsed well and
  patted dry, finely chopped
1 tablespoon Tomato Ketchup (page 313)
1½ tablespoons Worcestershire Sauce
  (page 315)
freshly ground black pepper
2 tablespoons extra-virgin olive oil
¼ cup salted baby capers, rinsed well
  and patted dry, chopped
¼ cup finely chopped red onion
1 Fermented "Pickle" (about 60 g)
  (page 111) or 4 cornichons,
  finely chopped
1 small handful flat-leaf parsley leaves,
  finely chopped
1 tablespoon lemon juice
14 ounces beef tenderloin, very finely
  chopped
1 handful watercress, to serve
finely snipped chives, to serve

To make the mustard vinaigrette, combine the mustard, honey, vinegar, and olive oil in a bowl and whisk well. Season with a little salt.

Bring a saucepan filled with water to a boil over medium heat. Reduce the heat to medium-low, carefully add the eggs, and cook for 5 minutes (for soft boiled), or adjust the cooking time to your liking. Remove the eggs with a slotted spoon, plunge into cold water to cool, then peel. Set aside until needed.

To make the tartare, combine the mustard and anchovies in a large stainless-steel bowl, and mix. Add the ketchup, Worcestershire sauce, and pepper, and mix well. Slowly whisk in the olive oil, then fold in the capers, onion, fermented cucumber or cornichons, parsley, lemon juice, and a little salt. Add the meat and mix well with a spoon or your hands.

To serve, using two spoons, shape 1½ tablespoons of tartare into quenelles. Repeat until you have 12 quenelles in total. Place three quenelles on each serving plate an inch or two apart. Cut the eggs in half lengthwise and place in between the quenelles. Add three dollops of mustard vinaigrette, scatter some watercress over, and sprinkle with the chives. To finish, season the egg yolks with a touch of salt and sprinkle with some pepper.

TIP

*To turn this into a more substantial meal,
add some fermented veg and a salad,
and you will be in culinary heaven.*

MAIN MEALS

CAULIFLOWER "STEAK" AND EGGS WITH SAUTÉED GREENS

GREEN PAPAYA SALAD WITH KING PRAWNS

PRAWN COCKTAIL WITH KIMCHI

PAN-FRIED SARDINES WITH SQUASH HUMMUS
AND SWEET AND SOUR ONIONS

INDIAN FISH CURRY

GRILLED FISH WITH SAUTÉED ONION AND BURNT LEMON

STEAMED SALMON WITH NORI AND ASIAN GREENS

CRISPY SKINNED SALMON WITH CELERY ROOT RÉMOULADE

SESAME-CRUSTED AVOCADO BOWL WITH CHICKEN AND SPROUTS

PORK-STUFFED BITTER MELONS
WITH CHICKEN AND GINGER BONE BROTH

CHICKEN LIVER AND PORK TERRINE

TERRY WAHL'S CHICKEN LIVERS WITH ONION AND BACON

CHICKEN, LEEK, BACON, AND EGG "PIE"

STUFFED SWEET POTATOES

CAULIFLOWER FRIED RICE WITH SAUSAGE

LEMONGRASS AND TURMERIC PORK CAKES
WITH THAI HERB SALAD

THAI MEATBALLS IN LETTUCE CUPS

SAUSAGES WITH ONION GRAVY

"SPAGHETTI" BOLOGNESE

THE PALEO MOM'S BURGERS

SPICED SIRLOIN WITH WILTED SWISS CHARD
AND ALMOND AND BACON VINAIGRETTE

BIBIMBAP

SIRLOIN WITH ROASTED BONE MARROW AND PARSLEY SALAD

TURKISH LAMB BURGER WITH LETTUCE WRAPS

SUNDAY ROAST LAMB WITH VEGGIES AND MINT JELLY

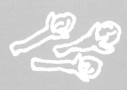

CAULIFLOWER "STEAK" AND EGGS WITH SAUTÉED GREENS

SERVES 4

This is my take on steak and eggs, but a modern version that incorporates vegetables and makes them the star. My favorite veggies for this dish are squash, broccoli, sweet potato, cabbage, mushroom, asparagus, zucchini, and Jerusalem artichoke. You can eat this for breakfast, lunch, or dinner, and it is great cold to take to work for lunch.

CAULIFLOWER STEAK

2 tablespoons coconut oil
1 large head of cauliflower (about
    2½ pounds), cut crosswise
    into 4 pieces about ½ inch thick
sea salt and freshly ground black pepper

BACON VINAIGRETTE

1 tablespoon coconut oil
2 shallots, finely chopped
5 ounces bacon, finely diced
3 tablespoons apple cider vinegar
1 teaspoon finely snipped chives
⅔ cup extra-virgin olive oil

SAUTÉED GREENS

2 bunches broccolini (about 13 ounces),
    trimmed and halved
3 tablespoons coconut oil
3 garlic cloves, sliced
1 bunch Swiss chard (about 10 ounces),
    stems removed (save for broths or
    soups), leaves torn
3 tablespoons hazelnuts (activated if
    possible*), toasted and roughly chopped,
    plus extra to serve

1 tablespoon coconut oil
4 eggs

* See Glossary

MAKE AIP FRIENDLY

Omit: eggs, black pepper, and hazelnuts

Preheat the oven to 350°F. Line two baking sheets with parchment paper.

For the cauliflower steak, melt 2 teaspoons of the coconut oil in a nonstick frying pan over medium-high heat. Add one cauliflower steak and cook, turning once, until golden, 2 minutes per side. Transfer to a prepared sheet and season with salt and pepper. Repeat this process with the remaining oil and cauliflower steaks. Place in the oven and roast until the cauliflower is tender, 12–15 minutes.

For the bacon vinaigrette, melt half the coconut oil in a small saucepan over low heat, add the shallots and gently cook until slightly softened, 1 minute. Remove from the pan, set aside, wipe the pan clean, and place over medium heat. Add the remaining oil and the bacon and fry until the bacon is crispy, 6–8 minutes. Add the vinegar and shallots and set aside to cool. Transfer to a bowl and whisk in the chives and olive oil. Season with salt.

For the sautéed greens, bring a saucepan of salted water to a boil. Blanch the broccolini until almost cooked through, 1 minute. Plunge into ice-cold water, then drain. Set aside. Melt the coconut oil in a large frying pan over medium heat. Add the garlic and cook until fragrant, 20 seconds. Stir in the Swiss chard, broccolini, and 2 tablespoons water, and cook, tossing occasionally, until the Swiss chard is slightly wilted and the broccolini is heated through, 1 minute. Toss in the hazelnuts and season.

Heat the coconut oil in a nonstick frying pan over medium heat. Fry the eggs for 2–3 minutes, or until cooked to your liking. Season, slide onto a plate, and keep warm.

Place the cauliflower steaks on warm serving plates, and top each with a fried egg. Add the sautéed greens, drizzle with some bacon vinaigrette, and serve the rest on the side.

TIPS

*For the bacon vinaigrette, if you prefer, you can use
½ red onion in place of the shallots, and 1 teaspoon finely
chopped flat-leaf parsley leaves instead of the chives.*

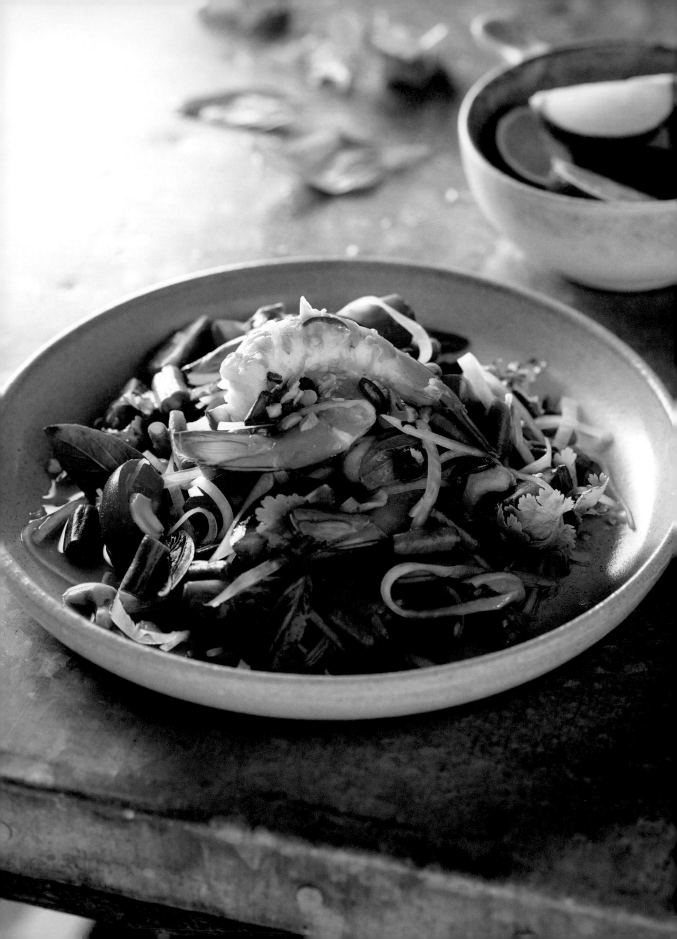

GREEN PAPAYA SALAD WITH KING PRAWNS

SERVES 4

In Asia, papaya is often eaten in its green or unripe state, when it is savory rather than sweet. As an enzyme-rich fruit, papaya is brilliant for breaking down proteins, which is basically what fermented foods do. Give this gut-healthy dish a go when you come across green papaya, or try green mango instead. You will be in for a real flavor explosion. If you cannot find green papaya or mango, swap in some cucumber and maybe a touch of green apple. You can use okra in place of the green beans and cooked chicken instead of the prawns, too.

---

2 tablespoons coconut sugar

3 tablespoons fish sauce

2 garlic cloves, crushed

1–2 long red chiles, seeded and sliced

1 tablespoon dried shrimp, chopped

1 green papaya, seeded and cut into
    matchsticks

¼ cup lime juice

10 cherry tomatoes, quartered

4 ounces green beans or haricots verts,
    cut into ½-inch lengths

12 cooked king prawns, peeled and
    deveined with tails intact

1 handful cilantro leaves

1 handful Thai basil leaves

3 tablespoons cashew nuts (activated if
    possible*), toasted and coarsely crushed

¼ cup Crispy Shallots (page 307)

1 lime, cut into wedges

* See Glossary

MAKE AIP FRIENDLY

Omit: coconut sugar, chile, cherry tomatoes,
green beans, and cashew nuts

Substitute: asparagus in place of green beans

Combine the coconut sugar, fish sauce, and 1 tablespoon water in a saucepan over low heat and cook until reduced to a shiny syrup (about 5 minutes). Set aside to cool.

Combine the garlic, chiles, and dried shrimp in a large mortar and lightly pound with the pestle. Add the papaya and continue to lightly pound. Add the coconut sugar and fish sauce syrup and the lime juice, and continue to gently pound so the mixture soaks up the flavors. Stir the tomato and beans through.

Tip the salad and dressing into a shallow serving bowl and toss through the prawns, cilantro, Thai basil, and cashews. Sprinkle with some crispy shallots, and serve with the lime wedges on the side.

PRAWN COCKTAIL WITH KIMCHI

SERVES 4 AS A STARTER

Growing up in Queensland (Australia's sunshine state) in the 1970s, I was initiated into the prawn cocktail club from a very young age. In those days the prawn cocktail was at its culinary peak, and in some parts of Oz it still is…and rightly so. Who doesn't love a wonderful salad that combines the best of paleo: good-quality wild-caught protein, plus an abundance of good fats in the form of avocado and a mayonnaise-based sauce? I've just added some fresh veggies flavored with gut-enriching kimchi.

DRESSING
1 garlic clove, very finely chopped
2 tablespoons extra-virgin olive oil
1 teaspoon lemon juice
1 teaspoon apple cider vinegar
1 teaspoon tamari
½ teaspoon finely chopped ginger

16 raw king prawns

SPICY AIOLI
2 teaspoons Sriracha Chile Sauce
   (page 313), or to taste
1½ teaspoons Tomato Ketchup (page 313)
1 teaspoon apple cider vinegar
1 cup Aioli (page 306)

½ iceberg lettuce, roughly shredded
½ cup Classic Kimchi (page 108)
1 handful dill fronds
1 avocado, sliced
white sesame seeds, toasted, to serve
lemon wedges, to serve

MAKE AIP FRIENDLY

Omit: kimchi, sesame seeds, tamari, and spicy aioli

Substitute: AIP friendly fermented cabbage in place of kimchi, coconut aminos instead of tamari, and puréed avocado instead of aioli

To make the dressing, combine all the ingredients in a bowl, and set aside.

Cook the prawns in boiling salted water until pink and firm, 2–3 minutes. Transfer the prawns to a bowl of ice-cold water and leave for 3–5 minutes, until they are completely cold. Peel and devein, leaving the tails intact.

Meanwhile, make the spicy aioli. Combine all the ingredients in a small bowl and mix until smooth. Add more aioli if the flavor is too spicy for your liking, or add more Sriracha if you prefer it extra spicy.

Combine the lettuce, kimchi, and dill in a mixing bowl. Add the dressing and toss through.

Place the salad in serving bowls and top with the avocado and prawns. Drizzle some of the spicy aioli over the prawns, sprinkle with sesame seeds, and serve with the lemon wedges.

> **TIP**
> *In this dish I have used kimchi, as I love how the spiciness goes with the rest of the dish, but it works equally well with kraut.*

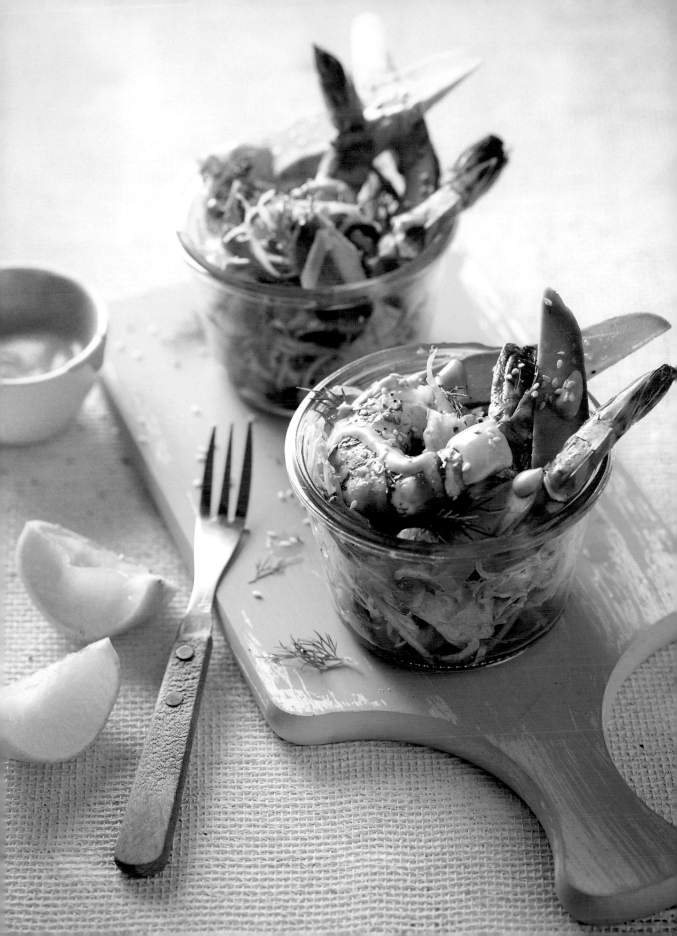

PAN-FRIED SARDINES WITH SQUASH HUMMUS AND SWEET AND SOUR ONIONS

SERVES 4

Sardines are probably the world's most sustainable and nutrient-dense fish, which gives them a huge plus. You can eat them nose to tail, bones and all, so nothing is wasted – another plus. Team them with some yummy accompaniments, as I've done here, or simply grill them and pop them on a salad with a simple dressing or some aioli, and you are in heaven.

SQUASH HUMMUS

1⅓ pounds butternut squash, cut into
   1-inch pieces
½ teaspoon ground cumin
sea salt and freshly ground black pepper
2 tablespoons coconut oil, melted
4 garlic cloves, peeled
2 tablespoons unhulled tahini*
1 teaspoon finely grated ginger
3 tablespoons lemon juice
¼ cup extra-virgin olive oil

SWEET AND SOUR ONIONS

1 tablespoon coconut oil or good-quality
   animal fat*
1 red onion, halved and thinly sliced
2 tablespoons raisins
2 teaspoons red wine vinegar

½ garlic clove, peeled
3 tablespoons pine nuts, toasted
1 teaspoon lemon juice
12–16 small sardines, cleaned and gutted
2 tablespoons coconut oil or good-quality
   animal fat*
1 handful mint leaves, torn, to serve
3 tablespoons pomegranate seeds, to serve
2 pinches of sumac*, to serve

* See Glossary

Preheat the oven to 375°F.

To make the squash hummus, arrange the squash in a single layer in an oiled roasting pan. Sprinkle with the ground cumin, salt, and pepper, and drizzle with the coconut oil. Mix with your hands to coat well, and roast until nicely colored, 20 minutes. Add the garlic cloves, then pour in ¾ cup water, cover with foil, and roast until the squash is very tender, 30 minutes more. Let cool. Combine the squash, garlic, and all the cooking juices in the bowl of a food processor, and process until smooth. Add the tahini, ginger, lemon juice, and olive oil, and whiz until smooth. Set aside.

To make the sweet and sour onions, melt the coconut oil or fat in a saucepan over low heat. Add the onion and a pinch of salt and cook, stirring frequently, until the onion softens but is still slightly crunchy, 5 minutes. Remove from the heat, stir in the raisins and vinegar, then cover and set aside to cool completely.

Using a mortar and pestle, crush the garlic with a pinch of salt. Add the pine nuts and crush to coarse crumbs. Mix through the lemon juice. Set aside.

Season the sardines with salt and pepper.

Heat a large nonstick frying pan over medium-high heat. Add the coconut oil or fat and swirl around the pan. Fry the sardines in batches for 30–40 seconds, then gently flip them over and fry until just cooked through, 30–40 seconds more.

To serve, smear 3 tablespoons of squash hummus on each serving plate and scatter with some sweet and sour onions. Top with 3–4 sardines, sprinkle with a generous teaspoon of crushed pine nuts, then finish with the mint, pomegranate seeds, and sumac.

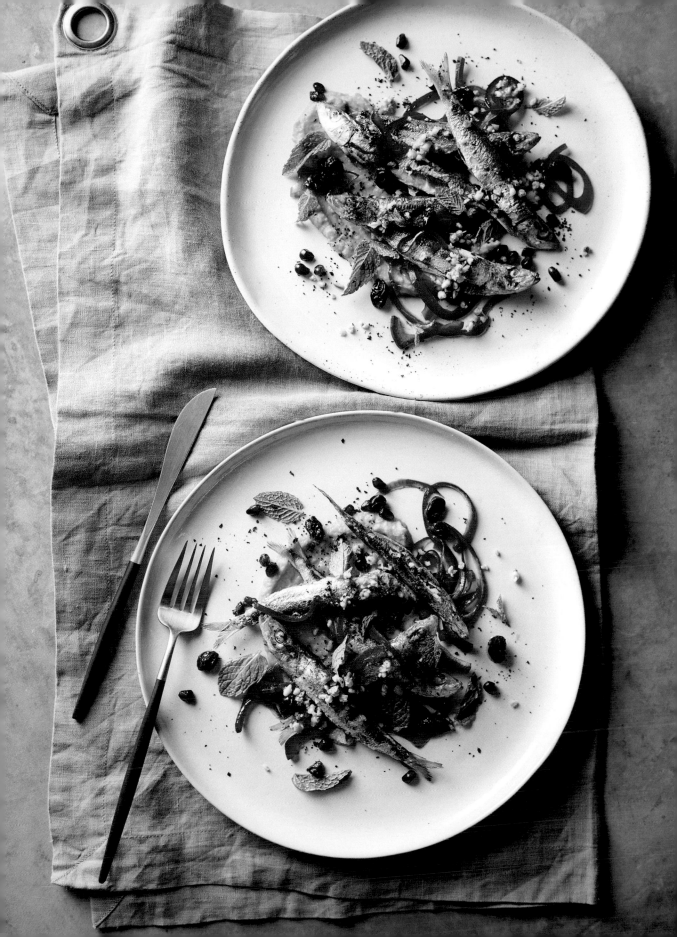

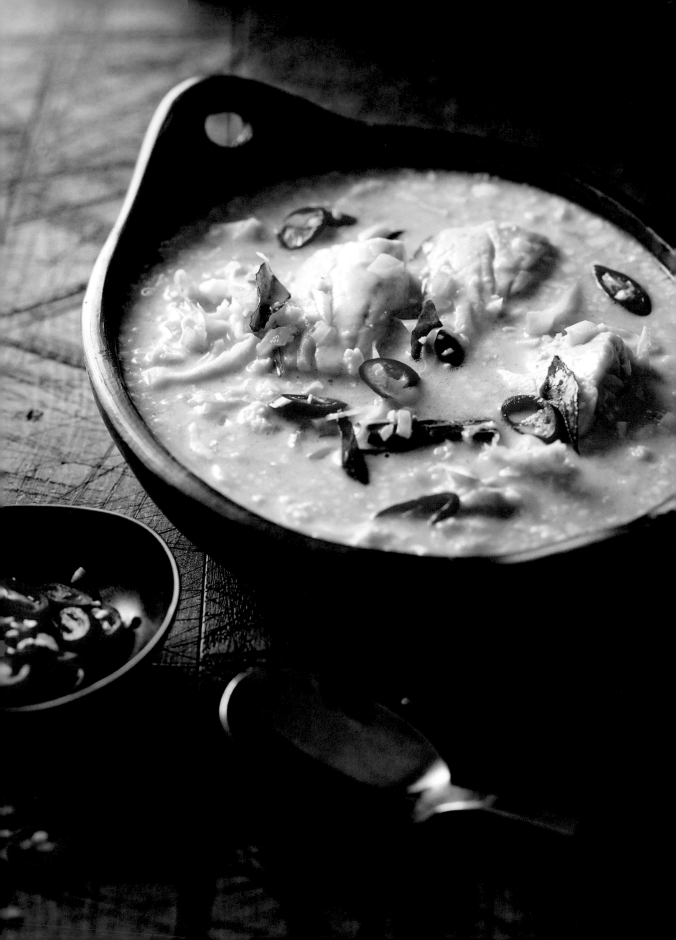

INDIAN FISH CURRY

SERVES 4-6

The tantalizing flavor and aroma of this curry come from the array of gently cooked spices that are synonymous with Indian cuisine and have been renowned for centuries the world over for their healing properties. I call it the one-two punch, as you are getting flavor and doing something wonderful for your body. Feel free to swap the fish for other seafood such as prawns, squid, mussels, or octopus, or even change it up with chicken, goat, lamb, or beef. Play around with different vegetables that are in season.

---

2 teaspoons ground turmeric

2 teaspoons ground coriander

¼ teaspoon ground cardamom

1 teaspoon ground cumin

½ head of cauliflower (about 14 ounces)
    broken into florets

1½ pounds snapper, Spanish mackerel,
    sea bass or bream (dorade), or
    black bass fillets, skin removed,
    cut into 1¼-inch pieces

¼ teaspoon sea salt

juice of 1 lemon

2 tablespoons coconut oil

1 onion, chopped

1 tablespoon finely grated ginger

3 garlic cloves, finely chopped

1 cinnamon stick

½ teaspoon red pepper flakes

12 fresh curry leaves

freshly ground black pepper

1 x 13.5-ounce can coconut cream

3 cups Fish Bone Broth
    (page 124)

1 long red chile, finely sliced (optional)

Mix the turmeric, coriander, cardamom, and cumin in a small bowl, and set aside.

Put the cauliflower in the bowl of a food processor and pulse into tiny, fine pieces that look like rice. Set aside.

Put the fish in a shallow bowl, season with the salt, and pour on half the lemon juice. Cover with plastic wrap and place in the refrigerator to marinate for 10 minutes.

Meanwhile, melt the coconut oil in a large frying pan over medium heat. Add the onion and sauté until softened, 5 minutes. Add the ginger and garlic and cook for 30 seconds, then stir in the spice mix, cinnamon, red pepper flakes, curry leaves, and a pinch of pepper, and cook until fragrant, 1 minute.

Pour the coconut cream and broth into the pan and bring to a simmer. Reduce the heat to low and cook until the flavors infuse, 10 minutes. Stir in the cauliflower, add the fish, and simmer until the fish is just cooked through, 8–10 minutes. To finish, season with salt, drizzle with the remaining lemon juice, and scatter the chile over (if using).

GRILLED FISH WITH SAUTÉED ONION AND BURNT LEMON

SERVES 4

Onions are one of the unsung heroes of the health world, as they provide the prebiotic inulin (a type of fiber) that gut flora convert to helpful short-chain fatty acids. Another wonderful thing about onions is that, when cooked slowly, they add a natural sweetness to dishes, which is why I love using them in my cooking. This simple dish is a lovely way to get dinner on the table quickly. Feel free to add a dollop of homemade mayo or aioli or some sliced avocado to enrich the dish.

2 tablespoons coconut oil or good-quality animal fat*, plus extra to rub
2 onions, sliced into rings
2 garlic cloves, finely chopped
½ bunch chives, snipped into ¾-inch lengths
sea salt and freshly ground black pepper
4 x 5-ounce snapper fillets (or any white-fleshed fish of your choice, such as tilapia, grouper, cod, mackerel), skin on
2 lemons, halved
extra-virgin olive oil, to serve
red pepper flakes, to serve

* See Glossary

MAKE AIP FRIENDLY

Omit: black pepper and chile
Substitute: fresh thyme or dill in place of chile

Melt the coconut oil or fat in a large frying pan over medium-high heat. Add the onions and cook, tossing frequently, until they start to caramelize, 8–10 minutes. Throw in the garlic and chives and sauté until the garlic is fragrant and just tender, 30 seconds. Season with salt and pepper.

Heat a grill pan or frying pan over high heat. Season the fish with salt and pepper and rub both sides with the extra coconut oil or fat. Place the fillets skin-side down in the pan, cover with foil, and cook until golden brown, about 3 minutes. Remove the foil, flip the fillets with a spatula, and cook until the fish is just cooked through, about 2–3 minutes. While the fish is cooking, add the lemon halves to the pan cut-side down and cook until nicely charred, 1½ minutes.

Arrange the fish on serving plates and add the sautéed onions. Drizzle with some olive oil, sprinkle with some red pepper flakes, then squeeze some burnt lemon juice over the top.

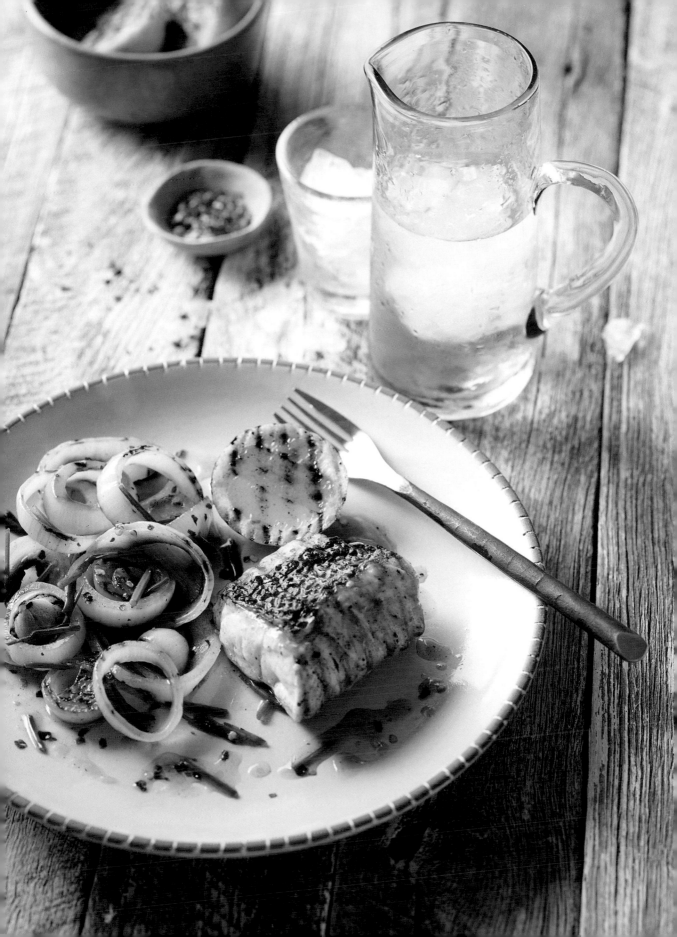

STEAMED SALMON
WITH NORI AND ASIAN GREENS

SERVES 4

We tend to steer clear of soy-based products, but from time to time I include small amounts of fermented organic soy in the form of miso paste and tamari, as I believe they have gut-healing properties. Here, we have a simple but very tasty miso broth with gently steamed seaweed-wrapped fish and veggies.

1 cup bonito flakes*, plus extra to serve
1 dried kombu seaweed* sheet, rinsed
3 tablespoons tamari or coconut aminos*
5 cups Fish or Chicken Bone Broth (pages 124 and 116)
1¼ nori seaweed* sheets
4 x 5-ounce salmon fillets, skin removed, pin-boned
1-inch piece of ginger, thinly sliced
1 tablespoon miso paste
1 bunch yau choy (choy sum) or other Asian greens (about ½ pound), trimmed and roughly chopped into large pieces
8 shiitake mushrooms, sliced
3 ounces shimeji mushrooms, trimmed
shiso leaves, to serve

* See Glossary

MAKE AIP FRIENDLY

Omit: tamari and miso
Substitute: coconut aminos in place of tamari, and a generous pinch of sea salt instead of miso paste

Combine the bonito flakes, kombu, tamari or coconut aminos, and fish or chicken bone broth in a large saucepan over medium-high heat. Bring to a boil, then take off the heat. Strain the broth into a clean saucepan.

Cut the nori into four 3 x 8–inch strips. Wrap a nori strip around each salmon fillet. Set aside.

Fill another saucepan with 1½ quarts (6 cups) of water, and add the ginger. Place a bamboo steamer over the pan and bring to a boil. Place the salmon in the steamer, cover, and cook until the fish is slightly pink in the center, 4–5 minutes.

Bring the broth back to a boil over medium heat. Stir in the miso, then add the yau choy and the shiitake and shimeji mushrooms and simmer until the vegetables are tender, 3–5 minutes.

Divide the vegetables among 4 serving bowls. Pour the broth over, then top with a piece of salmon. Finish with a scattering of shiso and extra bonito flakes, and serve.

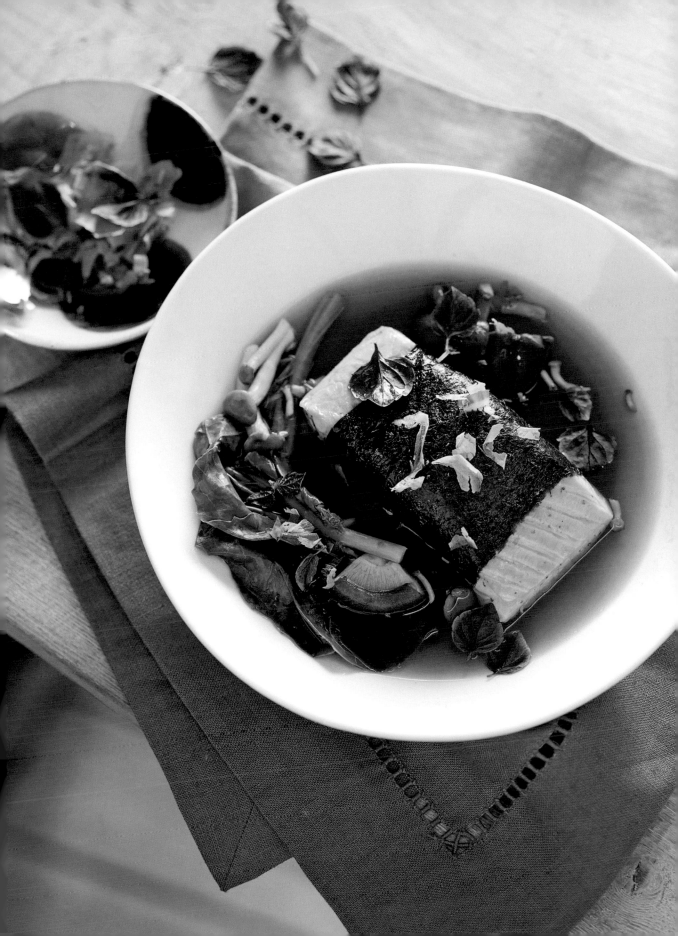

TIP

*Feel free to add some avocado, arugula
leaves, or zucchini noodles to the rémoulade.
You can also swap the salmon for another
type of fish or some meat.*

CRISPY-SKINNED SALMON
WITH CELERY ROOT RÉMOULADE

SERVES 4

Fish and salad is wonderfully healthy, but to many people doesn't seem like a meal that will leave you feeling satisfied. That is why I wanted to include this dish, as it is full of good fats – from the fish and the mayonnaise in the celery root – that truly satiate. Celery root is a wonderful vegetable to eat raw, and it's full of prebiotics. Serve with fermented veg or fold some through the rémoulade with the celery root. I guarantee this will become a new favorite recipe.

CELERY ROOT RÉMOULADE

1 celery root (about 470 g), peeled
¼ cup Mayonnaise in 30 Seconds
    (page 310)
1 tablespoon Fermented Mustard
    (page 309) or whole-grain mustard
1 tablespoon flat-leaf parsley leaves,
    chopped
1 tablespoon salted baby capers, rinsed well
    and patted dry, chopped
1 tablespoon chopped chervil
2 tablespoons snipped chives
1½ tablespoons lemon juice
sea salt and freshly ground black pepper

1 small handful chives, cut into batons
1 handful dill fronds
1 small handful mixed micro herbs
    (such as watercress, parsley, and
    red-vein sorrel) (optional)
extra-virgin olive oil
4 x 6-ounce salmon fillets, skin on,
    pin-boned
2 tablespoons coconut oil

> **MAKE** AIP FRIENDLY

Omit: mayonnaise, mustard, and black pepper
Substitute: apple cider vinegar and extra-virgin
olive oil in place of the mayonnaise and mustard

To make the rémoulade, cut the celery root into matchsticks using a mandoline. Celery root tends to discolor quickly, so place it in a bowl of cold water. Mix together the mayonnaise, mustard, parsley, capers, chervil, chives, and lemon juice in a bowl. Season to taste. Drain the celery root and pat dry with paper towel. Add the celery root to the mayo mixture, and mix well to combine. Taste and season again if necessary.

Mix together the chives, dill, and micro herbs (if using) in a small bowl, and drizzle with a little olive oil.

To score the salmon skin, make shallow slices about ¼ inch deep on the skin at intervals of about ½ inch. Sprinkle with a little bit of salt and pepper.

Melt half the coconut oil in a large nonstick frying pan over medium-high heat. Lightly brush the salmon skin with the remaining coconut oil to prevent any sticking. Place the salmon skin-side down in the pan, and very lightly press down for a few seconds. (Don't overcrowd the pan; you may need to cook the salmon in two batches.) Cook the salmon until it's a nice golden color, 2–3 minutes. Carefully slide a spatula under each salmon fillet to turn it over. Cook for 2–3 minutes more, or until the salmon is cooked to your liking.

To serve, divide the celery root among 4 serving plates. Add the salmon and some mixed herbs. Finish with a drizzle of olive oil.

SESAME-CRUSTED AVOCADO BOWL WITH CHICKEN AND SPROUTS

SERVES 2

Bowl food is becoming more and more popular, but, it is just a fancy way of serving a salad so it looks awesome. Here, I make the avocado look great by crusting it in sesame seeds and, to continue the theme, fill the cavity with a lovely tahini dressing. Then I simply add protein (chicken in this case, though tuna, prawns, and sardines would also work well), salad ingredients (you could also try cucumber, radish, cabbage, carrot, celery, green leaves, and seaweed) and some kraut.

TAHINI DRESSING
3 tablespoons hulled tahini*
3 tablespoons Coconut Yogurt
   (pages 86 and 88)
2 tablespoons lemon juice
1 garlic clove, finely chopped
sea salt

½ quantity of cooked Cauliflower Rice
   (page 307)
1 teaspoon finely chopped cilantro or
   flat-leaf parsley leaves
1 teaspoon extra-virgin olive oil
1 avocado, halved, pitted, and
   flesh scooped out intact
freshly ground black pepper
⅓ cup mixed white and black sesame seeds,
   toasted
1 cup leftover cooked chicken breast or
   thigh, shredded
loosely packed ¼ cup snow pea sprouts
⅓ cup alfalfa sprouts
2 teaspoons dried wakame seaweed*, soaked
   for 20 minutes in water, drained well
2 tablespoons (or to taste) fermented
   vegetables of your choice (see recipes,
   pages 94–111)

Put the cauliflower rice in a bowl, and stir in the chopped cilantro or parsley.

To make the tahini dressing, combine the tahini, coconut yogurt, lemon juice, and garlic in a small bowl, add 3 tablespoons water, and mix. Add a little salt to taste. Set aside.

Brush the olive oil on the avocado halves and season with salt and pepper. Coat the avocado halves with the sesame seeds.

Place the cauliflower rice in two serving bowls. Add a sesame-coated avocado half, cut-side up, then arrange the chicken, snow pea sprouts, alfalfa sprouts, wakame, and fermented veg on top. Spoon the dressing into the cavity of the avocado, drizzle with any remaining dressing as needed, and serve.

MAKE AIP FRIENDLY

Omit: black pepper, sesame seeds, and tahini dressing

Substitute: apple cider vinegar and extra-virgin olive oil dressing in place of the tahini dressing

TIP
Use broccoli rice in place of cauliflower rice if you prefer.

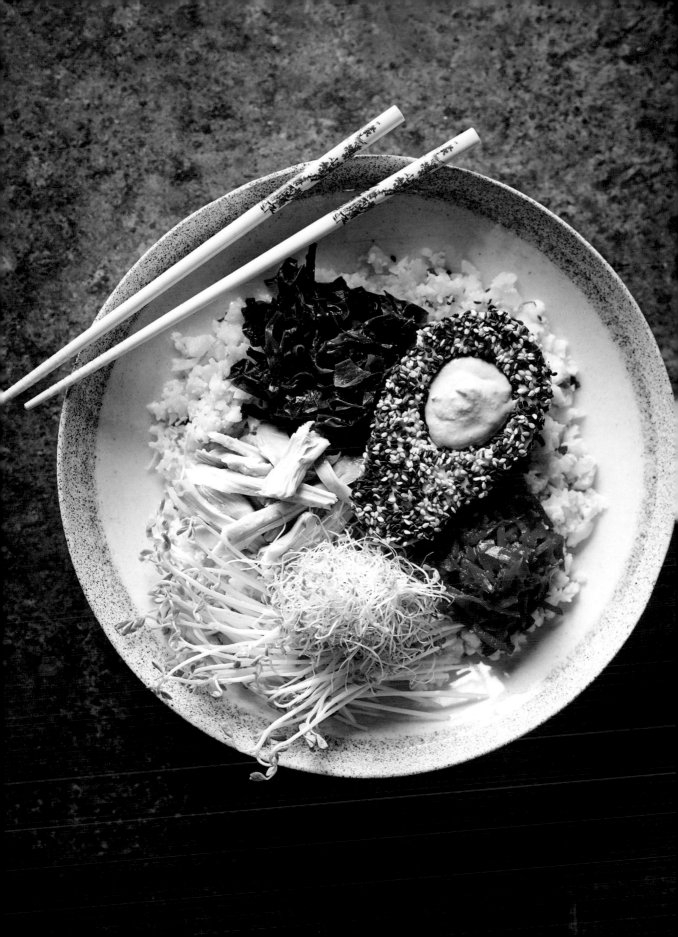

PORK-STUFFED BITTER MELONS WITH CHICKEN AND GINGER BONE BROTH

SERVES 4

I first discovered bitter melon about 15 years ago and was surprised that its powerful bitterness was quite addictive. It's also medicinal – traditionally being used as a natural remedy to help lower blood sugar levels for those with type 2 diabetes. This recipe is a great one to ease you into your bitter melon experience. Enjoy!

PORK STUFFING
1 pound ground pork
1½ ounces wood ear fungus* or shiitake
    mushrooms, chopped (optional)
3 teaspoons fish sauce
1 teaspoon freshly ground black pepper
1 shallot, finely chopped
2 garlic cloves, finely chopped
1 tablespoon chopped cilantro leaves
½ teaspoon sea salt

2 bitter melons*
2½ cups Chicken Bone Broth (page 116)
2-inch piece of ginger, thinly sliced
1 lemongrass stem, white part only,
    bruised with the back of a knife and
    roughly chopped
1 teaspoon fish sauce, or to taste
1 teaspoon lime juice
1 green onion, very thinly sliced on an angle

* See Glossary

MAKE AIP FRIENDLY

Omit: black pepper

To make the stuffing, combine the pork, fungus or mushrooms (if using), fish sauce, pepper, shallot, garlic, cilantro, and salt in a large bowl. Set aside until needed.

Fill a saucepan with water and bring to a boil. Add the bitter melons and blanch until they turn bright green, 1 minute. Remove from the pan and plunge straight into ice-cold water. When cool, cut the melons crosswise into 1-inch-thick slices. Using a tablespoon, scoop out the core and seeds.

Spoon 1½ tablespoons of the stuffing into the center of each bitter melon ring, pressing with your hands to firmly pack it in. Set aside.

Pour the broth into a large saucepan. Add the ginger, lemongrass, and fish sauce, and bring to a simmer over medium heat. Carefully add the stuffed bitter melon rings, cover, and cook until the filling is cooked through, 8 minutes.

Carefully place the stuffed bitter melon rings in a serving bowl. Stir the lime juice into the broth and add a little more fish sauce, if needed. Pour the broth over the bitter melon, scatter with the green onion, and serve.

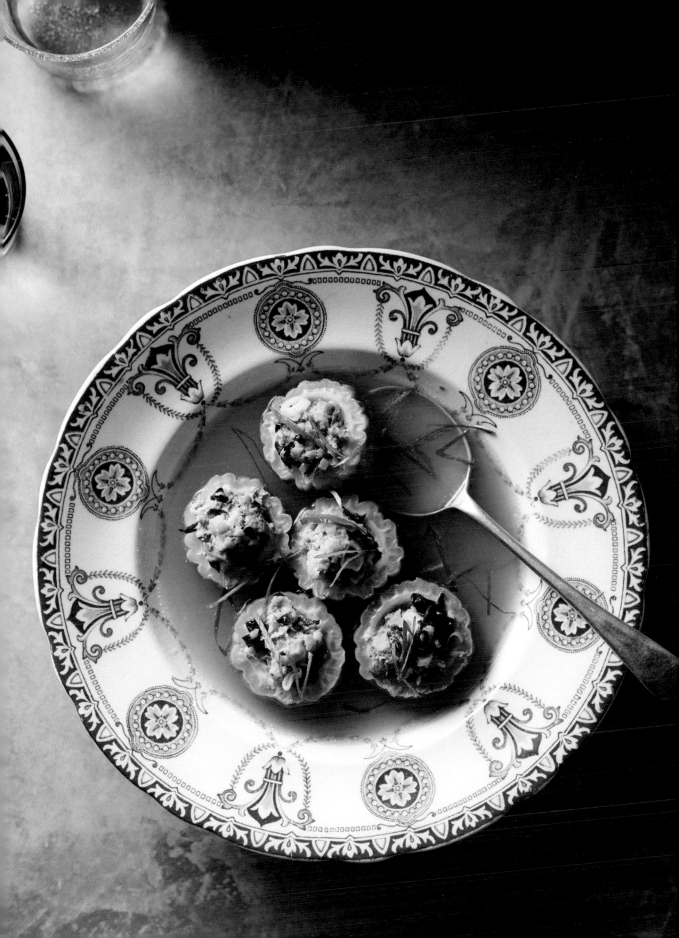

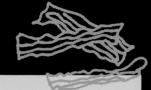

TIP

Make a big batch of this terrine, keep it in the fridge, and serve with seeded crackers and raw vegetables.

CHICKEN LIVER AND PORK TERRINE

SERVES 8

If you're not a fan of offal, I suggest you start with a classic like this delicious terrine – it will have even the staunchest offal-hater asking for more. So how can a terrine make offal taste so good? It all comes down to cooking the livers so they are still pink inside and retain their sweet and subtle taste. I urge you to give this a go for your next dinner party. It's perfect served with toasted seed and nut loaf, fermented vegetables, and the homemade condiments of your choice, such as mustard, pickles, and chutney.

---

3 tablespoons coconut oil or good-quality animal fat*

1 large onion, chopped

3 garlic cloves, chopped

1 teaspoon thyme leaves

½ cup organic dry red wine (such as Merlot)

1½ pounds chicken livers, trimmed of sinew and cut into ¾-inch pieces

14 ounces ground pork

1 tablespoon Dijon mustard

¼ cup Chicken Bone Broth (page 116)

3 egg yolks

pinch of freshly grated nutmeg

1½ teaspoons sea salt

2 teaspoons freshly ground black pepper

10–12 thin slices of prosciutto

* See Glossary

Preheat the oven to 275°F.

Melt the oil or fat in a frying pan over medium heat. Add the onion and cook until softened, 5 minutes. Add the garlic, thyme, and red wine, bring to a boil, and cook until reduced by half. Remove from the heat.

Combine the chicken livers, onion mixture, ground pork, mustard, broth, egg yolks, nutmeg, salt, and pepper in the bowl of a food processor, and blend until smooth and creamy.

Line a 2-quart terrine mold with 10 prosciutto slices, allowing enough overhang on the sides to enclose the top of the terrine. Tip the pork mixture into the mold. Smooth the top, then cover with the overhanging prosciutto. Add the remaining 2 slices of prosciutto if the top is not completely covered. Cover with a lid or some foil, and place the mold in a deep baking dish. Pour in enough boiling water to reach halfway up the sides of the mold. Bake until the terrine comes away from the sides of the mold, 2 hours. Remove the mold from the baking dish, and place in the refrigerator until set (about 5 hours).

Turn the terrine out onto a chopping board or platter, cut into thick slices, and serve. Stored in an airtight container, the terrine will keep in the fridge for 5 days, or in the freezer for 3 months.

TERRY WAHL'S CHICKEN LIVERS WITH ONION AND BACON

SERVES 2–4

This is without a doubt one of the yummiest and healthiest recipes in this whole book (well, they all are really, but I adore this one so much). Dr. Terry Wahls, author of *The Wahls Protocol*, cooked this dish with me in Texas recently, and paired it with her Rainbow Matchstick Salad on page 258. We were in gastronomic heaven. If you don't like liver, simply swap it for skin-on chicken thighs or a piece of steak.

---

1 pound chicken livers
2 tablespoons coconut oil or good-quality animal fat*
4 slices bacon, roughly chopped
1 onion, thinly sliced
1 tablespoon finely grated ginger
2 Swiss chard leaves, stems removed (save them for broths or soups), leaves torn
¼ cup Chicken or Beef Bone Broth (pages 116 and 121)
sea salt and freshly ground black pepper

* See Glossary

MAKE AIP FRIENDLY

Omit: black pepper

Rinse the chicken livers under cold water, pat dry with paper towels, and trim off any fat, sinew, and veins. Set aside.

Melt the oil or fat in a wok or large frying pan over medium heat. Add the bacon and onion and cook, stirring occasionally, until the onion is translucent and starting to caramelize, 8 minutes. Stir in the ginger and cook for 1 minute. Increase the heat to medium-high, add the chicken livers, and seal for 1 minute on each side until brown. Add the Swiss chard and broth and sauté until the Swiss chard is wilted and the livers are medium-rare, 1 minute more. Season with salt and pepper, and serve.

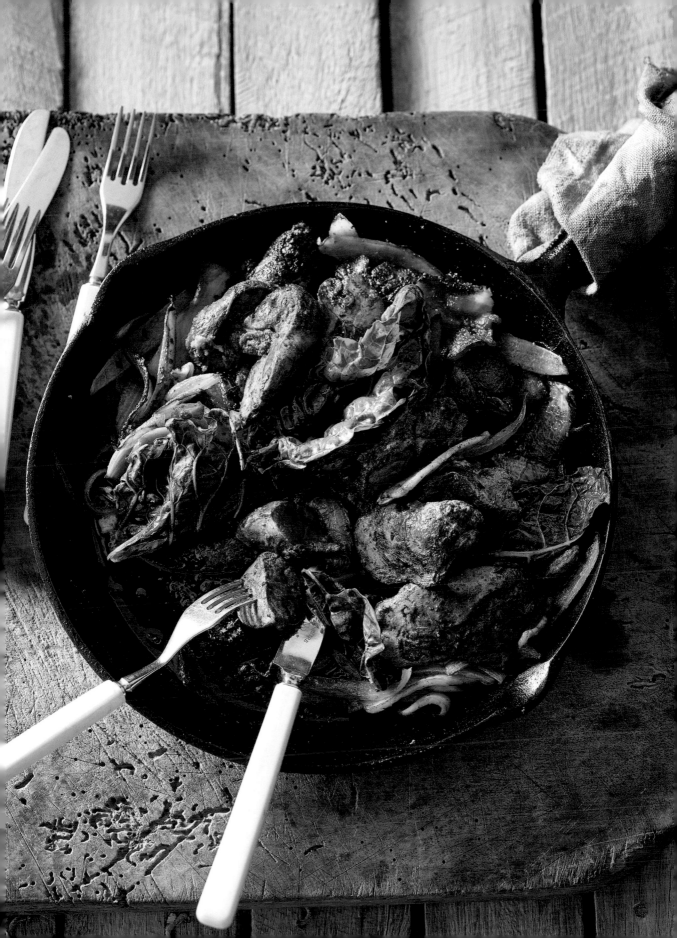

CHICKEN, LEEK, BACON, AND EGG "PIE"

SERVES 8

In the summer months, when it is 86 degrees outside, I love to eat gelatinous chicken bone broth straight from the fridge – which got me thinking about how I could turn that delicious chilled jelly into a meal to please the whole family. I came up with this wonderful take on the bacon and egg pie. This dish is a powerhouse on so many levels. Serve with a simple salad and some fermented cucumber (see recipe, page 111), and you are kicking goals.

---

2 pounds chicken feet
2 pounds chicken necks
1¾ pounds chicken winglets
1 tablespoon apple cider vinegar
1 onion, roughly chopped
1 celery rib, roughly chopped
6 garlic cloves, unpeeled
1 fresh or dried bay leaf
6 black peppercorns
sea salt and freshly ground black pepper
2 tablespoons coconut oil or good-quality
    animal fat*
1 leek, white part only, rinsed well,
    halved and sliced
4 slices bacon, chopped
1 boneless, skinless chicken breast or
    2 boneless, skinless thighs
3 large handfuls baby spinach leaves
2½ tablespoons powdered gelatin, soaked
    in ¼ cup water for 5 minutes
5 hard-cooked eggs, quartered

* See Glossary

MAKE AIP FRIENDLY

Omit: black peppercorns, black pepper, and eggs

Put the chicken pieces in a stockpot with 3½ quarts cold water, the vinegar, onion, celery, garlic, bay leaf, and peppercorns, and leave to stand for 30–60 minutes. Bring to a boil, skimming off the foam that forms on the surface. Reduce the heat to low and simmer for 12 hours, removing the chicken wings once tender, picking off and reserving the meat, then returning the bones to the stock. Season. Let cool slightly before straining through a fine sieve into a large saucepan (reserve the fat for cooking).

Heat 1 tablespoon of the oil or fat in a frying pan over medium heat. Add the leek and cook until softened, 6 minutes. Season with salt, remove from the pan, and set aside. Wipe the pan clean, place over medium heat, add the remaining oil and the bacon, and fry until golden, 5–6 minutes. Remove from the heat and set aside.

Bring the broth in the pan to a boil over high heat. Turn down the heat to medium, add the chicken breast or thigh, and simmer until the chicken is cooked through, 12 minutes. Remove the chicken from the broth and let cool. Add the spinach to the simmering broth and blanch for 3 seconds. Remove from the broth and let cool.

Remove the broth from the heat, let cool a little, and stir in the gelatin mixture. Mix until the gelatin is fully dissolved. Season to taste with salt and pepper.

Grease a 4 x 8-inch loaf pan with olive oil.

Cut the cooled chicken into pieces, and place in a bowl with the wing meat, spinach, leek and bacon. Season, then very gently fold the egg through. Place the mixture in the prepared pan and pour in enough gelatin broth to fill. Cover with plastic wrap and refrigerate until set, 6–10 hours.

Once the pie has set, carefully turn out onto a chopping board (see Tips). Cut into thick slices and serve.

TIPS

If you're having difficulty removing the pie from the pan, place the pan in hot water for a minute or two to loosen.

The remaining broth can be used for other recipes. Store in an airtight container in the refrigerator for up to 4 days, or in the freezer for up to 3 months.

Leftover pie will keep in the fridge for 4–5 days.

If you have any issues with eggs, then simply swap them for avocado.

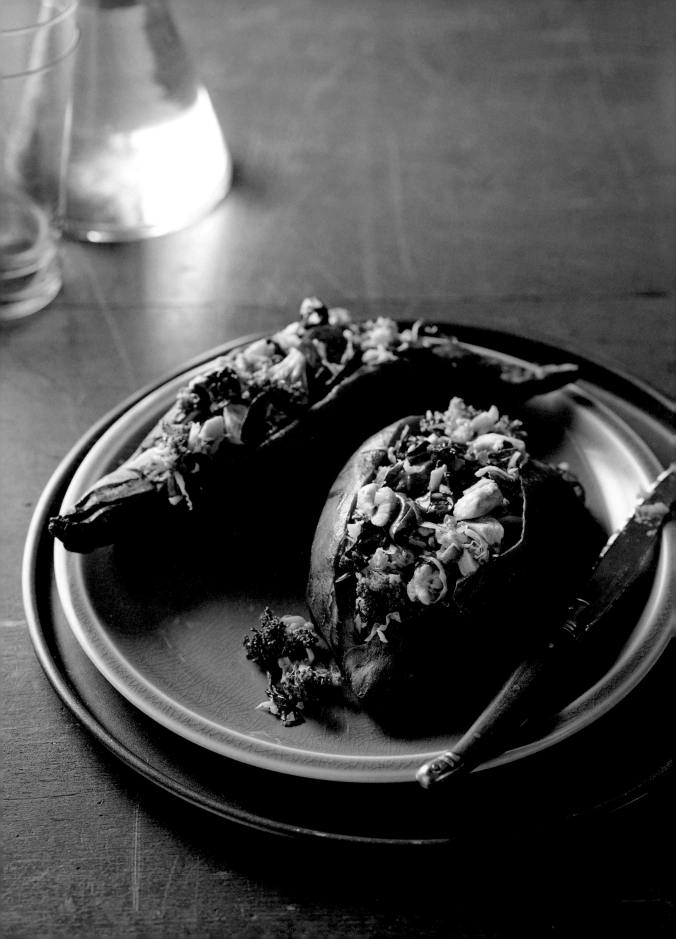

STUFFED SWEET POTATOES

SERVES 4

I fell in love with this recipe, created by Danielle Walker of Against All Grain, when filming *The Paleo Way* TV series at her house in San Francisco. You could also fill these beauties with anything from Mexican ground beef to leftover curry, or use small squashes instead of sweet potato. Serve with fermented veg on the side and a cup of broth.

---

2 tablespoons coconut oil
4 sweet potatoes (about 8 ounces each), scrubbed
1 teaspoon sea salt flakes
4 ounces bacon, chopped
2 boneless, skinless chicken breasts, diced
1 cup bite-sized broccoli florets
½ cup shredded Brussels sprouts
2 tablespoons Chicken Bone Broth (page 116)
2 packed cups baby spinach leaves
sea salt and freshly ground black pepper

MAKE AIP FRIENDLY

Omit: black pepper

Preheat the oven to 400°F and line a baking sheet with parchment paper.

Rub half the oil into the skin of the sweet potatoes and pat on the salt. Prick the sweet potatoes with a fork a few times, place on the prepared sheet, and roast until tender (about 40–50 minutes). Cut the sweet potatoes almost in half lengthwise, being careful not cut all the way through.

Heat the remaining oil in a large frying pan over medium-high heat. Add the bacon and sauté, stirring occasionally, until starting to crisp, 5 minutes. Add the chicken, broccoli, Brussels sprouts, and broth, and cook until the chicken is cooked through and the vegetables are softened, about 6 minutes. Stir in the spinach and cook for a further minute, then season with salt and pepper.

Slightly open up the cut center part of the sweet potatoes, spoon in the bacon and vegetable filling, and serve.

CAULIFLOWER FRIED RICE WITH SAUSAGE

SERVES 4

This is what I call a weeknight savior, as it can be whipped up in about ten minutes! These days it is pretty easy to find quality paleo sausages, made with good fat, good protein, and some seasoning – exactly how they used to be made in the old days. The whole family loves sausages and we eat them at least once a week. This is a great new and interesting way to use them – and it is full of veggies, too. Any leftovers make a perfect lunch for school or work the next day. Serve with some fermented veg on the side and a cup of broth.

1 head of cauliflower (about 2 pounds),
    separated into florets (discard the stalk
    or use it in another recipe)
¼ cup coconut oil
4 eggs, whisked
5 beef, chicken, or pork sausages
    (make sure they're free of black pepper
    if doing AIP – see below)
1 onion, finely chopped
½ red bell pepper, finely chopped
1 small red chile, seeded and finely chopped
1-inch piece of ginger, finely grated
2 garlic cloves, finely chopped
2 tablespoons tamari or coconut aminos*
2 green onions, thinly sliced
2 tablespoons chopped cilantro leaves,
    plus extra leaves to serve
sea salt and freshly ground white pepper
black and white sesame seeds, toasted,
    to serve
Sriracha Chile Sauce (page 313),
    to serve (optional)

* See Glossary

MAKE AIP FRIENDLY

Omit: eggs, bell pepper, chile, tamari, white pepper, sesame seeds, and chile sauce

Substitute: other vegetables (e.g., zucchini) in place of bell pepper, and coconut aminos instead of tamari

---

Put the cauliflower in the bowl of a food processor and pulse until it resembles grains of rice. Set aside.

Melt 1 tablespoon of the coconut oil in a wok or large frying pan over medium-high heat. Pour in the whisked egg and tilt the pan so they cover the base. Cook until the egg is set, 3 minutes. Remove, slice into thin strips, and set aside.

Wipe the wok or pan clean with paper towel, then melt 1 tablespoon of the remaining coconut oil over high heat. Add the sausages and cook until lightly golden and half cooked through, 5 minutes. Remove the sausages from the pan and, when cool enough to handle, cut into bite-sized pieces. Set aside.

Melt the remaining coconut oil in the wok or pan over medium-high heat. Add the onion, bell pepper, chile, ginger, and garlic, and stir-fry until softened, 5 minutes. Stir in the chopped sausage and cook until the sausage is almost cooked through, 3 minutes. Add the cauliflower and cook until tender, 2–3 minutes. Add the egg strips, tamari or coconut aminos, green onion, cilantro, and salt and white pepper, and stir-fry until everything is heated through and well combined, 2 minutes.

Spoon onto a platter and serve with the extra cilantro leaves, a sprinkling of sesame seeds, and the Sriracha chile sauce on the side (if using).

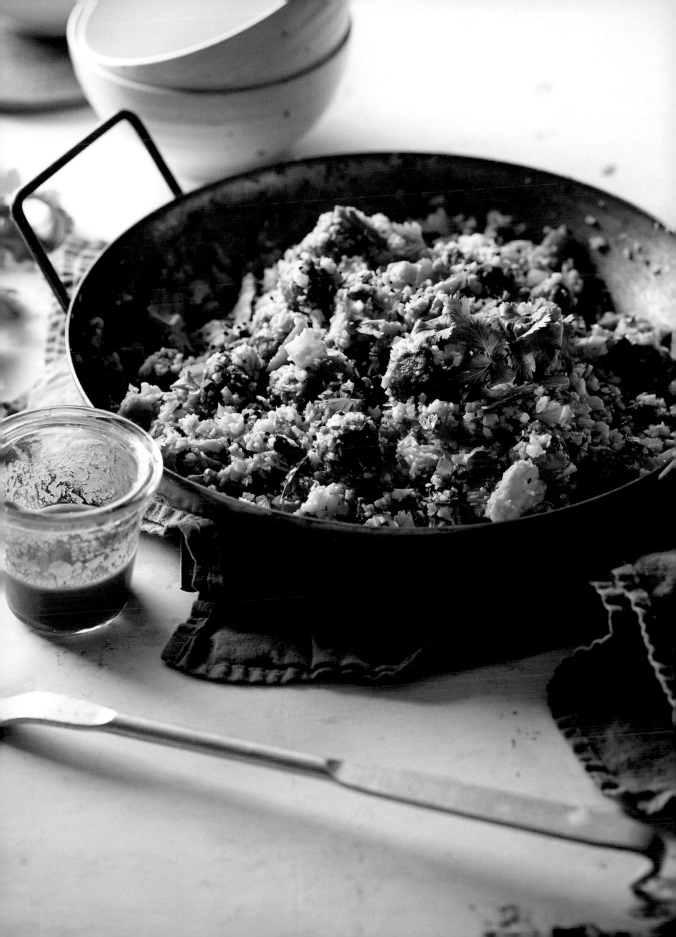

LEMONGRASS AND TURMERIC PORK CAKES WITH THAI HERB SALAD

SERVES 4

Ground meat has to be the easiest and cheapest way to add good-quality fat and protein to your diet. We often make mini meaty muffins with whatever ground protein we have on hand – pork, beef, lamb, chicken, or fish – and simply flavor them with whatever spices we are in the mood for. We then team them with some fermented veggies, as well as a salad or some cooked vegetables.

---

coconut oil or good-quality animal fat*,
   for greasing
1 teaspoon ground turmeric
3 garlic cloves, finely chopped
1 lemongrass stem, white part only,
   finely chopped
1 shallot, finely chopped
1 teaspoon finely grated ginger
3 teaspoons fish sauce
1 tablespoon chopped cilantro leaves
1 long red chile, seeded and finely chopped
   (optional)
3 tablespoons coconut cream
1 pound ground pork

ASIAN HERB SALAD
1 handful cilantro leaves
1 handful mint leaves
1 handful Thai basil leaves
1 red Asian shallot, thinly sliced
1 long red chile, seeded and finely sliced
3 tablespoons Nam Jim Dressing
   (page 312)

1 lime, halved, to serve
Fermented Hot Chile Sauce (page 308),
   to serve (optional)

* See Glossary

Omit: chile, chile sauce, and nam jim dressing

Preheat the oven to 350°F and lightly grease a 12-cup mini muffin pan with coconut oil or fat.

Combine the turmeric, garlic, lemongrass, shallot, ginger, fish sauce, cilantro, chile (if using), and coconut cream in the bowl of a food processor, and pulse a few times. Scrape down the sides of the bowl, add the ground pork, and process for 10 seconds to combine.

Spoon the pork mixture evenly into the prepared pan and bake until the pork cakes are cooked through, 8–10 minutes. Let cool slightly for 2 minutes. The pork cakes may release a little bit of liquid, so drain well before you turn them out of the pan.

To make the Asian herb salad, combine all the ingredients in a bowl and toss well.

Arrange the salad on a large platter or serving plates. Place the pork cakes on top and serve with the lime and fermented hot chile sauce (if using).

TIP

Double this recipe and make heaps, so the next day you can have pork cakes for breakfast, school or work lunches, or snacks.

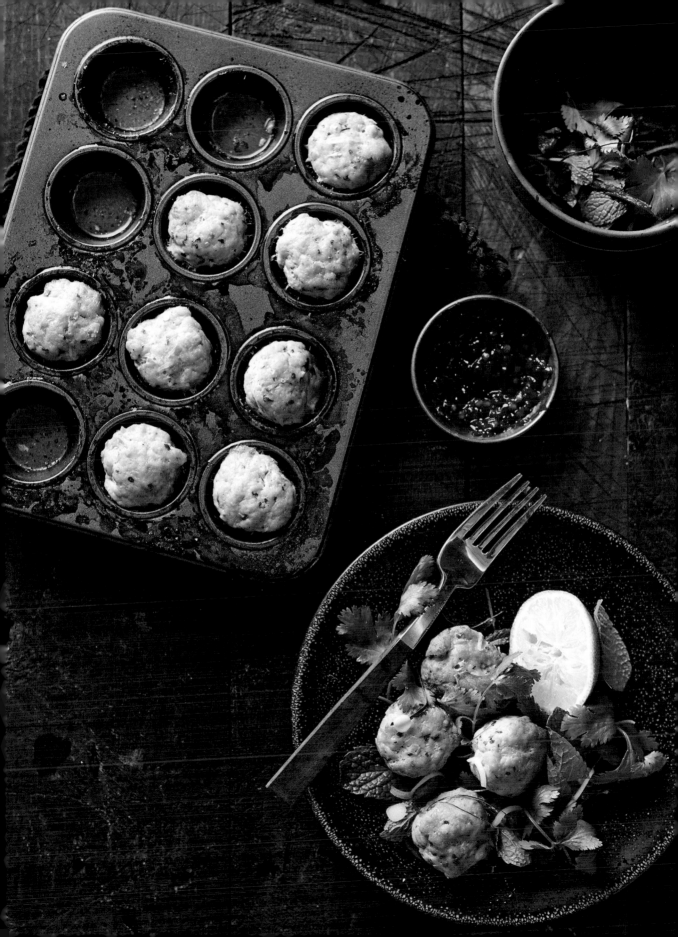

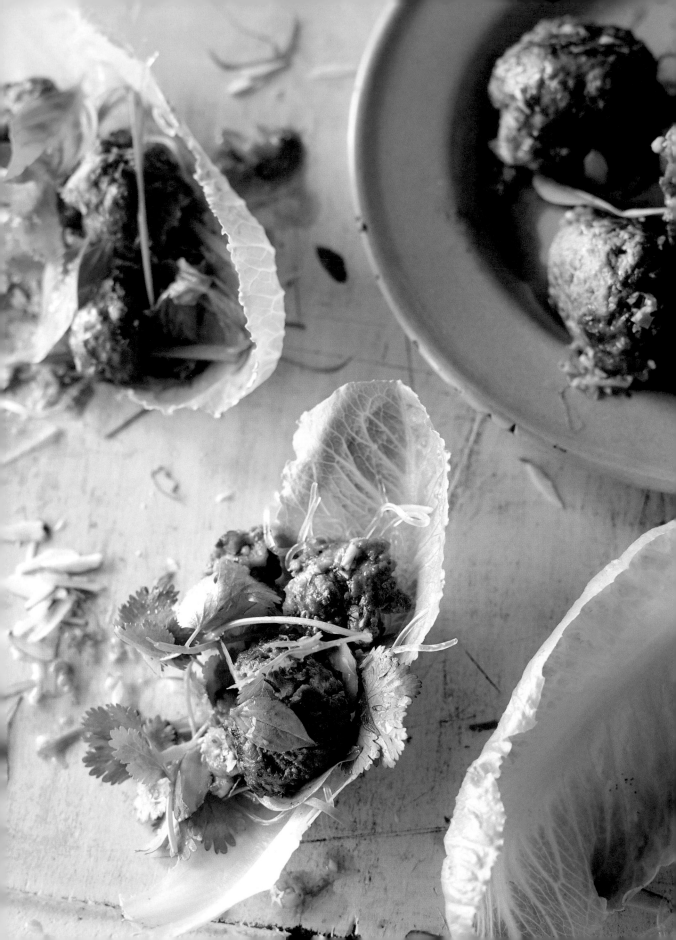

THAI MEATBALLS IN LETTUCE CUPS

SERVES 2–4

Let's face it, we all love putting food into lettuce or cabbage cups and popping them into our mouths. There is something so innocent and childlike when it comes to eating food with our hands that brings a smile to our faces. One night, my wife, Nic, and I made some Thai-flavored meatballs and wrapped them in cabbage leaves. We couldn't stop giggling as the sauce and juice dripped off our chins and down our hands and arms onto the plate. Break out the lettuce or cabbage cups, roll some meatballs and make a delicious dipping sauce, then push up your sleeves and eat with love and laughter.

---

7 ounces kelp noodles, roughly chopped

MEATBALLS
14 ounces ground pork
1½ tablespoons fish sauce
2 tablespoons green onions, finely chopped
1 tablespoon finely chopped lemongrass, white part only
2 tablespoons chopped cilantro leaves
2 tablespoons coconut oil

DRESSING
1 tablespoon finely grated ginger
1 tablespoon finely chopped cilantro roots and stalks
2 garlic cloves, finely chopped
1 tablespoon honey
2 tablespoons lime juice or apple cider vinegar
2 tablespoons tamari or coconut aminos*
1 lemongrass stem, white part only, sliced
1 teaspoon sesame oil
3 tablespoons extra-virgin olive oil

SALAD
3 green onions, thinly sliced on the diagonal
1 small handful Thai basil leaves
1 small handful mint leaves
1 carrot, cut into thin strips
1 kaffir lime leaf, thinly sliced
1 small handful cilantro leaves
2 tablespoons chopped almonds (activated if possible*)

8 baby romaine lettuce leaves

* See Glossary

Soak the kelp noodles in a bowl of warm water for 20–30 minutes until softened. Drain and set aside. Preheat the oven to 400°F.

To make the meatballs, combine the pork, fish sauce, chile (if using – see Tip), green onions, lemongrass, and cilantro in a bowl, then mix well. Roll 1 tablespoon of the pork mixture between the palms of your hands to form a 1¼-inch ball and set aside. Repeat until you've used all the pork mixture.

Melt the oil or fat in a large frying pan over medium heat. Cook the meatballs in batches until golden brown, 2–3 minutes. Transfer to a roasting pan and roast until the meatballs are cooked through, 5–10 minutes.

To make the dressing, combine the ingredients in a bowl and mix well.

Place the noodles and all the salad ingredients in a bowl. Pour on the dressing and gently toss to combine.

Arrange the salad in the romaine lettuce cups, top with the meatballs, and serve.

MAKE AIP FRIENDLY

Omit: almonds, honey, tamari, sesame oil, and chile
Substitute: 4 teaspoons freshly squeezed orange juice in place of honey, and coconut aminos instead of tamari

TIP
Add a seeded, finely chopped small red chile to the meatballs and a thinly sliced bird's eye chile to the dressing if you like it hot.

SAUSAGES WITH ONION GRAVY

SERVES 4

There is very little that needs to be said about this dish except that it is bloody good for you! Good fats, good protein, fresh salad with some fermented veg on the side, and a sauce made from bone broth ticks every single box in the paleo handbook. To make it even more exciting, you could add a fried egg, some blood pudding, a few chicken livers or slices of beef liver or lamb kidney to the pan, or roast some bone marrow or mushrooms and add to the gravy.

3⅓ cups Beef Bone Broth (page 121)
2 tablespoons coconut oil or good-quality
   animal fat*
8 pork or beef sausages (make sure
   they're free of black pepper if doing
   AIP – see below)
2 large onions, sliced
1 tablespoon tapioca flour*
5 thyme sprigs, leaves picked
1 tablespoon Worcestershire Sauce
   (page 315)
sea salt and freshly ground black pepper

SALAD

4 ounces cherry tomatoes
4 ounces yellow pear tomatoes
2 handfuls arugula leaves
1½ tablespoons extra-virgin olive oil
1½ teaspoons apple cider vinegar

Sauerkraut (page 94), to serve

* See Glossary

MAKE AIP FRIENDLY

Omit: tapioca flour, worcestershire sauce, cherry tomatoes, and black pepper

Substitute: to make a rich gravy, simply double the quantity of onions above and cook as per the recipe, then blend half the amount of the caramelized onion with the stock

---

Pour the broth into a saucepan, bring to a boil, and simmer until reduced by half, 10 minutes. Remove from the heat and set aside until needed.

Heat the oil or fat in a large frying pan over medium heat. Add the sausages and cook until browned on all sides and almost cooked through, about 8 minutes. Remove the sausages from the pan and set aside.

Add the onions to the same pan and cook over medium heat until softened and starting to caramelize, 5 minutes. Add the tapioca flour, stirring constantly for 1 minute, then add the thyme. Gradually pour in the broth and Worcestershire sauce, stirring constantly. Bring to a boil and simmer until the sauce is thickened, 5 minutes. Season with salt and pepper. Return the sausages to the pan and cook until they are completely cooked through, 2 minutes.

To make the salad, combine the salad ingredients in a bowl and gently toss. Season with salt and pepper.

Place two sausages on each serving plate, spoon the onion gravy over, and serve with the salad and a spoonful of sauerkraut on the side.

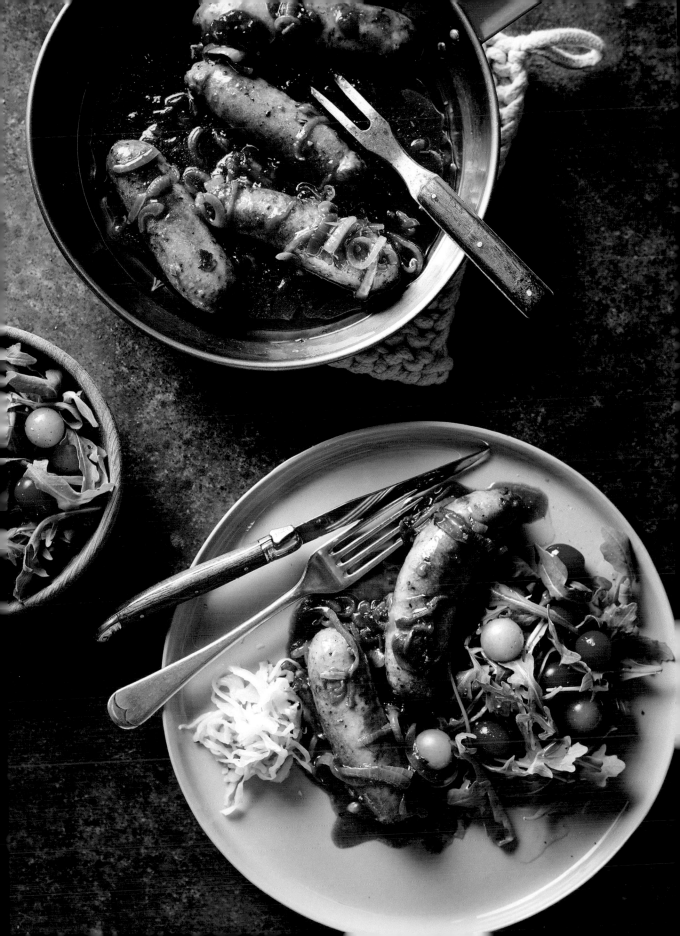

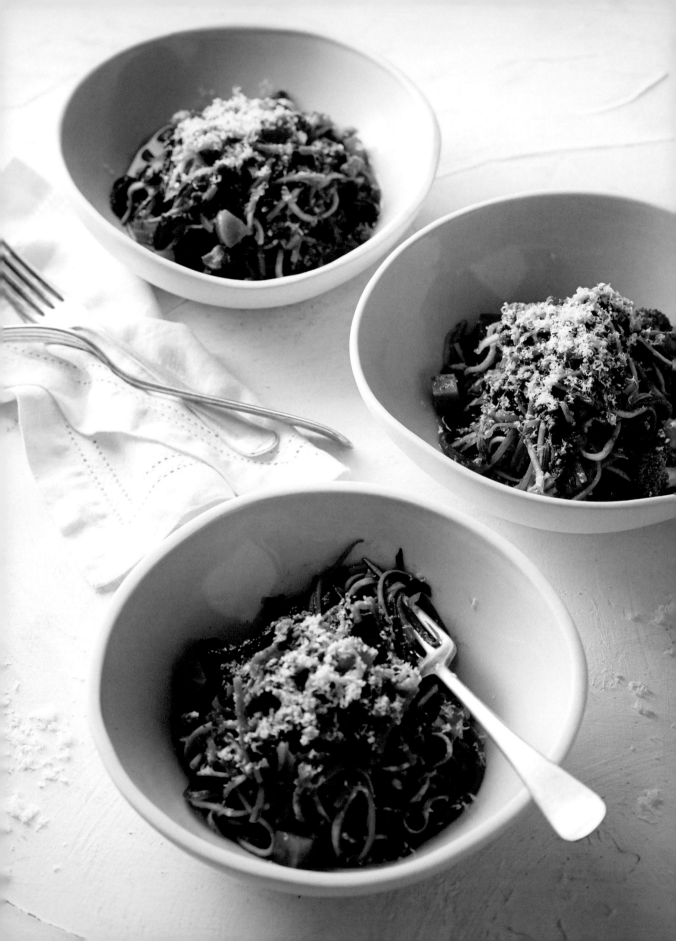

"SPAGHETTI" BOLOGNESE

SERVES 4

Replacing spaghetti with zucchini, carrot, and parsnip noodles has elevated this classic dish to new heights. Pasta can cause bloating and may potentially lead to inflammation of the gut, which makes these veggie noodles a healthier and more sensible choice for the whole family.

BOLOGNESE

2 tablespoons coconut oil or
    good-quality animal fat*
1 onion, chopped
1 carrot, diced
1 celery rib, finely diced
4 garlic cloves, finely chopped
1¼ pounds ground beef
1 teaspoon chopped oregano leaves
¾ cup organic dry red wine
    (such as Syrah; optional)
2 tablespoons tomato paste
2 cups canned tomatoes
1¼ cups Chicken Bone Broth (page 116)
1 pinch red pepper flakes (optional)
1 teaspoon chopped thyme
sea salt and freshly ground black pepper

2 carrots, ends trimmed, spiralized into
    thin noodles
2 parsnips, peeled and ends trimmed,
    spiralized into thin noodles
2 zucchini (about 14 ounces), ends
    trimmed, spiralized into thin noodles
2 tablespoons chopped flat-leaf parsley leaves
2 macadamia nuts (activated if possible*),
    finely grated

* See Glossary

MAKE AIP FRIENDLY

Omit: wine, tomato paste, canned tomatoes,
chile, and black pepper
Substitute: nomato sauce (omit black pepper)
(page 312) in place of omitted ingredients

To make the Bolognese, heat the oil or fat in a large frying pan over medium-high heat. Add the onion, carrot, and celery, and cook until softened, 4–5 minutes. Add the garlic and cook until fragrant and starting to brown, 1 minute. Stir in the ground beef and brown for 5–6 minutes, breaking up the lumps with a wooden spoon. Stir in the oregano and wine (if using) and cook until the wine has almost evaporated, 4–5 minutes. Stir in the tomato paste and cook for 1 minute. Add the tomatoes, chicken broth, red pepper flakes (if using), and thyme, and season with salt and pepper. Reduce the heat to low and simmer, stirring occasionally, until the meat is cooked through, 30 minutes.

Add the carrot and parsnip noodles to the Bolognese and cook for 1 minute. Add the zucchini noodles and parsley, toss to combine, and cook for another minute or so until the noodles are cooked through.

Spoon the Bolognese and noodles into 4 warm serving bowls, then sprinkle the grated macadamias on top.

TIPS

I love my spiralizer and always use it when making this dish. Spiralizers are inexpensive, simple to use and clean, and small enough to be stored easily.

I like to add offal to my Bolognese, burgers, and meatballs to make them even more nutritious (usually about 10 percent offal of the total meat quantity – in this recipe it would be about 2 ounces offal and 18 ounces ground beef). Try using ground liver, heart, marrow, or brain.

THE PALEO MOM'S BURGERS

SERVES 4–6

Recently, I was fortunate enough to spend the day with the amazing Sarah Ballantyne (also known as The Paleo Mom) filming some of her most famous recipes. This one is sure to be a big hit for kids of all ages. If you are concerned about how your kids will react to the flavor from the offal, simply reduce the amount and increase the ground beef. For adults, I suggest sticking to this recipe, as we all need to celebrate offal more. Serve with some fermented veg and maybe a cup of broth on the side.

---

14 ounces chicken, lamb, or beef liver, trimmed
14 ounces ground beef
14 ounces bacon, finely chopped
sea salt and freshly ground black pepper
2 tablespoons coconut oil or good-quality animal fat*
1 red onion, sliced into rings
8 slices of tomato
4 pickles, sliced
Beet Kraut with Wattleseeds (page 99)
8 butter lettuce leaves
Tomato Ketchup (page 313)
Fermented Mustard (page 309)

* See Glossary

MAKE AIP FRIENDLY

Omit: black pepper, tomato, tomato ketchup, and mustard

Substitute: nomato sauce (omit black pepper) (page 312) in place of tomato ketchup

Rinse the liver under cold water, place on paper towels, and pat dry to remove any excess moisture. Finely chop with a sharp knife.

Put the chopped liver in the bowl of a food processor. Add the ground beef and bacon and blitz for 15 seconds to combine. Alternatively, combine the ingredients in a bowl and mix with your hands (moisten them or wear gloves). Season with salt and pepper and shape into 8 patties.

Melt the coconut oil or fat in a large frying pan over medium-high heat. Add the patties in batches and cook for 3 minutes. Turn the patties over and continue to cook for a couple of minutes until they are cooked through. Remove from the pan and drain on paper towel.

Place the patties on a serving platter in the center of the table. Arrange the onion, tomato, pickles, kraut, lettuce leaves, ketchup, and mustard in bowls, and let everyone build his or her own burger.

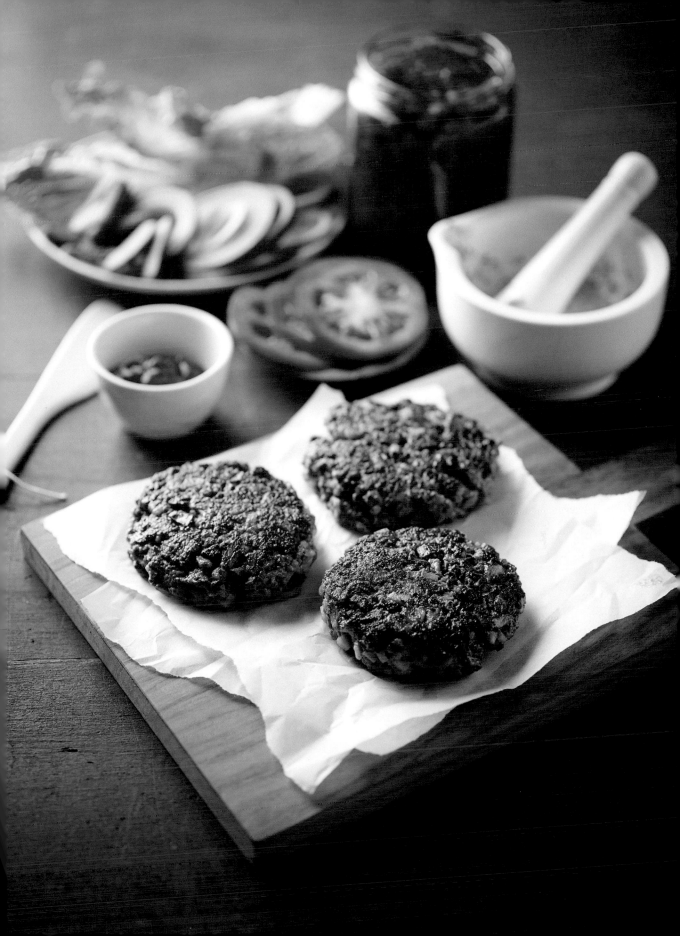

SPICED SIRLOIN WITH WILTED SWISS CHARD AND ALMOND AND BACON VINAIGRETTE

SERVES 4

If you can, choose grass-fed over grain-fed meat and eat only a palm-sized portion of animal protein per meal. For those with inflammation or trying to lose weight, an excess of protein turns to sugar in the body, so eat moderate amounts teamed with beautiful above-ground vegetables, good-quality fats, and, of course, include some fermented veg and bone broth on the side for good gut health.

SPICE MIX

2 teaspoons sea salt
2 teaspoons garlic powder
2½ tablespoons sweet paprika
1 teaspoon freshly ground black pepper
1 teaspoon onion powder
2 teaspoons dried oregano
2 teaspoons dried thyme

ALMOND AND BACON VINAIGRETTE

1 tablespoon coconut oil or good-quality animal fat*
1 shallot, finely chopped
4 ounces bacon, finely diced
1 cup almonds (activated if possible*), chopped
3 tablespoons apple cider vinegar
1 tablespoon Dijon mustard
½ cup extra-virgin olive oil

4 x 8-ounce sirloin steaks
¼ cup coconut oil or good-quality animal fat*
3 garlic cloves, finely chopped
10 ounces Swiss chard, stems removed (save for broths or soups), leaves torn

* See Glossary

MAKE AIP FRIENDLY

Omit: sweet paprika, black pepper, almonds, and Dijon mustard

---

To make the spice mix, combine all the ingredients in a bowl and mix until evenly blended.

To make the almond and bacon vinaigrette, heat half the coconut oil or fat in a small saucepan over low heat. Add the shallot and gently cook until softened, about 5 minutes. Remove from the pan and set aside. Wipe the pan dry with paper towels and place over medium heat. Add the remaining coconut oil or fat and the bacon and fry, stirring occasionally, until the bacon just starts to color, 6 minutes. Stir in the almonds and cook, stirring occasionally, until lightly golden, 2 minutes more. Add the vinegar and shallot and set aside to cool. Transfer to a bowl and whisk in the mustard and olive oil, and season with salt and pepper.

Lightly brush the steaks with 1 tablespoon of the coconut oil or fat, and then coat with 2 tablespoons of the spice mix.

Heat 1 tablespoon of coconut oil or fat in a large frying pan over high heat. Add the steaks, two at a time, and cook on one side for 2 minutes until browned. Turn over and cook for another 2 minutes (for medium-rare). Remove from the heat, place on a plate, cover loosely with foil, and allow to rest for 4 minutes. Repeat the process with the remaining steaks.

Wipe the pan clean with paper towel and place over medium heat. Add the remaining 2 tablespoons oil or fat and the garlic and cook until the garlic is softened and fragrant, 20 seconds. Toss through the Swiss chard and sauté for 1 minute. Add 3 tablespoons water and continue to cook, stirring occasionally, until the Swiss chard is slightly wilted, 3 minutes. Season with salt and pepper.

To serve, divide the Swiss chard among 4 warm serving plates, place a steak on each plate, then top with some almond and bacon vinaigrette.

TIP

You can store the leftover spice mix in an airtight container in the pantry for a few months.

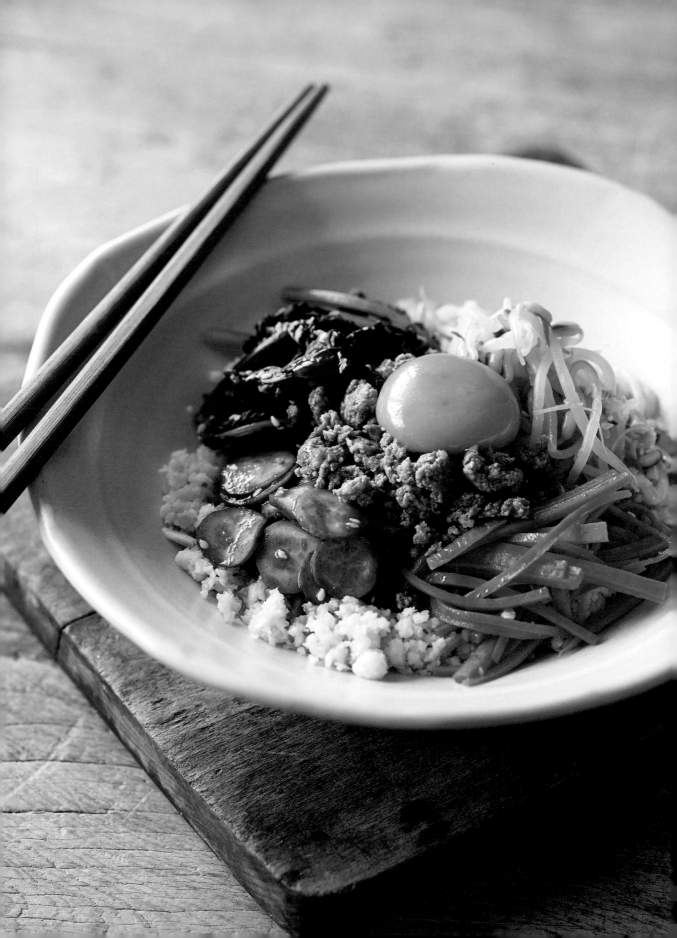

BIBIMBAP

SERVES 4

The Koreans really know about flavor and the importance of fermented vegetables. Here is one of their most-loved dishes that deserves to be part of everybody's cooking repertoire. The simple preparation means you can involve the whole family. Put the individual parts on the table for everyone to help themselves – I find the kids love to make their own – or you can, as we have done in the photo, plate it up. I put a kraut on the table for the kids, rather than a spicy kimchi. I am sure this will become a family favorite, once you give it a go.

SEASONED BEAN SPROUTS

7 ounces bean sprouts
1 teaspoon sea salt
1 teaspoon sesame oil

SEASONED CARROT

1 teaspoon coconut oil
1 large carrot, cut into matchsticks
¼ teaspoon sea salt, or more to taste
1 teaspoon sesame oil

SEASONED CUCUMBER

4 baby cucumbers, sliced
½ teaspoon sea salt
1 teaspoon Sriracha Chile Sauce (page 313)
pinch of sesame seeds, toasted

SEASONED SPINACH

14 ounces English spinach or baby spinach
1 teaspoon sesame seeds, toasted
1 teaspoon sesame oil
½ teaspoon sea salt

SEASONED BEEF

1⅓ pounds ground beef
4 garlic cloves, finely chopped
2 tablespoons tamari or coconut aminos
2 teaspoons honey
2 teaspoons coconut oil, melted
1 teaspoon sesame oil

2½ cups cooked Cauliflower Rice (page 307)
4 egg yolks
1¼ cups Classic Kimchi (page 108)
Sriracha Chile Sauce (page 313) (optional)

To make the seasoned bean sprouts, combine ½ cup water with the bean sprouts and salt in a saucepan, and bring to a boil. Reduce the heat to low, cover, and simmer for 5 minutes. Drain and transfer the sprouts to a bowl. Mix with the sesame oil, then set aside.

To make the seasoned carrot, melt the coconut oil in a frying pan over medium heat. Add the carrot and salt and stir-fry until just tender, 30 seconds. Drizzle with the sesame oil, transfer to a bowl, and set aside.

To make the seasoned cucumber, combine the cucumber and salt in a bowl, toss well, and set aside for 5 minutes. Gently squeeze the cucumber with your hands to remove any excess liquid. Transfer to another bowl, mix through the Sriracha and sesame seeds, and set aside.

To make the seasoned spinach, fill a large saucepan with water and bring to a boil. Add the spinach and cook for 1 minute. Drain the spinach and rinse with cold water. Then, taking a handful of spinach at a time, gently squeeze out the water. Place the spinach on a chopping board and chop into 2-inch pieces. Transfer to a bowl and add the sesame seeds, sesame oil, and salt. Mix well.

To make the seasoned beef, combine the ground beef, garlic, tamari or coconut aminos, and honey in a bowl and mix well. Set aside to marinate for 15 minutes. Melt the coconut oil in a wok or large saucepan over medium-high heat. Add the beef and marinade and stir-fry until cooked through, 5–6 minutes. Transfer to a bowl and top with the sesame oil.

Divide the cauliflower rice among four serving bowls, top with the seasoned salads, the beef, and an egg yolk. Place the kimchi and Sriracha (if using) in small serving bowls, and serve on the side.

SIRLOIN WITH ROASTED BONE MARROW AND PARSLEY SALAD

SERVES 4

People often ask me what foods are my guilty pleasures. And on thinking about what I like to indulge in, I can't go past bone marrow. The lusciousness of all that tasty fat when roasted with some quality salt and pepper is very, very hard to beat. Team with a simply grilled steak, a parsley salad, and some fermented vegetables, and, yes, you too will be indulging.

PICKLED ONION
½ red onion, sliced
¼ cup red wine vinegar

RED WINE JUS
2 tablespoons coconut oil or good-quality
   animal fat*, melted
4 ounces shallots, sliced
1 garlic clove, lightly crushed
4 thyme sprigs
3 tablespoons balsamic vinegar
1⅔ cup dry red wine (such as Syrah)
3⅓ cups Beef Bone Broth (page 121)
sea salt and freshly ground black pepper

2 x 5-inch pieces of beef bone marrow, halved
   lengthwise (ask your butcher to do this)
4 x 8-ounce sirloin steaks
2 tablespoons coconut oil or good-quality
   animal fat*, melted

PARSLEY SALAD
2 handfuls flat-leaf parsley leaves
1 tablespoon salted baby capers, rinsed
   and patted dry
1 green onion, green part only, thinly sliced
15 hazelnuts (activated if possible*),
   toasted and chopped
1½ teaspoons hazelnut oil or extra-virgin olive oil

* See Glossary

| MAKE AIP FRIENDLY |

Omit: black pepper, red wine, capers, and hazelnuts
Substitute: olive oil in place of hazelnut oil

To make the pickled onion, combine the onion and vinegar in a small saucepan and bring to a boil over medium-high heat. Remove from the heat and set aside to pickle for at least 1 hour (for best results, refrigerate overnight). Drain, reserving the vinegar for the parsley salad.

To make the jus, melt 1 tablespoon of the coconut oil or fat in a saucepan over medium-high heat. Add the shallot and sauté, stirring occasionally, until lightly caramelized, 5 minutes. Add the garlic and thyme and continue to cook for 3 minutes. Pour in the balsamic vinegar and reduce to a thick syrup. Stir in the wine, bring to a boil, and reduce by two-thirds. Pour in the broth and bring to a boil. Turn the heat down to medium and simmer until the jus is reduced by two-thirds to a sauce consistency. Add salt and pepper to taste. Keep warm.

Preheat the oven to 400°F.

Season the bone marrow with salt and pepper, place on a baking sheet, and roast for 15 minutes until brown.

Meanwhile, coat the steaks with the coconut oil or fat and season with salt and pepper. Heat a grill pan over high heat and cook the steaks on one side until browned, 2–3 minutes, then flip and cook for 2–3 minutes more (for medium-rare), or to your liking. Transfer to a plate, cover with foil, and leave to rest for 4–6 minutes. Reheat the grill pan over high heat, add the steaks, and cook for 30 seconds on each side. Set aside to rest in a warm place for 2 minutes, then thickly slice.

To make the salad, combine all the ingredients in a bowl. Add the pickled onion and 1½ teaspoons of the reserved pickling vinegar, and toss well. Season with salt and pepper.

To serve, place the steak and bone marrow on serving plates with a handful of parsley salad, and pour the jus over the steak.

TIPS

Serve a cup of bone broth on the side to up
the ante. Chicken Bone Broth (page 116)
also works well for the red wine jus.

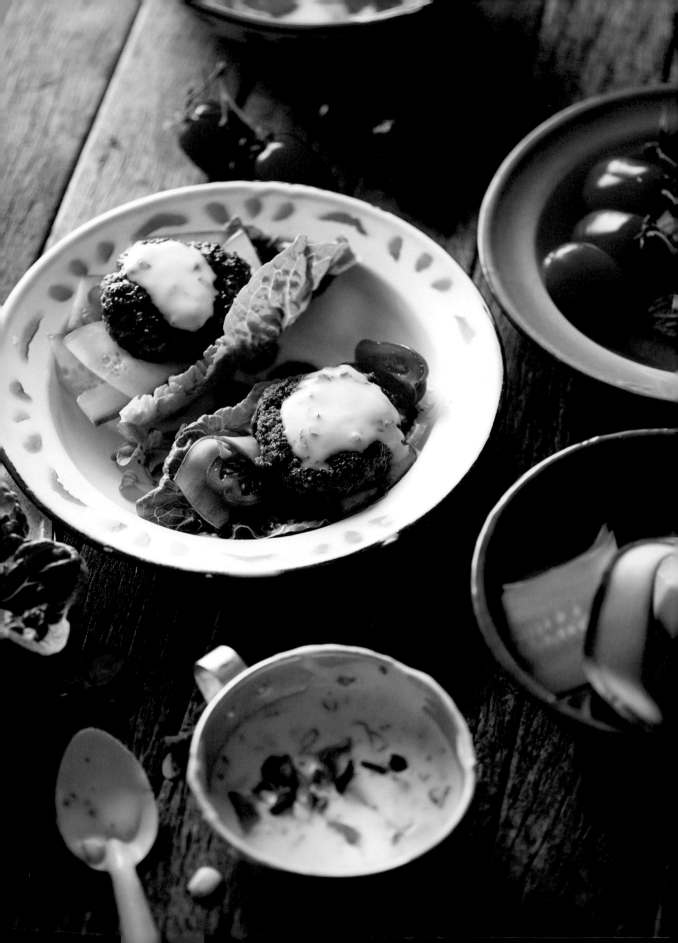

TURKISH LAMB BURGER WITH LETTUCE WRAPS

SERVES 4

These delicious burgers can be whipped up super quick and make a perfect breakfast, lunch, or dinner. Of course, feel free to swap the ground lamb for chicken, fish, beef, or pork, and to play with the spices, too. Serve with fermented veg, and you are well on your way to great gut health.

---

2 tablespoons coconut oil or
    good-quality animal fat*
1 onion, finely chopped
2 garlic cloves, finely chopped
1 pound medium-coarse ground lamb
5 ounces lamb or beef fat, ground
    (ask your butcher to do this)
1 tablespoon tomato paste
2 tablespoons Turkish Spice Mix
    (page 313)
1 teaspoon sea salt

TO SERVE

2 baby romaine lettuces, leaves separated
1 Persian cucumber, thinly sliced
    lengthwise
6 baby Roma or cherry tomatoes,
    thinly sliced
⅔ cup Tzatziki (page 314)

* See Glossary

MAKE AIP FRIENDLY

Omit: tomato paste, Turkish spice mix, and
Roma or cherry tomatoes

Melt 1½ tablespoons of the oil or fat in a large frying pan over medium heat. Add the onion and cook until softened and translucent, 8 minutes. Add the garlic and cook for a further 1 minute to soften. Let cool completely before mixing through the ground lamb.

To make the patties, combine the ground lamb, fat, tomato paste, Turkish spice mix, and salt in a large bowl, and mix well. Shape into 8 patties and flatten slightly.

Melt the remaining oil or fat in a large frying pan over medium-high heat. Add the lamb patties in batches and cook for 2–3 minutes on each side, or until just cooked through.

To serve, arrange the lettuce leaves on a platter, top each with slices of cucumber and tomato and a lamb patty, and spoon on some tzatziki.

SUNDAY ROAST LAMB
WITH VEGGIES AND MINT JELLY

SERVES 8

Roasts are hands down my favorite dish to tell people to make when swapping to a paleo way of life. Everyone loves them; they are familiar and super easy. And, thankfully, you don't have to forgo your gravy addiction, as you can easily make a paleo version. Simply add bone broth to the pan and reduce and thicken it by blending in some of your roasted veg. Or, you can serve your roast lamb with its traditional sidekick: the legendary mint jelly.

SPICE PASTE
2 tablespoons sweet paprika
½ teaspoon ground cumin
½ teaspoon ground coriander
2 teaspoons freshly ground black pepper
2 teaspoons sea salt
6 garlic cloves, finely chopped
1½ tablespoons lemon juice
3 tablespoons good-quality animal fat*

coconut oil, for greasing
1 leg of lamb (about 5½ pounds)
6 garlic cloves, unpeeled
2 large fennel bulbs, trimmed and cut
    into quarters
2 large red onions, cut into wedges
1⅓ pounds kabocha squash, unpeeled,
    cut into 2-inch pieces
6 rosemary sprigs
3 cups Beef or Chicken Bone Broth
    (pages 121 and 116)
Mint Jelly (page 310), to serve

* See Glossary

MAKE AIP FRIENDLY

Omit: spice paste
Substitute: salt, lemon juice, animal fat, garlic, and rosemary in place of the spice paste

---

To make the spice paste, combine the ingredients in a bowl and mix to form a paste. Set aside until needed.

Preheat the oven to 350°F. Grease a large roasting pan with coconut oil.

Using the tip of a sharp knife, make ¼-inch deep incisions over the leg of lamb. Pre-cut 6–8 lengths of kitchen string long enough to go around the lamb, and tie into a knot. Run a length of string under the lamb and tie the ends into a tight knot. Make it snug, but not so tight that the string cuts into the lamb during cooking. Repeat at 2-inch intervals along the leg of lamb.

Scatter the garlic, fennel, onions, and squash over the base of the prepared pan and sit the lamb on top. Rub the spice paste evenly over the lamb and tuck the rosemary sprigs under the strings. Tip 1 cup broth into the spice paste bowl and stir to incorporate any remaining paste. Pour over the lamb. Roast for 1¾ hours, basting the meat occasionally with the cooking juices. If you prefer your lamb to be well done, cook for a further 15 minutes.

Transfer the roast lamb to a carving board, cover loosely with foil, and let rest for 15 minutes. Transfer the vegetables to a serving dish and cover to keep warm.

Place the roasting pan over medium heat on the stove top. Pour in the remaining broth and bring to a boil. Using a wooden spoon, stir to dislodge any cooked-on bits, and simmer the jus until reduced by two-thirds to a saucelike consistency. If you prefer the sauce to be thicker, put the jus in a blender and add a couple of pieces of onion and fennel and blend until smooth. Season with salt if needed.

Carve the lamb and serve with the roasted vegetables, lamb jus, and mint jelly.

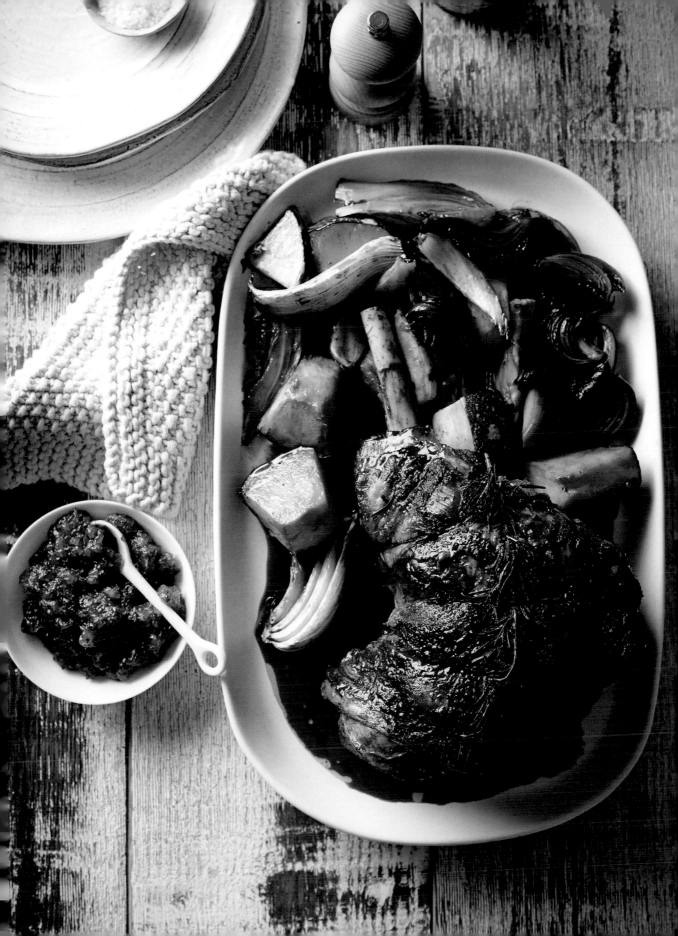

SIDES

DANIELLE'S STRAWBERRY AND ARUGULA SALAD
ASPARAGUS SALAD WITH TARATOR DRESSING AND POMEGRANATE
BROCCOLINI WITH GARLIC, CHILE, AND LEMON
NIC'S ROASTED SQUASH, CASHEW CHEESE, AND POMEGRANATE SALAD
TERRY'S RAINBOW MATCHSTICK SALAD
BROCCOLI AND SESAME SALAD

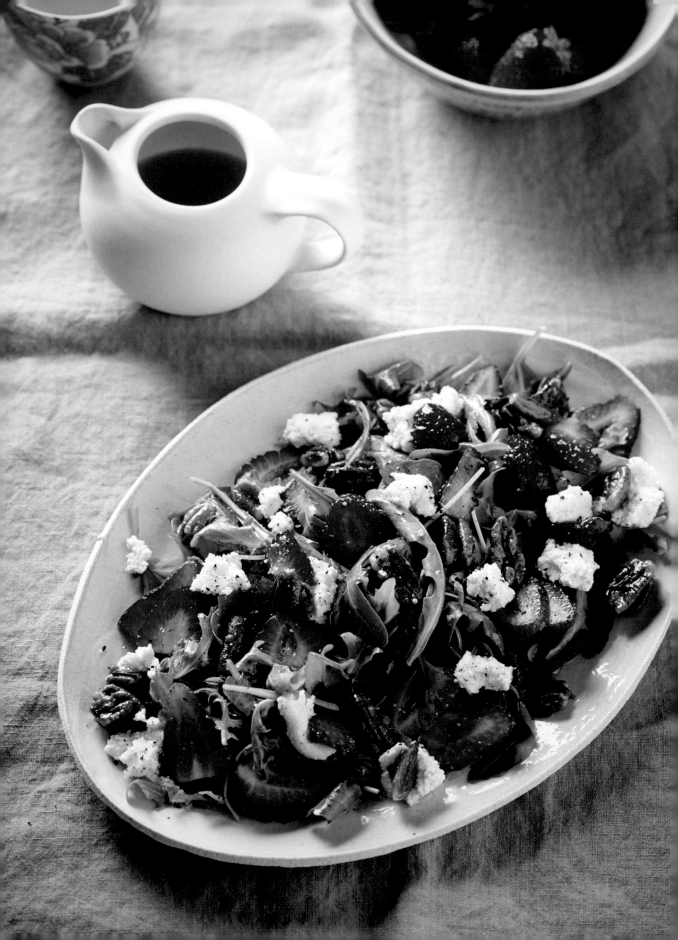

DANIELLE'S STRAWBERRY AND ARUGULA SALAD

SERVES 4

Danielle Walker of Against All Grain lovingly prepared this salad with me while we were filming together. The whole crew fell in love with its freshness. I recommend making this when strawberries are at their peak – popping it on the table at a picnic or Fourth-of-July celebration – and serving it alongside ham or roast chicken or turkey and some fermented veg.

---

3 handfuls arugula
1½ cups strawberries, hulled and sliced
1 cup Spiced Pecans (page 312)

LIME VINAIGRETTE
juice of 1 lime (about 1½ tablespoons)
2 tablespoons extra-virgin olive oil
freshly ground black pepper

sea salt and freshly ground black pepper
½ cup Cashew Cheese (page 307)

Toss the arugula, strawberries, and pecans together in a large bowl.

To make the lime vinaigrette, combine the lime juice, olive oil, and a pinch of pepper in a bowl and mix well.

Drizzle the dressing over the salad and gently toss through. Season with salt and pepper. Arrange the salad on a platter, and crumble the cashew cheese over the top. Sprinkle on a little extra pepper, if you wish.

MAKE AIP FRIENDLY

Omit: spiced pecans, black pepper, and cashew cheese

Substitute: coconut yogurt in place of cashew cheese

ASPARAGUS SALAD WITH TARATOR DRESSING AND POMEGRANATE

SERVES 4–6

I like to think of my approach to eating as being vegetable-based with a moderate portion of meat, some healthy fats on the side, and some broth and fermented veg to round it all off. Play around with this formula to create your meals, and you'll see how easy it is to eat for health. This delicious salad is perfect with grilled or steamed seafood or leftover roast chicken.

TARATOR DRESSING

2 cups walnuts, soaked in boiled water
   for 30 minutes
2 tablespoons hulled tahini*
3 garlic cloves, finely chopped
2 tablespoons apple cider vinegar
juice of 1 lemon
¼ cup extra-virgin olive oil
sea salt and freshly ground black pepper

3 bunches of asparagus (about 1 pound),
   woody ends trimmed, cut in half
   lengthwise
14 ounces okra pods, cut in half lengthwise
¼ cup extra-virgin olive oil
½ cup pomegranate seeds
⅓ cup pumpkin seeds (activated
   if possible*), toasted
1–2 pinches of sumac*

* See Glossary

To make the tarator dressing, drain the walnuts, put them in the bowl of a food processor, and process to fine crumbs. Add the remaining dressing ingredients, along with 2 tablespoons water, and blitz for 10 seconds to combine (it should be quite thick). Set aside.

Steam the asparagus and okra until just tender, 3–4 minutes, then place in ice-cold water to cool. Drain well and shake off as much excess water as possible.

Combine the asparagus and okra in a bowl, season with salt, and toss with the olive oil. Arrange the vegetables on a serving platter, dollop with the dressing, then scatter with the pomegranate and pumpkin seeds. Finish with a sprinkle of sumac, and serve.

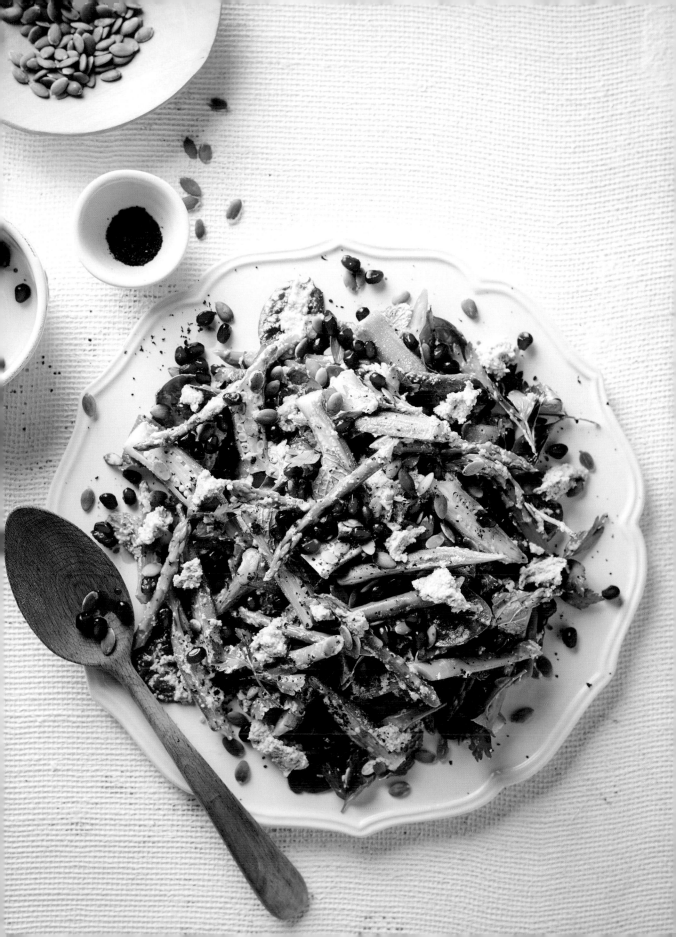

BROCCOLINI WITH GARLIC, CHILE, AND LEMON

SERVES 4

Could this be the yummiest way to serve broccolini? It doesn't get much better than this winning formula of fresh veggies, good fats from the oils, sharpness from the vinegar, heat from the garlic and chile, and saltiness from the anchovies. To make it a meal, add grilled or steamed seafood, or sausage and fried egg.

---

2 bunches of broccolini (about 13 ounces), trimmed

3 tablespoons coconut oil

3 garlic cloves, finely chopped

1 long red chile, halved lengthwise, seeded and finely chopped

2 salted anchovy fillets, rinsed well and patted dry, finely chopped (optional)

2 tablespoons finely chopped flat-leaf parsley leaves

zest and juice of 1 lemon

sea salt and freshly ground black pepper

3 tablespoons extra-virgin olive oil

Blanch the broccolini in boiling water until tender, 3–4 minutes. Drain well.

Meanwhile, melt the coconut oil in a large frying pan over medium heat. Add the garlic, chile, and anchovies, and cook until the garlic starts to color slightly and becomes fragrant (about 1 minute).

Add the broccolini and parsley to the pan and sauté for 2 minutes. Stir in the lemon zest and juice, and season with salt and pepper.

Place the broccolini mixture on a platter, and drizzle with the olive oil. Serve immediately.

MAKE AIP FRIENDLY

Omit: chile and black pepper

TIP

You can also make this dish with any vegetable that is in season: try okra, asparagus, cauliflower, squash, mushrooms, zucchini, carrots, sweet potato, eggplant, green beans, Brussels sprouts, or chargrilled lettuce.

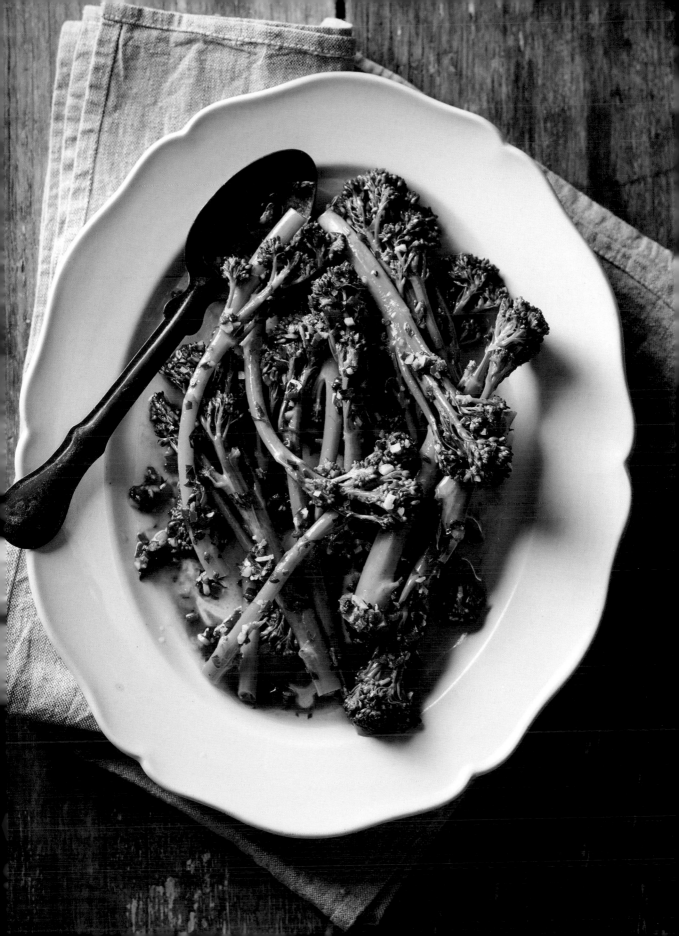

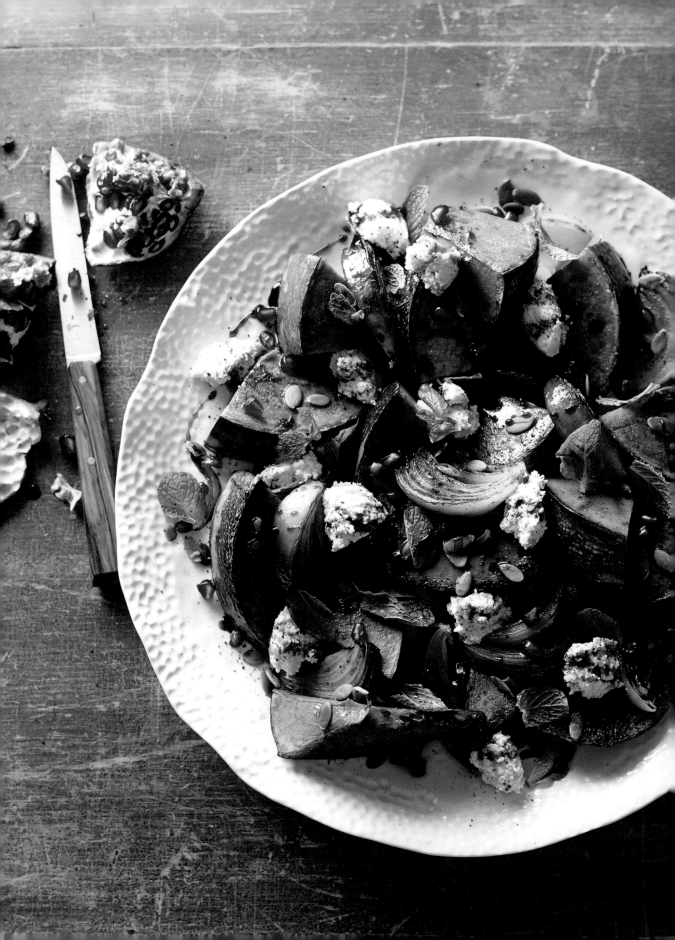

NIC'S ROASTED SQUASH, CASHEW CHEESE, AND POMEGRANATE SALAD

SERVES 4

Squash has got to be my all-time favorite vegetable to roast. Once you get the hang of how easy it is to roast veg in bulk, you can cook up a different assortment a few times a week. Sometimes we keep it simple – just one or two veggies, some onion, garlic, and spices with a healthy fat, and, voilà, 30 or so minutes later we have the most delicious way to eat vegetables ever. Serve them as is with a dressing or mayonnaise, bake them in a frittata, or add a side of seafood, meat, or eggs, and you are done.

1½ pounds kabocha squash, unpeeled, seeded and chopped into large chunks
1 red onion, cut into wedges
pinch of ground cumin
pinch of red pepper flakes
sea salt and freshly ground black pepper
1 tablespoon coconut oil, melted
1 large handful mint leaves
2 tablespoons pumpkin seeds (activated if possible*)
5½ oz/150 g Cashew Cheese (page 307)
3 tablespoons extra-virgin olive oil
2–3 tablespoons pomegranate molasses*
3 tablespoons pomegranate seeds

* See Glossary

Preheat the oven to 350°F.

Combine the squash and onion in a roasting pan and toss with the cumin, red pepper flakes, and salt and pepper. Drizzle on the coconut oil, gently toss, and roast until the squash and onion are golden and cooked through, 35–40 minutes.

Gently toss the roasted vegetables with the mint and pumpkin seeds, then transfer to a serving platter. Scatter the cashew cheese over, drizzle with the olive oil and pomegranate molasses, and sprinkle with the pomegranate seeds before serving.

TERRY'S RAINBOW MATCHSTICK SALAD

SERVES 4

Dr. Terry Wahls and I cooked the most amazing meal together recently while we were filming for our *Food is Medicine* documentary. Dr. Wahls is very well known in the paleo and gut health community as, through diet and a lot of research, she has managed to get on top of her MS. If you want to know more, I urge you to read *The Wahls Protocol.* It was a great honor to spend quality time in the kitchen with her. Serve this salad with Terry's chicken livers (see recipe on page 220).

---

1 large beet, cut into matchsticks
2 turnips, cut into matchsticks
2 carrots, cut into matchsticks
1½ tablespoons finely grated ginger
2 tablespoons chopped flat-leaf parsley
    or cilantro leaves or a mixture of both
1 teaspoon finely grated lime zest
juice of 2 limes, plus extra if needed
3 tablespoons extra-virgin olive oil or
    flaxseed oil (or 1½ tablespoons of each)
sea salt and freshly ground black pepper

Place the beet in ice-cold water for 10 minutes. (This helps stop the beet from bleeding into the salad, and gives it a crisper texture.) Drain and shake off as much excess water as possible.

Place the turnips, carrots, ginger, and parsley and/or cilantro in a bowl. Add the lime zest and juice, olive and/or flaxseed oil, and beet, and gently mix. Season with salt and pepper, and add more lime juice if you prefer a tangier flavor. Arrange the salad on a platter, and serve.

MAKE AIP FRIENDLY

Omit: black pepper
Substitute: extra-virgin olive oil in place of flaxseed oil

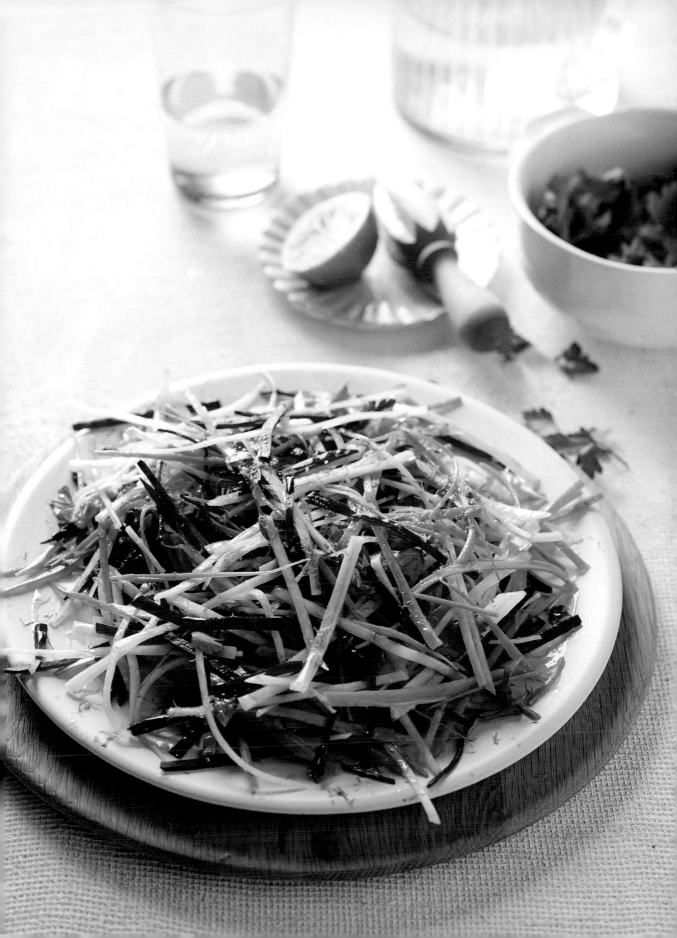

BROCCOLI AND SESAME SALAD

SERVES 4–6

Here is an utterly delicious dish that deserves to be eaten at any time of the year. It will leave you wanting to have it again and again and again. When we make this at home we simply add in some protein in the form of leftover roast chicken, pork, or lamb, or sometimes we add prawns, crabmeat, or flaked fish. Serve with some fermented veg tossed through the salad.

DRESSING
¼ cup hulled tahini*
3 tablespoons apple cider vinegar
1 garlic clove, finely chopped
sea salt and freshly ground black pepper

7 ounces broccoli, broken into florets, stems reserved
1 bunch (about 6 ounces) broccolini
2 green onions, thinly sliced
2 handfuls arugula
1 small handful mint leaves, torn
½ cup almonds (activated if possible*), toasted and chopped
2 tablespoons extra-virgin olive oil
1 teaspoon sesame seeds, toasted

* See Glossary

MAKE AIP FRIENDLY

Omit: almonds, sesame seeds, tahini, and black pepper

To make the dressing, combine the tahini, vinegar and garlic with 3 tablespoons water in a bowl. Season with salt and pepper, and mix well.

Thinly slice the broccoli stems lengthwise using a mandoline, or peel into strips with a vegetable peeler, and place in a bowl. Slice the broccolini lengthwise, chop into ¾-inch pieces, and combine with the sliced broccoli stems. Add the broccoli florets, green onion, arugula, mint, and half the almonds. Pour on the olive oil, season with salt and pepper, and gently toss to combine.

Arrange the salad in a serving bowl, drizzle on the dressing, and sprinkle with the remaining almonds and the sesame seeds.

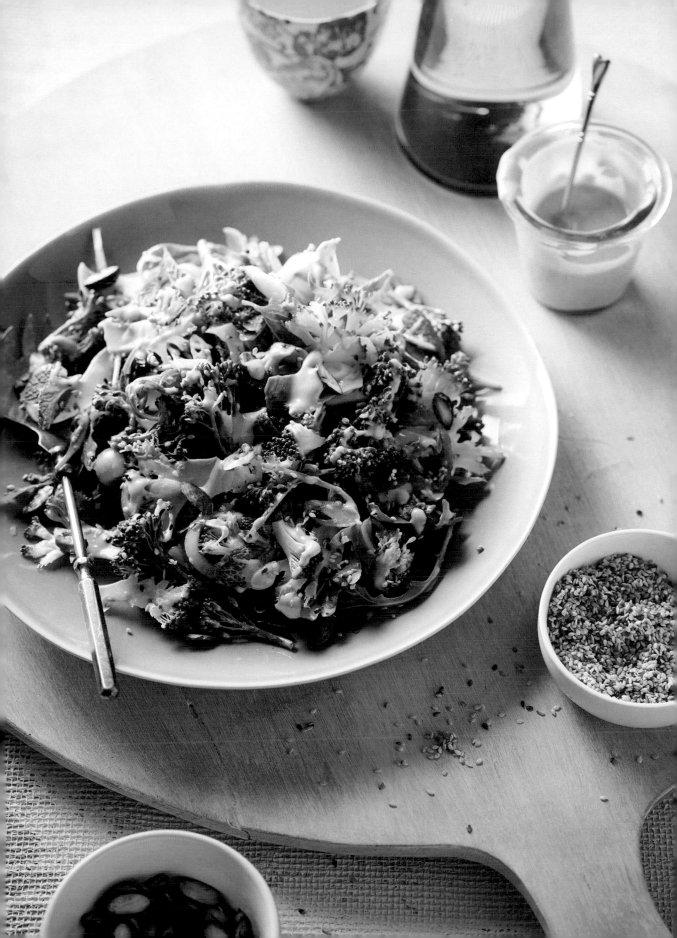

TREATS

TULSI JELLIES

NIC'S CHIA SLAB

SUNSHINE MYLK ICE POPS

CHILLI AND INDII'S PROBIOTIC JELLIES

COCONUT AND GINGER KEFIR ICE POPS WITH FRESH MINT

CINNAMON ICE CREAM

HELEN'S LAVENDER PANNA COTTA

CHOCOLATE PUDDINGS

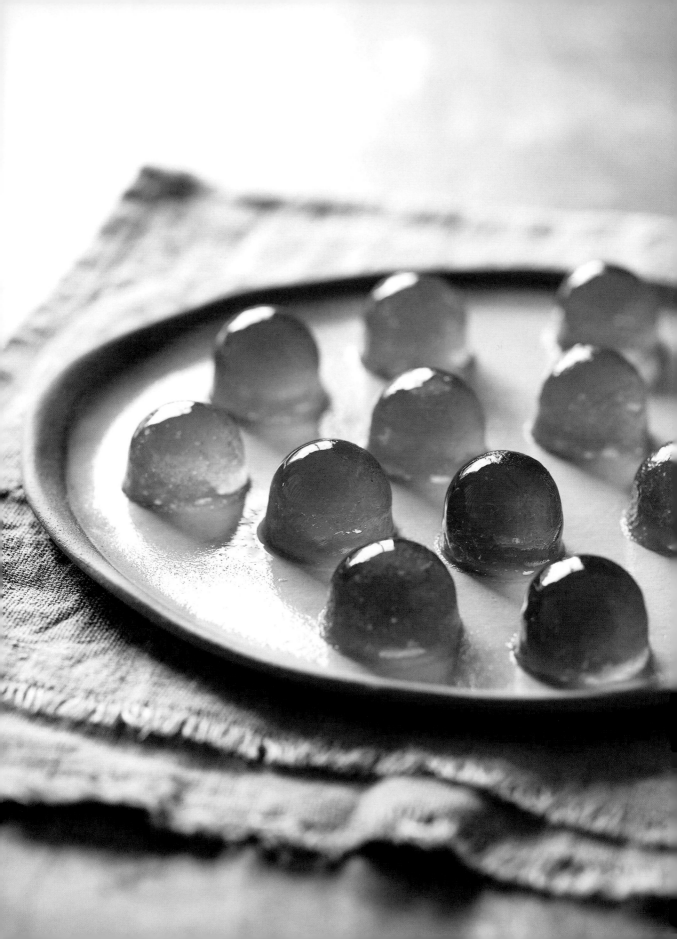

TULSI JELLIES

MAKES 30

Tulsi, or holy basil, is known in India as the queen of herbs – and for good reason. It is full of antioxidants, and is believed to promote well-being. Drinking the tea of this healing herb is said to boost the immune system, support liver function – which is essential for digestive health – and relieve stress. I recommend having a pot of tulsi tea every day, and making these delicious jellies to enjoy as treats.

2½ tablespoons powdered gelatin
3 tablespoons tulsi tea leaves (see Note)
1-inch piece of ginger, sliced
2 cups boiling water
2 tablespoons honey (optional)
pinch of sea salt

MAKE AIP FRIENDLY

Omit: honey
Substitute: ¼ cup freshly squeezed apple or pear juice in place of honey

Put the gelatin in a small bowl. Add ¼ cup water and set aside for 5 minutes to allow the gelatin granules to expand and soften.

Combine the tulsi tea leaves and ginger in a large heatproof bowl, and pour in the boiling water. Whisk in the gelatin mixture, cover with plastic wrap, and allow to steep for 30 minutes.

Strain the mixture into a jug. Stir and add the honey (if using) and salt. Pour into silicone molds and place in the fridge until set, about 4 hours. Store the jellies in an airtight container in the fridge for up to 2 weeks.

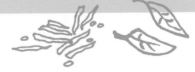

NOTE
You can find tulsi tea leaves at health-food stores and some supermarkets.

NIC'S CHIA SLAB

MAKES 20 PIECES

I am a very lucky man! I have the most wonderful wife, Nic; a beautiful human being who is a whiz in the kitchen and who nourishes me with her creative cooking skills. Now, Nic doesn't use recipes and never makes the same dish twice, as she lets intuition guide her. When she made this, I begged her to create a recipe so that I could share it with you. And here it is in all its gut-healthy glory! Thanks, angel – we make a great team.

---

2 tablespoons powdered gelatin
2 x 13.5-ounce cans coconut cream
3 tablespoons honey (optional)
1⅔ cups chia seeds
zest of ½ lemon
3½ cups mixed fresh or frozen berries

Grease an 8 x 12-inch baking pan and line the base and sides with parchment paper.

Put the gelatin in a small bowl. Add ¼ cup water and set aside for 5 minutes to allow the gelatin granules to soften and expand.

Heat the coconut cream in a saucepan over medium heat until just starting to simmer. Remove from the heat, add the gelatin mixture, and stir until the gelatin has dissolved. Stir in the honey (if using).

Pour the warm coconut cream mixture into a bowl, sprinkle in the chia seeds a little at a time, and mix through. Fold in the lemon zest and half the mixed berries, and pour into the prepared pan. Smooth the top with a spatula, then sprinkle on the remaining berries. Cover with plastic wrap and place in the fridge to set for 4 hours.

When the chia slab is firm, remove from the pan and cut into 2-inch squares. Place on a platter and serve. Store leftovers in an airtight container in the fridge for 1 week.

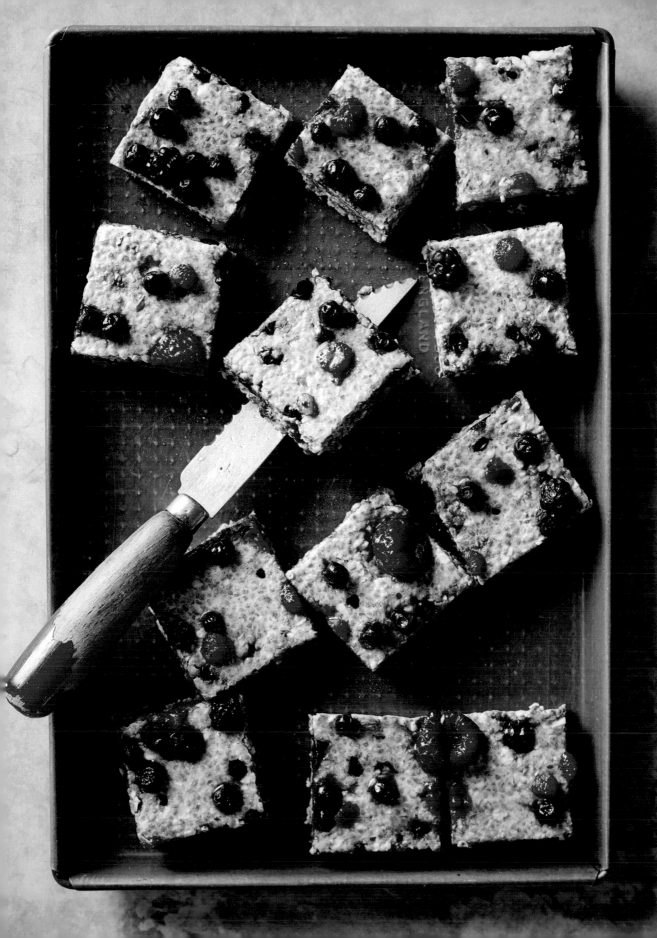

SUNSHINE MYLK ICE POPS

MAKES 6

A turmeric latte is a wonderful Indian-inspired drink of spice-infused hot milk (I like to use nut or coconut). Enjoying a latte or two is a great way to get more turmeric into your diet. When the weather is warm and you don't feel like a hot drink, you can simply make a cold version by turning your latte into a smoothie or ice pop, as I have done here. You can use banana or dates to sweeten, if you prefer.

TURMERIC PASTE

¼ cup ground turmeric

1½ teaspoons coconut oil
5 cardamom pods, crushed
2 cups Almond or Macadamia Milk
   (pages 306 and 309) or coconut milk
   or coconut cream
pinch of freshly ground black pepper
½ teaspoon vanilla powder
¼ teaspoon ground cinnamon
maple syrup, to taste (optional)

MAKE AIP FRIENDLY

Omit: cardamom, nut milk, black pepper, vanilla, and maple syrup

Substitute: coconut milk or cream in place of nut milk, and 1 teaspoon grated ginger instead of vanilla

To make the turmeric paste, combine the turmeric with 1 cup water in a small saucepan. Simmer over low heat, stirring occasionally, until you have a creamy and smooth paste, about 15 minutes.

Combine the coconut oil and cardamom in a saucepan and cook over medium heat until fragrant, about 1 minute. Reduce the heat to medium-low and add the milk, pepper, vanilla, cinnamon, maple syrup (if using), and 1½ teaspoons of the turmeric paste. Stir until just simmering, 3 minutes. Remove from the heat, cover with plastic wrap, and set aside to infuse for 30 minutes. Add more maple syrup if you like, then strain through a fine sieve.

Pour the sunshine mylk into six ⅓-cup ice pop molds, insert an ice pop stick into each mold, and freeze until solid, 6–8 hours.

TIP
Leftover turmeric paste will keep for 2–3 weeks in an airtight glass container in the fridge.

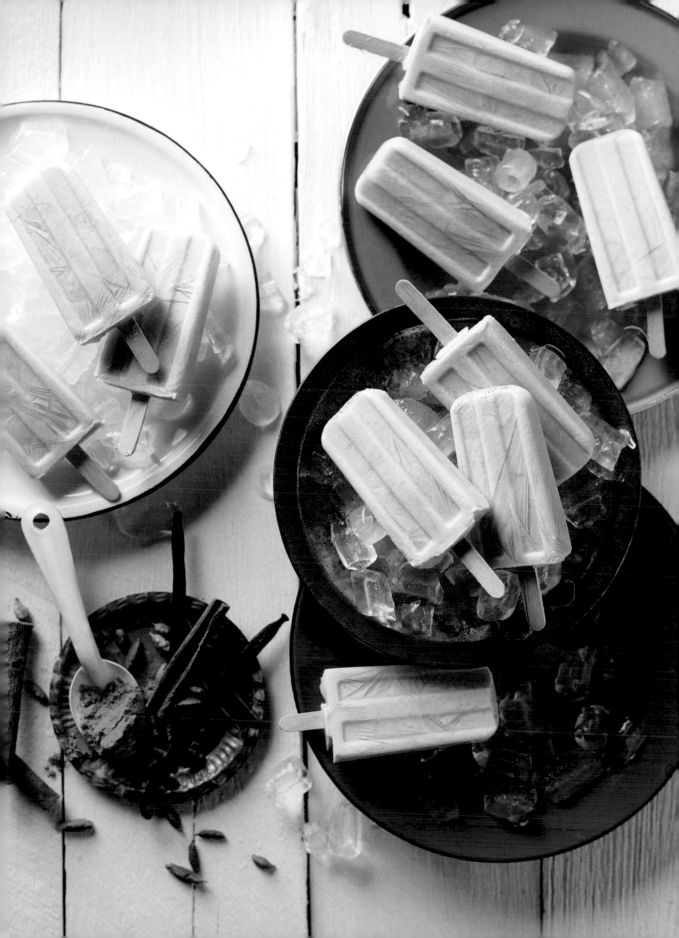

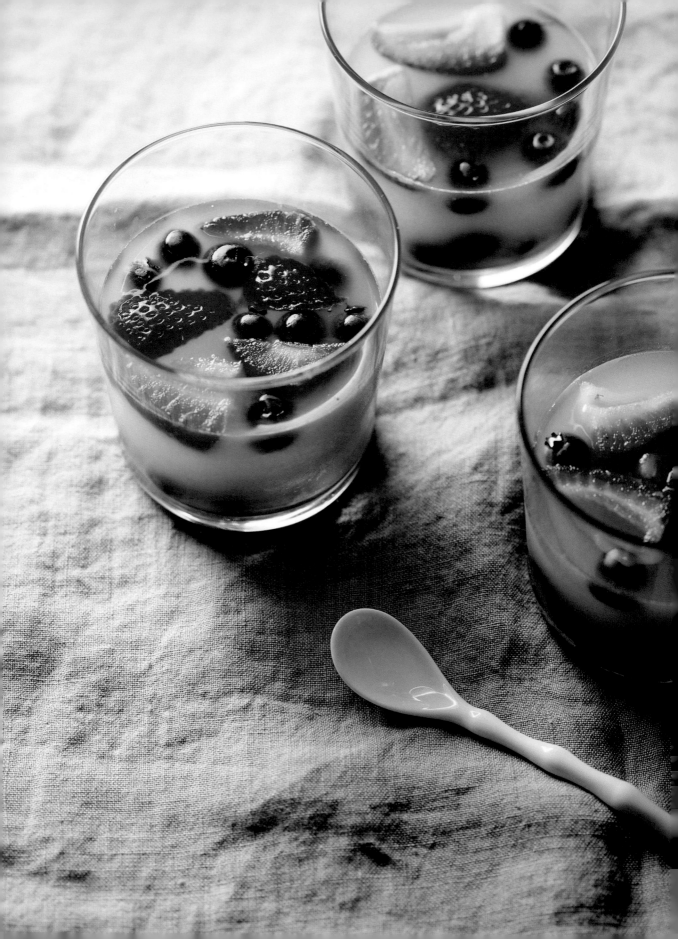

CHILLI AND INDII'S PROBIOTIC JELLIES

SERVES 8

When people consider changing their diets to a paleo-inspired one, they often worry how they will cope without sugary sweets. As a way to make the transition easier, we have created some gut-healthy treats, such as these probiotic jellies, that the whole family will love. Now, that isn't an open invitation to eat these for breakfast, lunch, and dinner, but rather to indulge in them from time to time. These are my daughters' favorites.

---

1 tablespoon powdered gelatin
2 cups Coconut and Ginger Kefir
   (page 296)
honey, to taste (optional)
¾ cup strawberries, hulled and quartered
1 cup blueberries

MAKE AIP FRIENDLY

Omit: honey

Put the gelatin in a small saucepan. Add 3 tablespoons water and set aside for 5 minutes to allow the gelatin granules to soften and expand.

Place the pan over low heat and bring just to a simmer, stirring continuously until the gelatin dissolves. Remove from the heat and set aside to cool to lukewarm.

Whisk the kefir and honey (if using) into the lukewarm gelatin mixture. Pour the mixture into eight ½-cup glasses, filling the glasses three-quarters of the way full. Add the strawberries and blueberries, and chill the jellies until set, 4 hours. The jellies will keep in the fridge for a week in an airtight container.

TIP

You can use kombucha or coconut water in place of the Coconut and Ginger Kefir, if you prefer.

COCONUT AND GINGER KEFIR ICE POPS WITH FRESH MINT

MAKES 8

My kids absolutely adore ice pops – and to tell the truth, they are my favorite as well. They remind me of hot summer days on the Gold Coast when I'd crave something cold after spending hours at the beach surfing. These days we make our ice pops full of probiotic goodness by using homemade kefir. Play around with different flavors and fruits, and enjoy.

2⅔ cups Coconut and Ginger Kefir
(page 296)
1 large handful mint leaves, torn
(or use whole micro mint leaves)

AIP FRIENDLY

Pour the kefir into eight ⅓-cup ice pop molds, add some mint leaves to each mold, and place in the freezer for 1 hour. After 1 hour, insert an ice pop stick into each mold (this will help keep the sticks fixed in the center – if you have a support lid for the sticks, the sticks can go straight in after pouring the liquid into the molds). Return to the freezer until completely frozen, 4–8 hours.

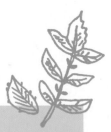

TIPS

You can enjoy your ice pops plain, or you can mix in some fresh juice of your choice.

Swap the Coconut and Ginger Kefir for the same quantity of kombucha or coconut water, if you prefer.

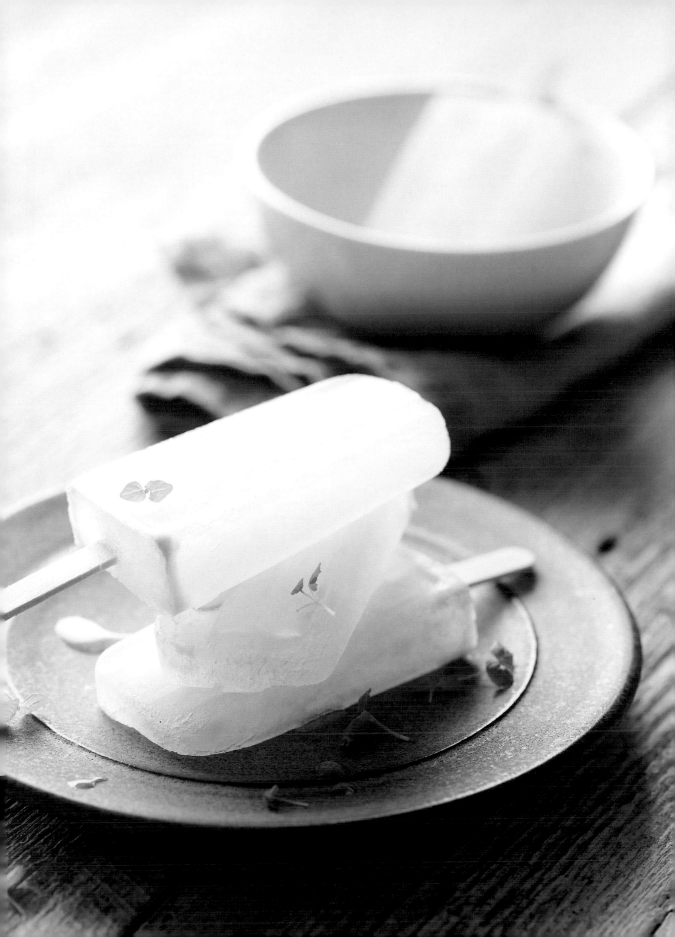

CINNAMON ICE CREAM

MAKES 5 CUPS

Cinnamon is a wonder spice in anyone's book. It is such a versatile and powerful ingredient that adds not only flavor, but also medicinal value to dishes. Holistic health practitioners have long known that cinnamon helps with digestion and to break down the fats in food. And that's why cinnamon ice cream makes a lot of sense. Eat it on its own, add it to your favorite smoothie, or serve it with a paleo apple pie – but remember that this is a treat because of the sugar (honey or maple syrup) in it.

---

1 x 13.5-ounce can coconut cream
4 egg yolks
1 cup honey or maple syrup
1¾ cup Coconut Yogurt (pages 86 and 88)
1½ tablespoons ground cinnamon

Put the coconut cream in a saucepan and bring to a boil, stirring occasionally to prevent the coconut from sticking to the bottom of the pan.

Whisk the egg yolks and honey or maple syrup in a large bowl until pale and fluffy. Pour in half of the hot coconut cream, whisking well. Whisk in the remaining hot coconut cream, then pour the mixture into a clean saucepan. Cook, stirring with a wooden spoon or spatula, over medium heat until the mixture thickens slightly and coats the back of the spoon, 3–5 minutes. Strain the mixture through a fine sieve into a bowl. Cover with plastic wrap and chill for at least 1 hour.

Remove the coconut cream custard from the freezer and mix in the coconut yogurt and cinnamon. Pour into an ice-cream maker and churn according to the manufacturer's instructions. Transfer to a container, cover, and freeze until firm. If the ice cream is too firm, place in the refrigerator to soften a little before serving.

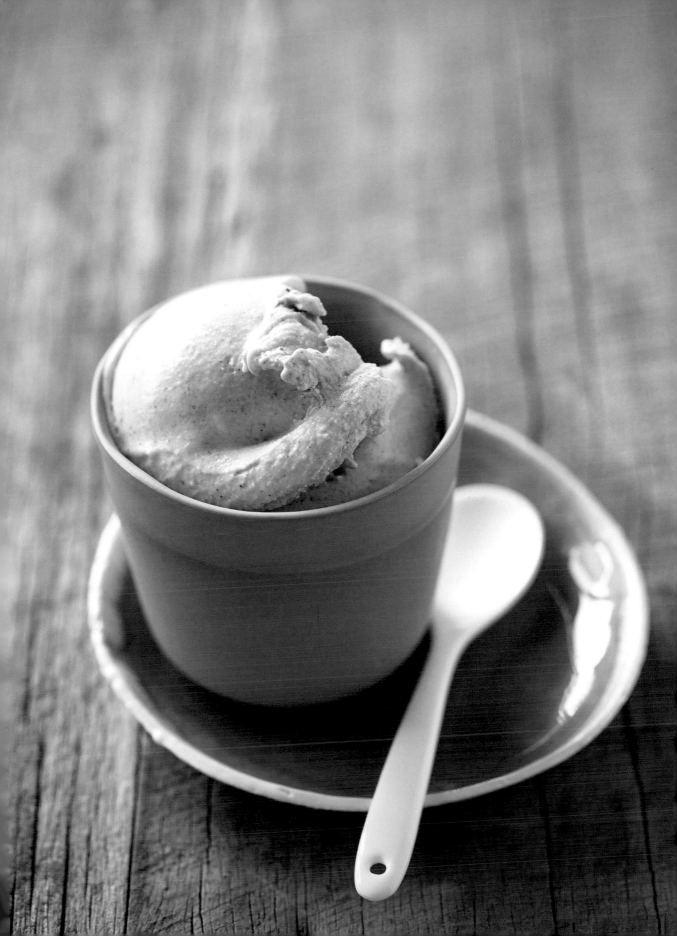

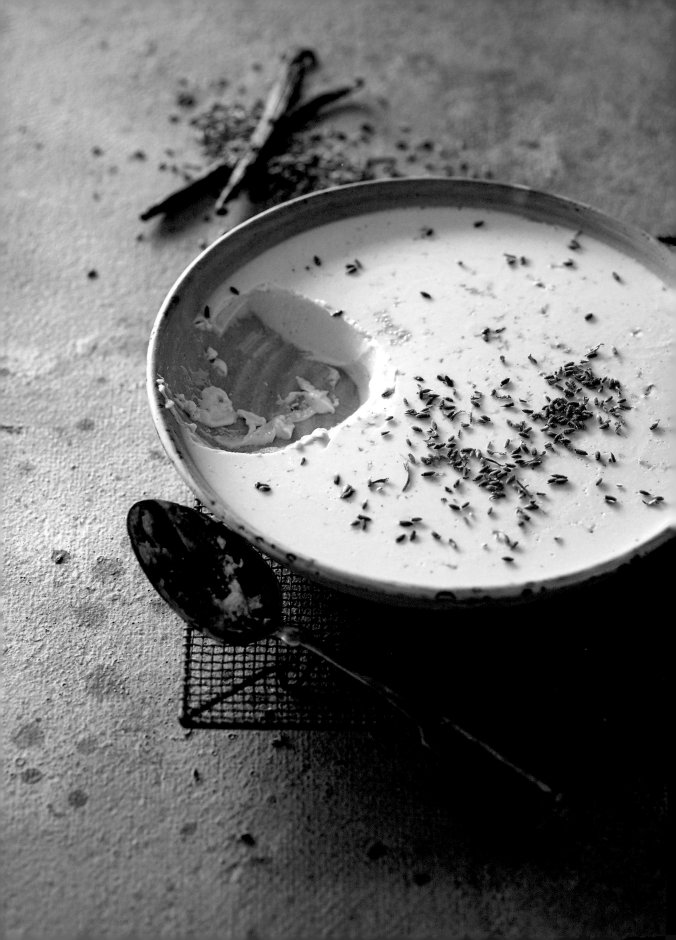

HELEN'S LAVENDER PANNA COTTA

SERVES 2–3

This amazing dish makes a perfect treat for a special occasion. Rich with gut-healing gelatin, this recipe features fragrant lavender – a soothing, calming herb that is also great for stimulating digestion.

---

2 cups coconut cream
½ cup honey
½ vanilla pod, split lengthwise and seeds scraped
2½ tablespoons dried edible lavender, plus extra to serve
finely grated zest of ½ lime, plus extra to serve
1½ teaspoons powdered gelatin

Combine the coconut cream, honey, vanilla pod and seeds, lavender, and lime zest in a saucepan over medium heat and bring to a boil, stirring to dissolve the honey. Remove from the heat, cover, and set aside for 1 hour to allow the flavors to infuse.

Pour 2 tablespoons water into a small cup, sprinkle in the gelatin, and set aside for 5 minutes to allow the gelatin granules to expand and soften.

Place the coconut cream mixture over low heat and bring just to a simmer. Remove from the heat, pour in the gelatin mixture, and whisk until the gelatin dissolves. Strain and let cool to room temperature.

Pour the cooled panna cotta into a serving dish. Place in the refrigerator to set until firm with a slight wobble, 4 hours. Sprinkle with some extra lavender and lime zest to decorate.

NOTE
Edible lavender can be found at health-food stores or online.

CHOCOLATE PUDDINGS

SERVES 4

What can I say about these chocolate puddings except that they are super yummy! You can substitute the cacao with carob if you are giving this to youngsters, as cacao can have a stimulating effect whereas carob is a lot gentler.

1 tablespoon powdered gelatin
1 x 13.5-ounce can coconut milk
generous ½ cup raw cacao powder, plus extra for dusting
¼ teaspoon ground cinnamon
3 tablespoons honey or maple syrup
2 cups Whipped Coconut Cream (page 315), to serve
toasted coconut chips, to serve
toasted crushed hazelnuts (activated if possible*), to serve

* See Glossary

Mix the gelatin with 3 tablespoons water in a small bowl and set aside for 5 minutes to allow the gelatin granules to expand and soften.

Combine the coconut milk, cacao powder, cinnamon, and honey or maple syrup in a saucepan over medium heat, and whisk. Bring to just below a simmer, and remove from the heat.

Add the gelatin mixture to the warm coconut milk mixture and stir until the gelatin dissolves. Transfer to four 5-ounce (⅔-cup) ramekins or dishes, and place in the fridge for 1 hour to set (or freezer for 20 minutes for faster setting).

To serve, spoon some whipped coconut cream over, then sprinkle with some toasted coconut chips and hazelnuts and finish with a dusting of extra cacao.

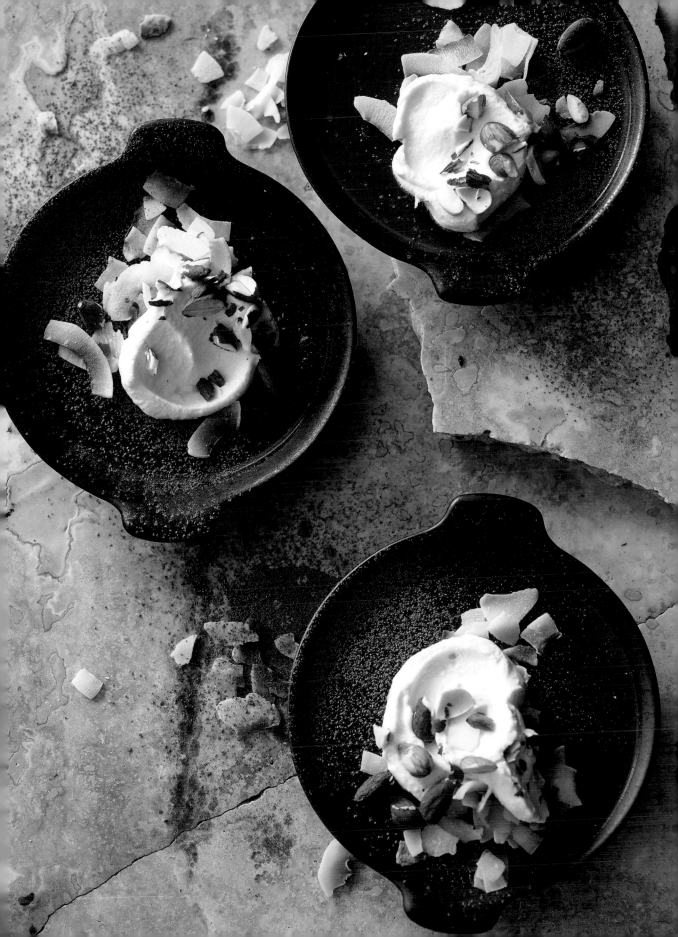

DRINKS

GUT-SOOTHING TEA

HELEN'S CHAI-BIOTIC

DIGESTIF TEA

GUT AND LIVER CLEANSE TEA

CHARCOAL MOP-UP

CHAMOMILE AND LICORICE TEA

GREEN SMOOTHIE

COCONUT AND GINGER KEFIR

COCONUT AND TURMERIC KEFIR WITH GINGER AND CAYENNE

BEET, GINGER, AND TURMERIC KVASS

FIRE TONIC

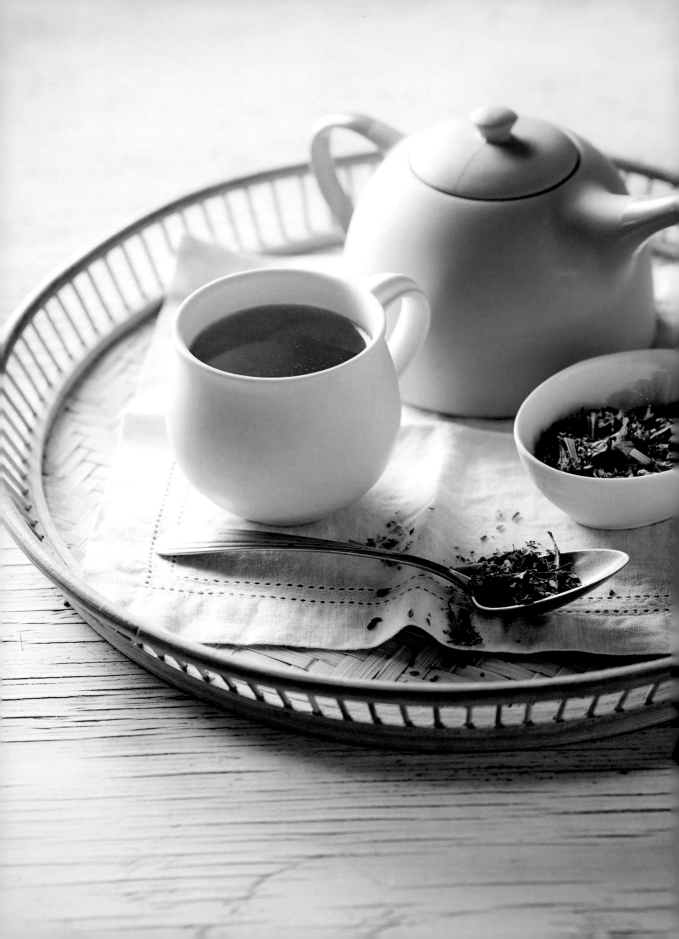

GUT-SOOTHING TEA

SERVES 8

Just as the name suggests, this tea is like a gentle hug for your gut. All of the ingredients have wonderful anti-inflammatory properties – licorice and slippery elm are both demulcent herbs that soothe an inflamed gut wall, calendula helps heal it by increasing the proliferation of cells required for wound repair, lemon balm calms the central nervous system, and lemongrass and ginger provide anti-inflammatory effects while stimulating circulation.

---

1 teaspoon slippery elm powder*

1 tablespoon licorice root sticks*

1 tablespoon dried calendula flowers or calendula tea leaves (see Note)

1 tablespoon dried lemon balm leaves

1 tablespoon lemongrass tea (see Note)

1 tablespoon ginger tea (see Note)

* See Glossary

AIP FRIENDLY

Mix all the ingredients in a bowl to combine. Place in an airtight container and store for up to 3 months.

For each cup of tea, steep 1 heaping teaspoon of the dried herb mixture in 1 cup boiling water until cool enough to drink. Sip slowly.

NOTE

You can buy dried calendula flowers, lemongrass tea, and ginger tea from health-food stores or online.

Feel free to replace the lemongrass tea and ginger tea with the same amount of finely chopped lemongrass and finely grated ginger. Just add these fresh ingredients to each brew (you can prepare them ahead and store them in the freezer).

HELEN'S CHAI-BIOTIC

SERVES 2

Tea (chai) for life (biotic). This absolutely delicious, warming, and comforting tea is fantastic for helping to keep your gut and immune system in good shape. It's particularly great if you are experiencing any yeast problems, as the spices used are strong antifungals. They also stimulate blood circulation, which is wonderful if your fingers and toes are a bit cold or if your brain is a bit foggy.

---

1 teaspoon pau d'arco bark or powder*
1 teaspoon cat's claw bark or powder*
   (see Note)
1 teaspoon ground cinnamon
½ teaspoon freshly grated nutmeg
3 cardamom pods or ¼ teaspoon
   ground cardamom
1–2 star anise
¼ teaspoon licorice root powder*
¼ teaspoon ground turmeric
1 cup Almond Milk (page 306)
   or coconut milk

* See Glossary

> **MAKE** AIP FRIENDLY

Omit: nutmeg, cardamom, star anise,
and almond milk

Substitute: coconut milk in place of almond milk

Combine the pau d'arco, cat's claw, and spices in a saucepan, add 1 cup filtered water, and simmer for 5 minutes. Add your chosen milk, and strain through a sieve. Serve and savor. Yum!

NOTE

Leave out the cat's claw if you are pregnant or hoping to become pregnant in the next 2 months. Cat's claw has traditionally been used as a contraceptive, and while there is no conclusive evidence as to its effectiveness, it is best to play it safe.

TIP

The spice mix in this recipe can be made up in big batches and stored in an airtight container ready to go – it's lovely to give to friends and family.

DIGESTIF TEA

SERVES 8

This is the perfect drink to sip and enjoy 20 minutes after meals to support and ease your digestion. A quarter or half a cup is all you need to avoid disrupting your gut enzymes' doing their work.

1 tablespoon fennel seeds
3 tablespoons dried chamomile flowers*
3 tablespoons cardamom pods
3 tablespoons spearmint tea leaves

* See Glossary

MAKE AIP FRIENDLY

Omit: fennel seeds and cardamom
Substitute: ginger in place of fennel seeds, and cinnamon instead of cardamom

Mix all the ingredients to combine and store in an airtight container.

For each cup of tea, steep 1 heaping teaspoon of the dried herb-and-spice mixture in 1 cup boiling water until cool enough to drink. Sip slowly.

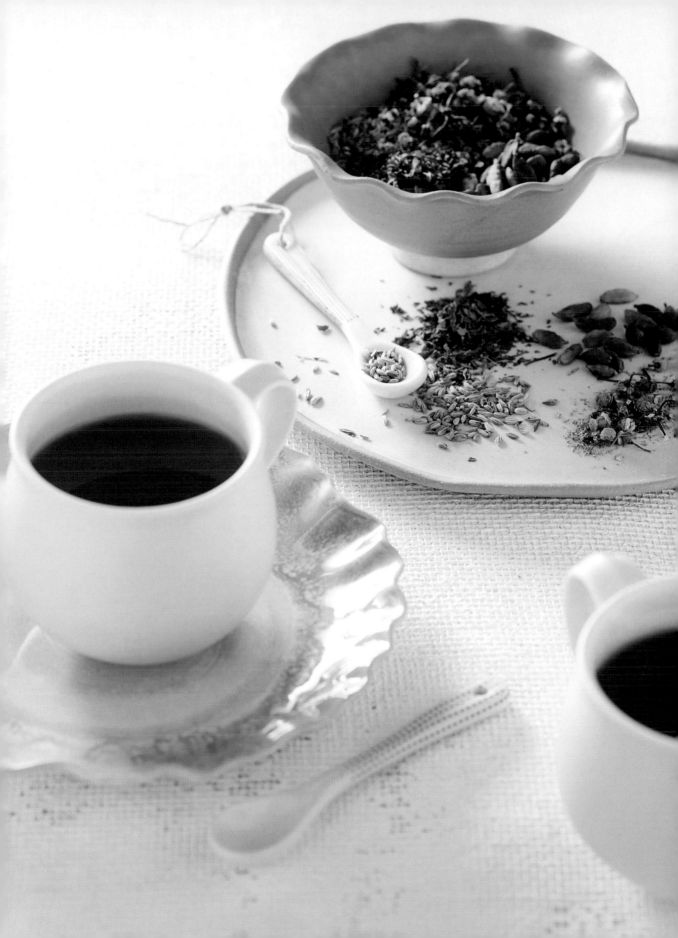

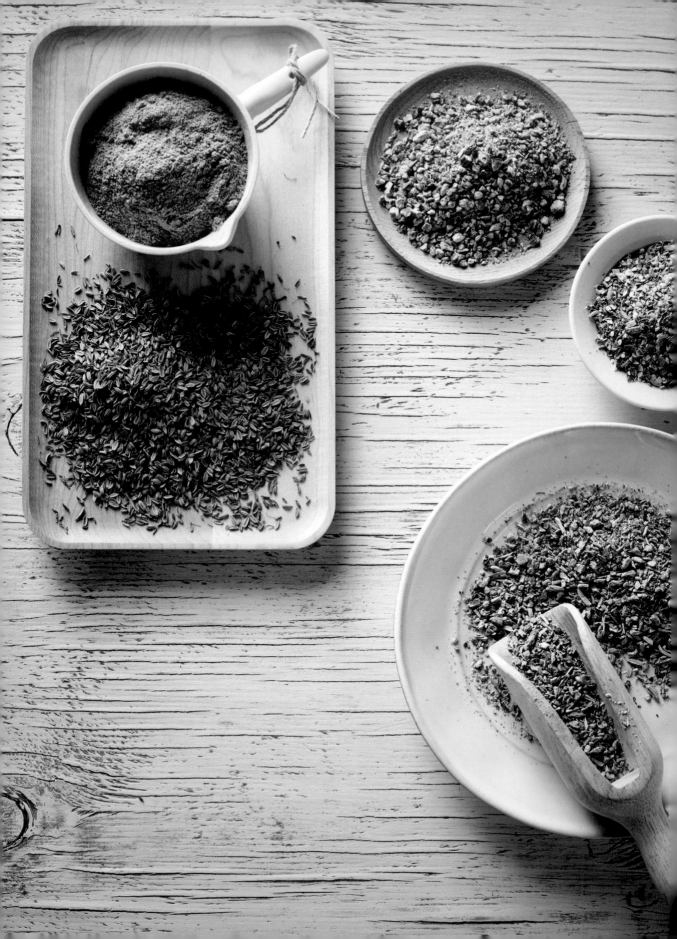

GUT AND LIVER CLEANSE TEA

SERVES ABOUT 10

This tea is not a laxative, but naturopaths use it to help improve regularity because it contains yellow dock and burdock to stimulate bile flow, St. Mary's thistle to stimulate liver detoxification, fennel to ease cramping and spasms, and slippery elm to soothe the gut. This is also excellent if you experience skin problems like pimples or eczema.

---

2 tablespoons yellow dock tea leaves
2 tablespoons burdock root tea
1 tablespoon fennel seeds
2 tablespoons St. Mary's thistle tea
2 tablespoons slippery elm powder*

* See Glossary

MAKE AIP FRIENDLY

Omit: fennel seeds and St. Mary's thistle
Substitute: spearmint or peppermint in place of fennel seeds, and dandelion root instead of St. Mary's thistle

Combine all the ingredients in a bowl, mix well, and store in an airtight container.

For each cup of tea, steep 1 heaping teaspoon of the dried herb mixture in 1 cup boiling water until cool enough to drink. Sip slowly.

CHARCOAL MOP-UP

SERVES 1

If at any stage during your four-week gut health program (see page 72) and beyond you experience significant gas or bloating, using charcoal can provide great relief. Charcoal is super *ad*sorbent (that's right, *not* absorbent) and binds to waste and toxins in the gut and carries them through and out the bowels, easing discomfort. Note that it will bind to good stuff too (like minerals), so don't drink it close to meals, supplements, and medications. It is best taken on an empty stomach roughly 1–2 hours after eating, and no sooner than 20 minutes before eating. Take 1–3 times daily as needed.

1¼ cups filtered, remineralized water
    (see Note)
1 tablespoon activated charcoal powder
juice of ¼ lemon

Mix the water, charcoal, and lemon juice and drink immediately on an empty stomach. Wait at least 30 minutes before eating. When finished, sip on a glass of plain filtered, remineralized water.

AIP FRIENDLY

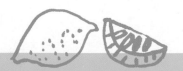

NOTE

Most water filters remove substances from water, but not just the undesirable stuff. They also remove minerals that act as electrolytes to facilitate water absorption. Remineralized water is filtered water with the beneficial minerals added back in.

Activated charcoal powder is readily available from health-food stores, pharmacies, or online.

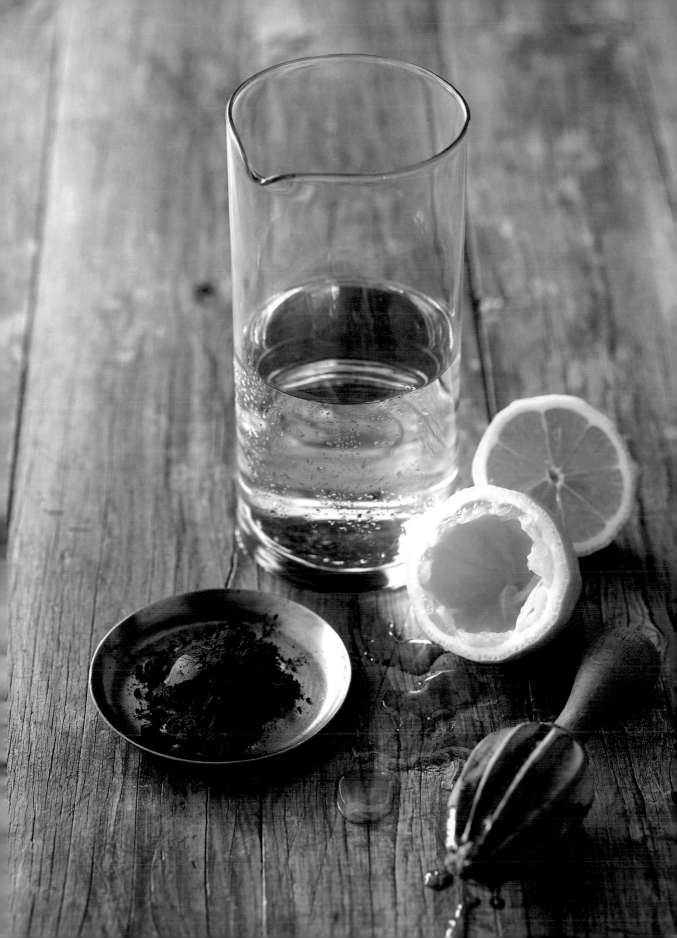

CHAMOMILE AND LICORICE TEA

SERVES 2

A super-simple soothing tea for the gut and central nervous system. Chamomile is anti-inflammatory, great for easing digestive cramps and spasms, and it also very gently stimulates digestion. Licorice is anti-inflammatory and demulcent, making it extra soothing for the gut.

---

2 tablespoons dried chamomile flowers*
1 tablespoon licorice root sticks*

* See Glossary

AIP FRIENDLY

Fill two mugs with boiling water from the kettle. Evenly divide the chamomile flowers and licorice root between the mugs, stir, and leave to infuse for 3 minutes. Strain and serve.

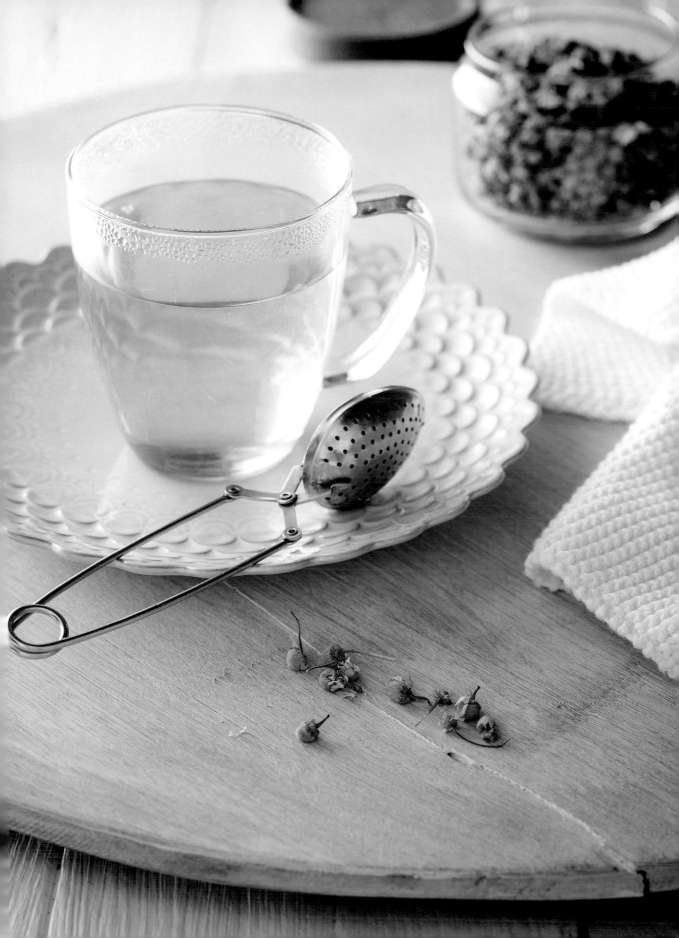

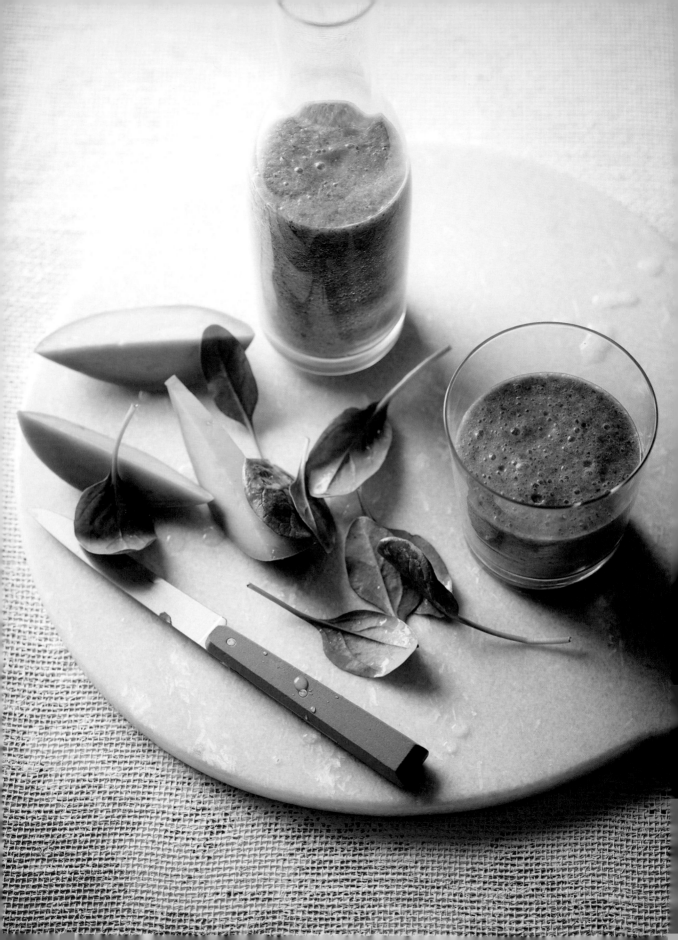

GREEN SMOOTHIE

SERVES 1

Here is one tasty example of how to build a really good green smoothie: combine minimal fruit (just enough to make it taste good) with fresh leafy greens (including herbs), anti-inflammatory spices, good fats, and easy-to-utilize protein. Mango and basil make a delicious combo.

---

2 mango halves, peeled
1½ cups baby spinach and/or basil leaves
1 teaspoon ground cinnamon
½ teaspoon ground turmeric
½ teaspoon ground ginger
¼ avocado
1 tablespoon powdered collagen
½ teaspoon maca powder* (optional)

* See Glossary

AIP FRIENDLY

Combine all the ingredients in a blender, pour in 1 cup filtered water, and blend until smooth. Add more filtered water slowly until you reach your desired consistency, blend again, and serve immediately.

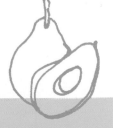

NOTE

It is super important to remember that smoothies are like meals, so you need to "chew your smoothies" or, at the very least, swish each mouthful around your mouth before swallowing.

Powdered collagen sourced from organic, grass-fed beef can be purchased at health-food stores or online.

COCONUT AND GINGER KEFIR

SERVES 2-4

Here is another favorite of mine, and it's a favorite with many kids, too. Aside from its probiotics and enzymes to help improve digestion, coconut and ginger kefir is a yummy tonic for those with bloating, allergies, candida, and sugar cravings. The ginger makes it taste like ginger beer.

---

3 young coconuts*
1–2 probiotic capsules or 2 tablespoons
    water kefir grains*
1 tablespoon finely grated ginger

* See Glossary

AIP FRIENDLY

TIPS

It is imperative to sterilize all materials that come into contact with the kefir. You want only good bacteria to flourish, so boil all utensils and wash your hands very well.

Glass jars and storage bottles are preferable to plastic, since kefir eats away at plastic. If the kefir eats the plastic, you in turn consume plastic. Limited contact is fine, but prolonged exposure is discouraged.

Use only coconut water from young coconuts. Store-bought coconut water will not work, as the product is pasteurized.

Never add probiotics or water kefir grains to refrigerated water, as it will drastically slow or stunt the fermentation process.

You will need a 1-quart glass bottle or jar for this recipe. Wash the bottle or jar, a nonmetallic spoon, and a grater in very hot soapy water, then run them through the dishwasher on a hot rinse cycle to sterilize. Alternatively, place the bottle or jar, spoon, and grater in a large saucepan filled with water, and boil for 10 minutes, then place on a baking sheet in a 300°F oven to dry.

Open the coconuts by cutting off the tops. Strain the coconut water into your sterilized jar, and set aside. If using a probiotic capsule, open up the capsule. Add the probiotic powder or water kefir grains to the coconut water, then add the ginger and, using the sterilized spoon, stir well (or secure the lid and give it a good swish if using a bottle). Cover with a piece of cheesecloth and a rubber band. Place in the pantry or in a dark spot for 24–48 hours to ferment. The kefir is ready when the water turns from relatively clear to cloudy white.

Taste the kefir after 24–30 hours. Pour some into a glass – it should taste sour, with no sweetness left, like ginger beer. Some batches are fizzier than others, but all are beneficial. If it still tastes sweet, place it back in the pantry for the remaining recommended fermentation time. When you're happy with the flavor, pour through a sterilized sieve to remove the water kefir grains (if using), and return the kefir to the jar. Keep in the fridge for up to 2 months. The water kefir grains can be stored in coconut water in the fridge until you make your next batch of kefir (refresh the coconut water every 5 days or so).

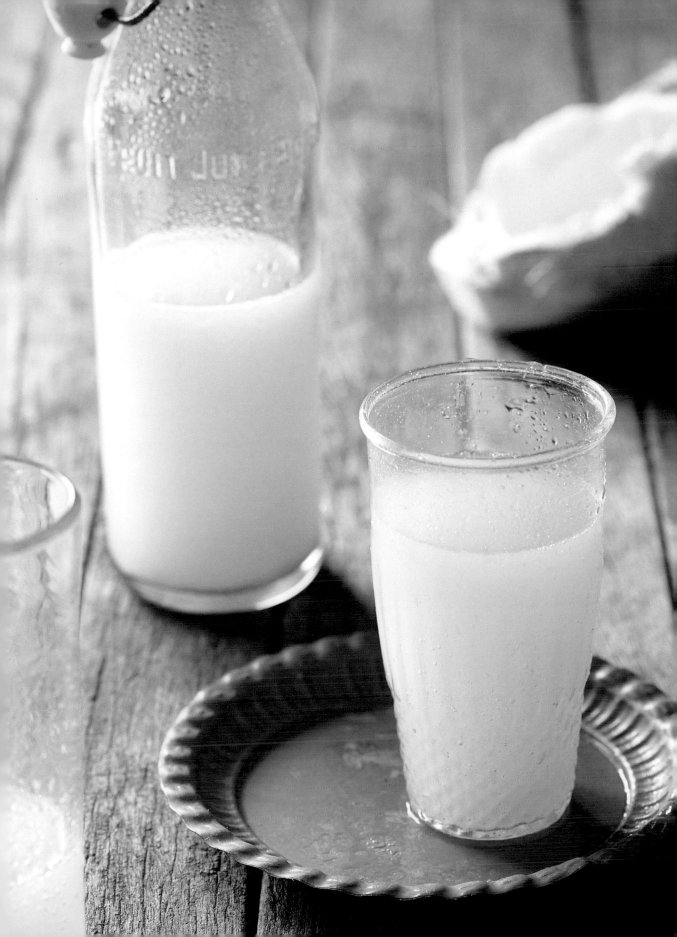

COCONUT AND TURMERIC KEFIR
WITH GINGER AND CAYENNE

SERVES 4

This is supercharged water kefir. It has all the probiotic and enzymic benefits of water kefir, with the added digestive-stimulating and anti-inflammatory properties of turmeric and cayenne pepper. If you are sensitive to chile or doing AIP, just leave out the cayenne.

3 young coconuts*
1–2 probiotic capsules or water kefir grains*
1½ tablespoons finely grated fresh turmeric or 1½ teaspoons ground turmeric
1½ tablespoons finely grated ginger
pinch of cayenne pepper (or to taste)

* See Glossary

MAKE AIP FRIENDLY

Omit: cayenne

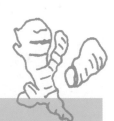

TIPS

It is imperative to sterilize all materials that come into contact with the kefir. You want only good bacteria to flourish, so boil all utensils and wash your hands very well.

Glass jars and storage bottles are preferable to plastic, since kefir actually eats away at plastic. If the kefir eats the plastic, you in turn consume plastic. Limited contact is fine, but prolonged exposure is discouraged.

Only use coconut water from young coconuts. Store-bought coconut water will not work, as the product is pasteurized.

Never add probiotics or water kefir grains to refrigerated water, as it will drastically slow or stunt the fermentation process.

You will need a 1-quart glass bottle or jar for this recipe. Wash the bottle or jar, a nonmetallic spoon, and a grater in very hot soapy water, then run them through the dishwasher on a hot rinse cycle to sterilize. Alternatively, place the bottle or jar, spoon, and grater in a large saucepan filled with water, and boil for 10 minutes, then place on a baking sheet in a 300°F oven to dry.

Open the coconuts by cutting off the tops. Strain the coconut water into your sterilized jar. If using a probiotic capsule, open up the capsule. Add the probiotic powder or water kefir grains to the coconut water. Add the turmeric, ginger, and cayenne. Stir well using the sterilized spoon (or secure the lid and give it a good swish if using a bottle). Cover with a piece of cheesecloth and a rubber band. Place in the pantry or in a dark spot for 24–48 hours to ferment. The kefir is ready when the water turns from relatively clear to cloudy white.

Taste the kefir after 24–30 hours. Pour some into a glass – it should taste sour, with no sweetness left, like coconut "beer." Some batches are fizzier than others, but all are beneficial. If it still tastes sweet, place it back in the pantry for the remaining recommended fermentation time. When you're happy with the flavor, pour through a sieve to remove the water kefir grains (if using), and return the kefir to the jar. Keep in the fridge for up to 2 months. The water kefir grains can be stored in coconut water in the fridge until you make your next batch of kefir (refresh the coconut water every 5 days or so).

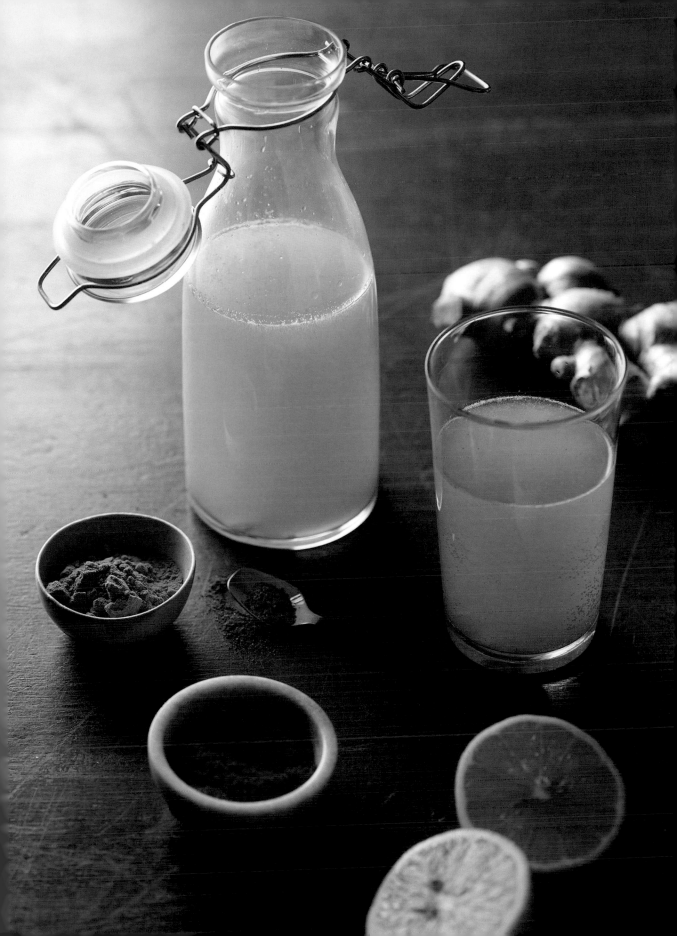

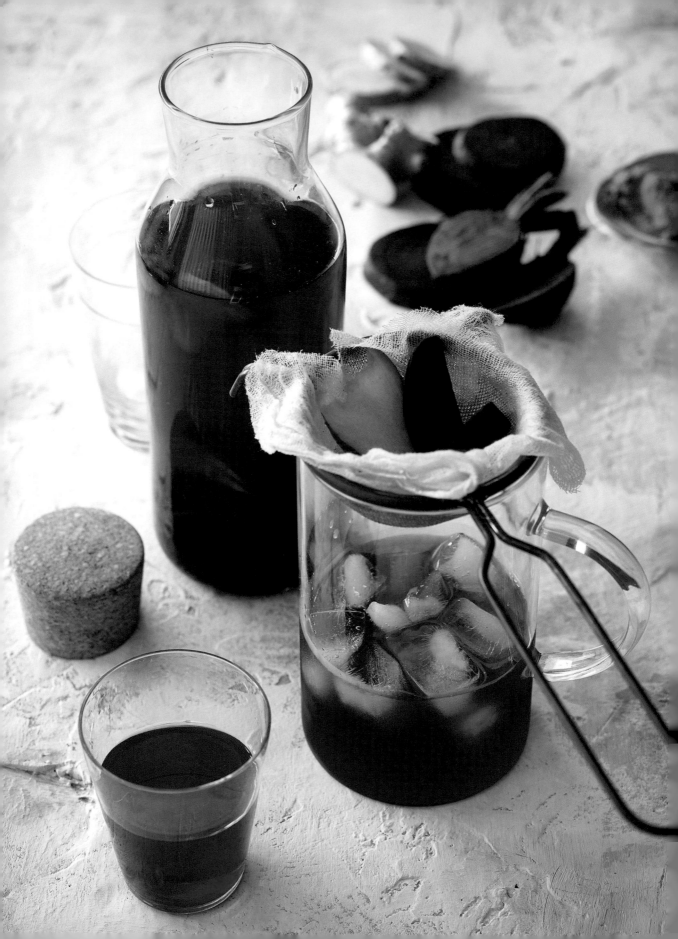

BEET, GINGER, AND TURMERIC KVASS

SERVES 4-6

One of my all-time favorite ferments, this earthy, liver-loving tonic is rich in iron and betaine (which helps increase oxygen delivery to muscle cells), and is great for supporting liver detoxification.

2–4 beets
2-inch piece of ginger, sliced
1 tablespoon sea salt or Himalayan salt*
1 teaspoon ground turmeric or
   1-inch piece of fresh turmeric, sliced
⅓ packet vegetable starter culture*
   or 3 tablespoons sauerkraut brine
   (to make your own sauerkraut,
   see page 94)

* See Glossary

AIP FRIENDLY

You will need a sterilized 1½-quart preserving jar with an airlock lid for this recipe. You will also need to sterilize the knife, chopping board, glass measuring cup, and stainless-steel spoon you will be using. To do this, wash the jar and utensils in very hot soapy water, then run them through a hot rinse cycle in the dishwasher.

Wash and scrub the beets (peel them if they are not organic). Chop the beets into ½-inch cubes and combine the beets and ginger in the jar. Mix the salt, turmeric, 1 cup filtered water, and the starter culture or sauerkraut brine in a glass measuring cup, then pour into the jar.

Fill the jar with filtered water, leaving ¾ inch free at the top. Cover the jar with a piece of cheesecloth held down with an elastic band (so you can strain the liquid out later) and secure the lid. Leave on the kitchen counter at room temperature for 3–5 days to ferment. Chill before drinking. The kvass will keep for 2 weeks in the fridge once opened.

TIPS

If you don't have sauerkraut brine or starter culture, you can double the amount of salt, though this will take double the amount of time to ferment.

For a basic beet kvass recipe, simply omit the ginger and turmeric.

FIRE TONIC

SERVES 12–15

Our fire tonic is a powerful combination of warming, digestive-stimulating herbs in a base of unpasteurized apple cider vinegar. This is a tonic to stoke your digestive fire (acid and enzyme production). Unlike other fire tonic recipes, this one does not contain any chile, which can irritate the gut.

---

2 cups apple cider vinegar,
    plus extra if needed
10 garlic cloves, roughly chopped
4 ounces fresh horseradish, roughly
    chopped
4 ounces ginger, roughly chopped
1 celery rib, chopped
1 carrot, chopped
1 onion, chopped
1-inch piece of fresh turmeric, chopped,
    or 1 teaspoon ground turmeric
1 tablespoon mustard seeds
a few flat-leaf parsley stalks,
    roughly chopped
a few rosemary sprigs, roughly chopped
a few oregano sprigs, roughly chopped
a few thyme sprigs, roughly chopped
1 tablespoon juniper berries*
1 tablespoon black peppercorns
3 fresh bay leaves
1 tablespoon licorice root sticks*
1 teaspoon sea salt

* See Glossary

MAKE AIP FRIENDLY

Omit: mustard seeds, juniper berries, and black peppercorns

You will need a 1½-quart preserving jar with an airlock lid for this recipe. Wash the jar and utensils thoroughly in very hot soapy water, then run them through the dishwasher on a hot rinse cycle to sterilize. Alternatively, place them in a large saucepan filled with water and boil for 10 minutes, then place on a baking sheet in a 300°F oven to dry.

Combine all the ingredients in a glass or stainless-steel bowl and mix well. Fill the jar with the vegetable and herb mix, pressing down well with a large spoon or potato masher to remove any air pockets. The vegetables and herbs should be completely submerged in the liquid, so add more vinegar if necessary. Add a small glass weight (a shot glass is ideal) to keep everything submerged. Close the lid, then wrap a kitchen towel around the jar to block out the light.

Store the jar in a dark place with a temperature of 60–73°F for 14 days. (You can place the jar in a cooler to maintain a more consistent temperature.)

Strain the tonic into a clean jar with a lid. Discard the vegetables, herbs, and spices. Chill the fire tonic before serving. Refrigerate, unopened, for up to 12 months. Once opened, the tonic will last for 6–9 months in the fridge.

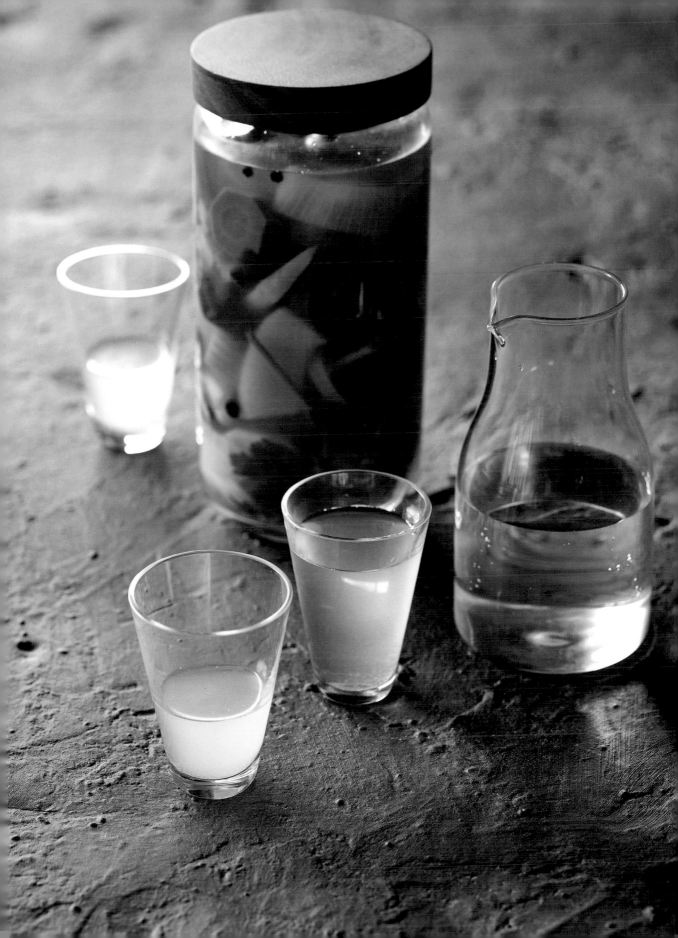

BASICS

AIOLI

MAKES ABOUT 1⅔ CUPS

2 roasted garlic cloves
2 egg yolks
1 teaspoon Dijon mustard
1 tablespoon apple cider vinegar
juice of ½ lemon
1⅓ cups extra-virgin olive oil,
   plus extra if needed
sea salt and freshly ground black pepper

Combine the garlic, egg yolks, mustard, vinegar, lemon juice, and olive oil in a glass jug or jar and, using a handheld blender, blend until thick and creamy. Alternatively, place the garlic, egg yolks, mustard, vinegar and lemon juice in the bowl of a food processor and process until combined. With the motor running, slowly pour in the olive oil in a thin stream and process until the aioli is thick and creamy. Add extra olive oil if the aioli is too thick. Season with salt and pepper. Store in an airtight container in the fridge for 4–5 days.

ALMOND MILK

MAKES 1 QUART

1 cup almonds (activated if possible*)

*See Glossary

You will need a 1-quart glass bottle for this recipe. Wash the bottle well in very hot soapy water, then run it through the dishwasher on a hot rinse cycle to sterilize.

Place the almonds in a blender, add 1 quart filtered water and blend for a couple of minutes until smooth.

Line a bowl with a piece of cheesecloth so that the cheesecloth hangs over the rim (alternatively, use a nut milk bag). Pour the blended almonds and water into the cheesecloth-lined bowl. Pick up the edges of the cheesecloth, bring together, and twist to squeeze out all the milk. (The leftover solids can be used to make bliss balls or in place of almond meal or other nut meals in baking recipes.)

Pour the almond milk into the sterilized bottle, cover, and place in the fridge. Give the bottle a good shake each time you want to use it. Almond milk will last, stored in the refrigerator, for 3–4 days.

CASHEW CHEESE

MAKES ⅔ CUP

1 cup cashew nuts
2 teaspoons lemon juice
½ teaspoon sea salt
pinch of freshly ground black pepper

Soak the cashews in 3 cups filtered water for 1–4 hours. Drain and rinse well.

Place the cashews in the bowl of a food processor, add the lemon juice, salt, and pepper and pulse for a minute to combine. Add 3 tablespoons filtered water and continue to process until smooth. Store in an airtight glass container in the fridge for 5–7 days.

CAULIFLOWER RICE

SERVES 4

1 head of cauliflower, florets and stems
    roughly chopped
2 tablespoons coconut oil
sea salt and freshly ground black pepper

Put the cauliflower in the bowl of a food processor and pulse into tiny pieces that look like rice.

Melt the coconut oil in a large frying pan over medium heat. Add the cauliflower and cook until softened, 4–6 minutes. Season with salt and pepper, and serve.

MAKE AIP FRIENDLY

Omit: black pepper

CRISPY SHALLOTS

MAKES 2–4 TABLESPOONS

1 cup coconut oil or good-quality animal fat*
4–8 shallots, thinly sliced

*See Glossary

Melt the oil in a small saucepan over medium heat. Add the shallots and cook until golden, 2–3 minutes. Remove with a slotted spoon and drain on paper towels. (You can re-use the oil for sautéing vegetables or cooking meat, chicken, or fish.)

AIP FRIENDLY

FERMENTED HOT CHILE SAUCE

MAKES 1 x 1½-QUART JAR

1 packet vegetable starter culture*
3–3½ pounds long red chiles
5 garlic cloves, peeled
2 tablespoons honey
2 teaspoons sea salt

* See Glossary

You will need a 1½-quart preserving jar with an airlock lid for this recipe. Wash the jar and all the utensils you will be using in very hot water, then run them through a hot rinse cycle in the dishwasher to sterilize.

Dissolve the starter culture in filtered water according to the packet instructions (the amount of water will depend on the brand).

Place the starter culture and all the remaining ingredients in the bowl of a food processor, and process to a fine paste. Spoon into the preserving jar, close the lid to seal, then wrap a kitchen towel around the jar to block out the light, leaving the airlock exposed.

Store in a dark place with a temperature of 60–73°F for 5–7 days. (You can place the jar in a cooler to maintain a more consistent temperature.)

After the chile paste has bubbled and brewed for about a week, set a fine sieve over a bowl, tip the chile paste into the sieve, and press down with a wooden spoon to extract as much chile sauce as possible.

Pour the sauce from the bowl into a clean 1-quart jar, seal, and store in the refrigerator. The sauce will keep for several months in the fridge.

FERMENTED MUSTARD

MAKES 1 CUP

¾ cup sauerkraut brine (to make your own sauerkraut, see page 94)

1 cup mixed brown and yellow mustard seeds (brown seeds are spicier)

1 shallot, peeled

2 garlic cloves, peeled

1 tablespoon maple syrup

sea salt

You will need a 1-cup preserving jar with an airlock lid for this recipe. Wash the jar and your utensils thoroughly in very hot water, then run them through a hot rinse cycle in the dishwasher.

Combine the sauerkraut brine, mustard seeds, shallot, and garlic in a glass or stainless-steel bowl, cover with a plate, and allow to soak at room temperature overnight.

The next day, combine the soaked seed mixture with the maple syrup in the bowl of a food processor. If you like whole seeds in your mustard, process for about 30 seconds; if you like a smoother mustard, process for longer. Add salt to taste. Store in the preserving jar in the fridge for up to 3 months.

MACADAMIA MILK

MAKES 1 QUART

1 cup macadamia nuts

You will need a 1-quart glass bottle for this recipe. Wash the bottle well in very hot soapy water, then run it through the dishwasher on a hot rinse cycle to sterilize.

Place the macadamia nuts in a bowl, cover with 1 quart filtered water, and soak for 8 hours or overnight. Drain and rinse well.

Place the nuts and 1 quart filtered water in a high-powered blender and blend until smooth. Line a bowl with a piece of cheesecloth so that the cheesecloth hangs over the edge of the bowl (alternatively, use a nut milk bag). Pick up the edges of the cheesecloth, bring them together, and twist to squeeze out all the milk. (The leftover solids can be used to make bliss balls or in place of almond meal or other nut meals in baking recipes.) Pour the nut milk into the sterilized bottle, then refrigerate until ready to use. Shake the bottle before each use, as the milk will settle and separate over time. Macadamia nut milk will keep in the fridge for 3–4 days.

MAYONNAISE IN 30 SECONDS

MAKES ABOUT 2 CUPS

4 egg yolks
2 teaspoons Dijon mustard
1 tablespoon apple cider vinegar
1 tablespoon lemon juice
1⅔ cup extra-virgin olive oil or macadamia
    oil, or a combination of both
sea salt and freshly ground black pepper

Place the egg yolks, mustard, vinegar, lemon juice, olive oil, and a pinch of salt in a glass jug or jar, and blend with a handheld blender until smooth and creamy. Season with salt and pepper. Alternatively, place the egg yolks, mustard, vinegar, lemon juice, and a pinch of salt in the bowl of a food processor, and process until combined. With the motor running, slowly pour in the olive oil in a thin stream and process until the mayonnaise is thick and creamy. Season with salt and pepper. Store in a sealed glass jar in the fridge for 4–5 days.

MINT JELLY

MAKES 2 CUPS

2 Granny Smith apples, cored and chopped
    but not peeled
1 tablespoon lemon juice
2 large handfuls mint leaves
1½ tablespoons powdered gelatin, soaked
    in 3 tablespoons water to allow the
    granules to soften and expand
3 tablespoons honey, or to taste

MAKE AIP FRIENDLY

Omit: honey
Substitute: 2½ tablespoons freshly squeezed
pear juice in place of honey

Place the apples, 2 cups filtered water, the lemon juice, and 1 handful of the mint leaves in a saucepan, and bring to a simmer. Cook over medium-low heat until the apple is soft, 10 minutes. Remove from the heat, add the gelatin mixture and honey, and stir until the gelatin dissolves. Let cool completely. Place the apple mixture in the bowl of a food processor, and blend until smooth. Pass through a fine sieve and discard the leftover pulp.

Finely chop the remaining mint and mix into the apple mixture. Pour into a glass jar, cover, and refrigerate until set to a wobbly jelly consistency, 4 hours. Give it a good mix before serving.

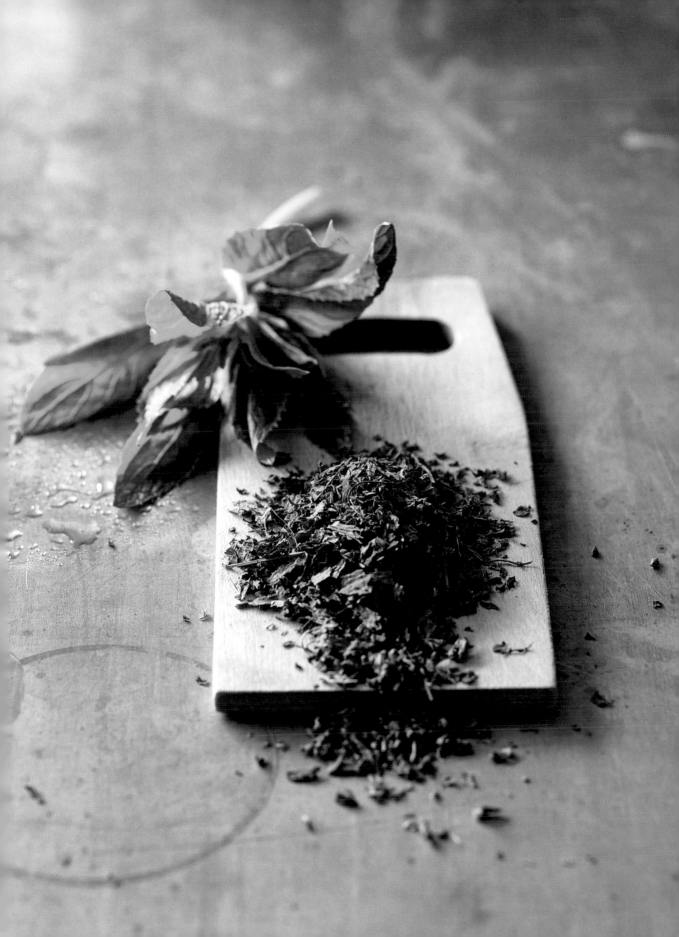

NAM JIM DRESSING

MAKES ABOUT ¾ CUP

4 red Asian shallots, chopped

2 long red chiles, halved lengthwise, seeded, and chopped

2 garlic cloves, chopped

1-inch piece of ginger, chopped

1 teaspoon chopped cilantro root

⅔ cup lime juice

1 tablespoon coconut sugar

2½ tablespoons fish sauce

Pound the shallots, chiles, garlic, ginger, and cilantro root to a paste using a large mortar and pestle. Add the lime juice and mix well. Mix in the coconut sugar and fish sauce, taste, and adjust the seasoning if necessary, so that the dressing is a balance of hot, sour, salty, and sweet. Strain through a sieve and discard the pulp. Store in an airtight glass jar in the fridge for 3–4 weeks.

NOMATO SAUCE

MAKES 2½ QUARTS

1 tablespoon coconut oil

½ large onion, chopped

2 garlic cloves, finely chopped

6 large carrots, chopped

2 large beets (about 1⅓ pounds), chopped

1 quart (4 cups) Chicken or Beef Bone Broth (pages 116 and 121) or water

2 teaspoons dried Italian herbs

1 bay leaf

2 tablespoons lemon juice

sea salt and freshly ground black pepper

Melt the oil in a large saucepan over medium heat. Add the onion and cook, stirring occasionally, until soft. Add the garlic, carrot, and beets and cook, stirring occasionally, for 5 minutes. Pour in enough broth or water to just cover the vegetables, then add the dried herbs, bay leaf, and lemon juice. Stir well. Bring to a boil, reduce the heat to low, and simmer until the veggies are very soft, 30–40 minutes. Remove the bay leaf. Allow the sauce to cool, then blend with a handheld blender until smooth. Add more broth or water if needed, and season to taste. Store in an airtight container in the refrigerator for up to 4–5 days, or freeze for up to 3 months.

SPICED PECANS

MAKES ABOUT 1 CUP

1 tablespoon coconut oil

2 teaspoons honey

1 cup pecan halves (activated if possible*)

1 teaspoon freshly grated nutmeg

½ teaspoon ground allspice

¼ teaspoon ground cinnamon

¼ teaspoon ground cardamom

Heat a frying pan over medium-high heat. Add the coconut oil and honey and cook until melted. Stir in the pecans, sprinkle with the spices, and toss to coat evenly. Cook, stirring constantly, until the pecans are fragrant and brown, about 5 minutes. Watch carefully to make sure they don't burn! Pour out onto a plate and let cool.

* See Glossary

SRIRACHA CHILE SAUCE

MAKES 2⅓ CUPS

1½ pounds long red chiles, seeded and
    roughly chopped
8 garlic cloves, crushed
¼ cup apple cider vinegar
3 tablespoons tomato paste
1 large medjool date, pitted
2 tablespoons fish sauce
1½ teaspoons sea salt

Combine all the ingredients in the bowl of a food processor and process until smooth. Pour into a saucepan and bring to a boil over high heat, stirring occasionally. Reduce the heat to low and simmer, stirring now and then, until the sauce is vibrant and red, 5–10 minutes. Remove from the heat and let cool. Transfer to a large airtight glass jar and refrigerate for up to 2 weeks.

TOMATO KETCHUP

MAKES ABOUT 1¼ CUPS

⅔ cup tomato paste
1 tablespoon apple cider vinegar
1 teaspoon garlic powder
1 teaspoon onion powder
½ teaspoon ground cinnamon
¼ teaspoon freshly grated nutmeg
1 teaspoon honey
⅛ teaspoon ground cloves

Mix the tomato paste with ½ cup filtered water in a small saucepan and place over medium heat. Bring to a simmer, then remove from the heat and stir in the remaining ingredients until fully incorporated. Cool and store in an airtight glass jar in the fridge for 4 weeks.

TURKISH SPICE MIX

MAKES ¾ CUP

3½ tablespoons ground cumin
3 tablespoons dried mint
3 tablespoons dried oregano
2 tablespoons sweet paprika
2 tablespoons freshly ground
    black pepper
2 teaspoons hot paprika

Combine all the ingredients in a bowl and mix well. Store in an airtight container in the pantry for up to 12 months.

TURMERIC OIL

MAKES ½ CUP

½ cup coconut oil, macadamia oil,
 or good-quality animal fat*
1 teaspoon ground turmeric

* See Glossary

MAKE AIP FRIENDLY

Omit: macadamia oil
Substitute: coconut oil or animal fat in place of
macadamia oil

Melt the oil or fat in a saucepan over low heat. Mix in the turmeric and gently simmer for 10 minutes (do not bring to a boil). Set aside and let cool completely before using. Store the turmeric oil in an airtight container and melt before using. If using animal fat, you will need to store your turmeric oil in the fridge.

TZATZIKI

MAKES ABOUT 2¾ CUPS

2 cups Coconut Yogurt (pages 86 and 88)
1 Persian cucumber (about 8 ounces),
 peeled, seeded, and finely chopped
2 garlic cloves, finely chopped
½ teaspoon sea salt
30 mint leaves, finely chopped
1½ tablespoons lemon juice

AIP FRIENDLY

Mix all the ingredients in a bowl to combine. Store in an airtight container in the fridge for 5–6 days.

WHIPPED COCONUT CREAM

MAKES 3 CUPS

2 x 13.5-ounce cans coconut cream
2 tablespoons honey, or to taste

Place the unopened cans of coconut cream in a stainless-steel bowl and refrigerate overnight.

Open the cans of chilled coconut cream, scoop out the hardened cream layer, and place in the chilled bowl with the honey. Store the leftover coconut water in a sealed container in the fridge for another use.

Use an electric mixer to whip the coconut cream and honey on high until soft peaks form (about 3 minutes). Allow to set for 40 minutes in the fridge.

MAKE AIP FRIENDLY

Omit: honey

WORCESTERSHIRE SAUCE

MAKES ½ CUP

½ cup apple cider vinegar
2 ½ tablespoons tamari or coconut aminos*
½ teaspoon ground ginger
½ teaspoon mustard powder
½ teaspoon onion powder
½ teaspoon garlic powder
¼ teaspoon ground cinnamon
¼ teaspoon freshly ground black pepper

* See Glossary

Combine all the ingredients with 2 tablespoons filtered water in a saucepan and, stirring occasionally, bring to a boil over medium heat. Turn down the heat to low and simmer for 10 minutes. Remove from the heat and let cool. Pour into a sterilized bottle and store in the fridge for up to 1 month.

MAKE AIP FRIENDLY

Omit: tamari, mustard powder, and black pepper
Substitute: coconut aminos in place of tamari

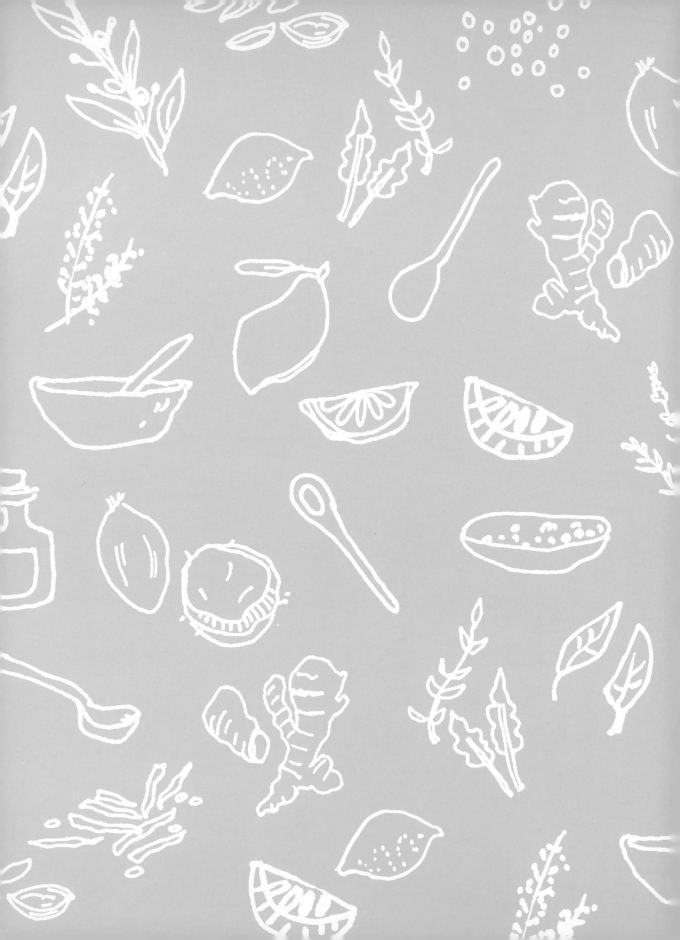

HOME REMEDIES

ENLIVEN-ME BATH SALTS

SWEET DREAMS BATH SALTS

ESSENTIAL OILS USED IN NATUROPATHY
TO PROMOTE GUT HEALING

THE TUMMY COMFORTER

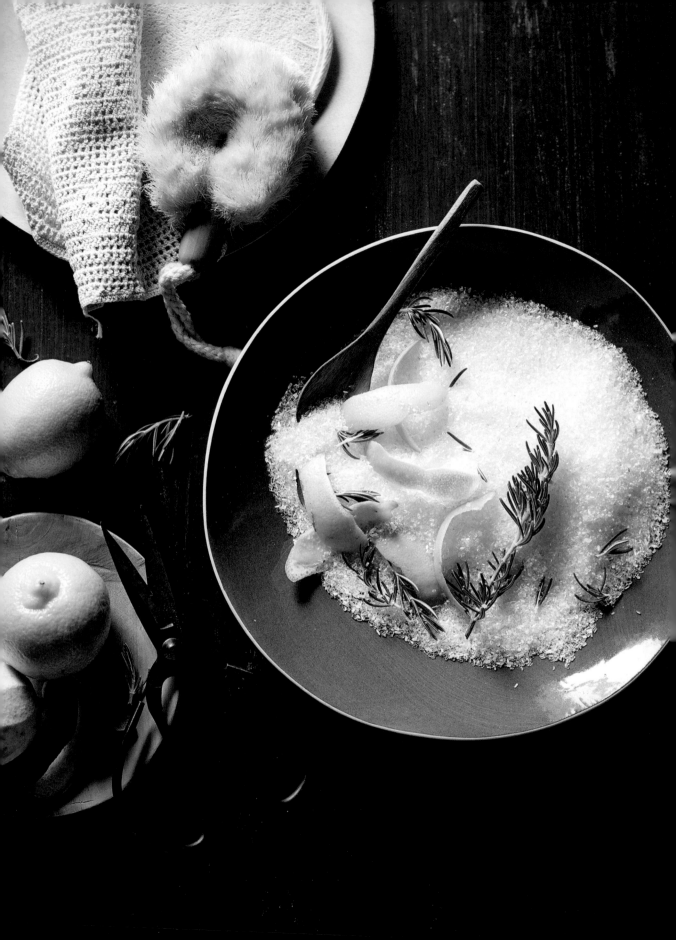

ENLIVEN-ME BATH SALTS

MAKES 2¼ CUPS

The perfect way to detox, relax, and lift your energy levels all at once. Epsom salts provide magnesium for relaxation of nerves and muscles and sulphate to support detoxification. Lemon and rosemary essential oils uplift the senses and are wonderful to use as a simple pick-me-up on days where you are feeling down in spirit or dull in mind.

---

3 tablespoons chopped rosemary leaves
zest of 1 lemon
6–8 drops of lemon essential oil (optional)
6–8 drops of rosemary essential oil
  (optional)
2 cups Epsom salts

Mix all the ingredients together to combine. Store in an airtight container for up to 6 months.

When ready to use, add ¼ cup of bath salt mixture to your hot bath, and feel your body unwind.

SWEET DREAMS BATH SALTS

MAKES 1⅓ CUPS

The benefits of detoxification and relaxation from Epsom salts combined with the petals of calming herbs. Let the aroma infuse your senses and carry you off to a blissful sleep.

---

1 cup Epsom salts
2 tablespoons dried chamomile flowers*
2 tablespoons dried lavender buds
1 tablespoon dried rose petals

* See Glossary

Mix all the ingredients together until well combined. Store in an airtight container for up to 6 months.

When ready to use, add ¼ cup of bath salt mixture to your hot bath, and feel your body unwind.

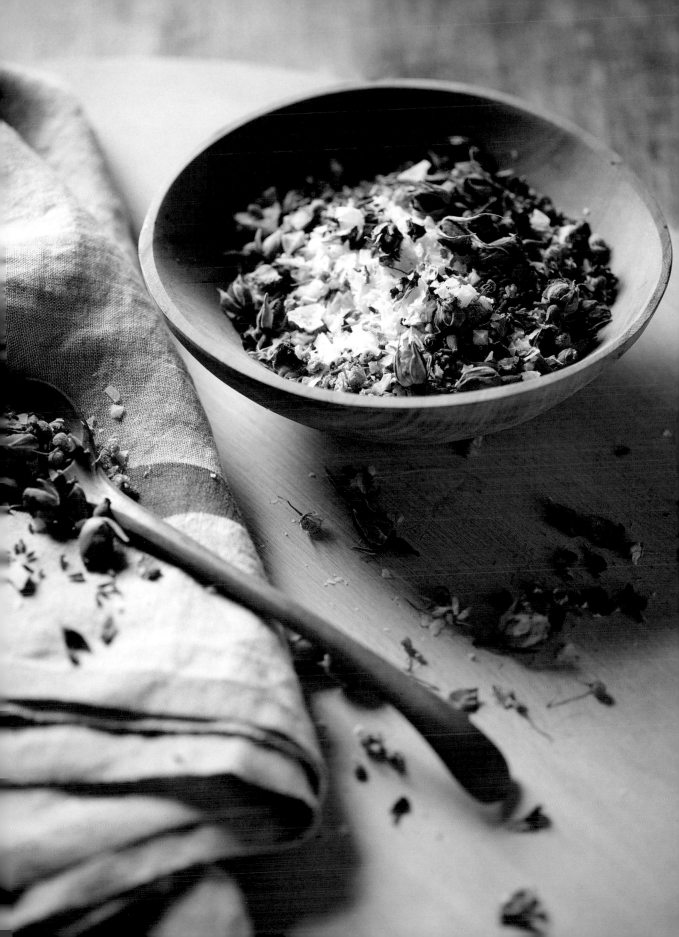

Essential oils used in naturopathy to promote gut healing

Essential oils are an incredibly potent extract of the volatile oils from plants. They have useful therapeutic properties and should only be used externally, as they can be toxic if ingested.

It may seem strange to inhale or apply something to your skin in order to heal your gut, but these are both rapid routes of absorption into the bloodstream. In fact, substances we inhale and rub onto our skin can actually be more potent than those we ingest. When we consume food, drinks, supplements, and medications, molecules from these are absorbed into the bloodstream sent straight to the liver via the hepatic artery, where some breakdown of the molecules takes place, before they are sent around the rest of the body. On the other hand, when inhalants and topical preparations are absorbed into the bloodstream, they make their way around the body untouched before getting to the liver for breakdown. This is why I also suggest that all your skincare should be free of toxic chemicals and synthetic fragrances!

When applying essential oils to the skin, they should be diluted in a carrier oil such as coconut, jojoba, macadamia, rosehip, or olive oil (all cold-pressed, extra-virgin, and organic). Note the difference below between massaging the stomach (top center of the abdomen just below the sternum) and the whole abdomen. For abdominal massage, always stroke upwards on the right-hand side, across the top, and down the left-hand side (as this is the direction food/waste is moving in).

SYMPTOM	OIL	APPLICATION
Nausea	2 drops ginger + 1 drop lemon in 1 teaspoon carrier oil	Inhale, or gently massage over stomach
	2 drops peppermint + 1 drop ginger in 1 teaspoon carrier oil	Inhale, or gently massage over stomach
	2 drops peppermint + 2 drops lemon balm in 1 teaspoon carrier oil	Inhale, apply to a tissue to sniff, or place in a bowl of piping hot water, then place your head above the bowl and pop a towel over your head to create a steam tent
Irritable Bowel Syndrome	1 drop peppermint + 2 drops chamomile in 1 tablespoon coconut oil	Massage into abdomen
Bloating and gas	2 drops peppermint + 1 drop ginger in 2 tablespoons activated charcoal powder	Inhale, or gently massage over stomach
Candida / Thrush	1 drop thyme + 1 drop clove + 1 drop oregano + 1 drop tea tree in 2 teaspoons coconut oil	Massage into abdomen, or add to a bath
Anxious tummy	2 drops lavender in 2 tablespoons coconut oil	Massage into abdomen

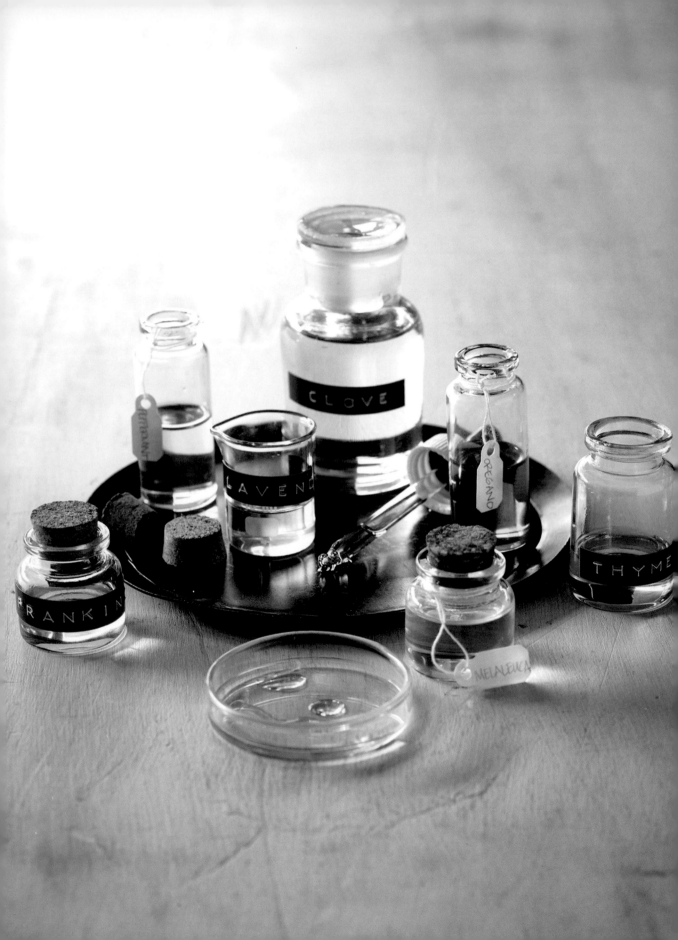

THE TUMMY COMFORTER

MAKES ¼ CUP

Essential oils are absorbed very effectively through the skin into the bloodstream. Abdominal massage with essential oils of chamomile and peppermint (in a base or carrier oil) is effective for helping to relieve intestinal bloating and gas. Always massage the abdomen in a circular motion, stroking up on the right-hand side, across the top to the left, and then down the left-hand side (this follows the same direction as food moving through your system).

2½ tablespoons coconut oil, melted, or sesame oil
50 drops of chamomile essential oil
10–15 drops of peppermint essential oil

Mix the ingredients together in a small glass container (a clean lip balm jar is perfect). Store, tightly sealed, at room temperature for 6 months.

Use about a teaspoon or two to massage in a circular motion on your abdomen.

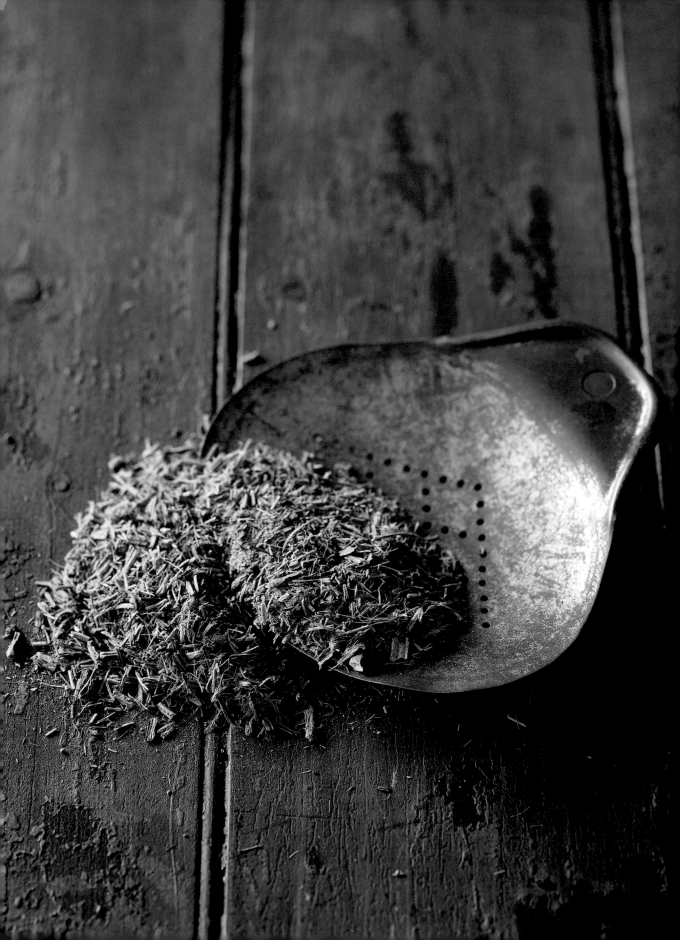

GLOSSARY

ACTIVATED NUTS AND SEEDS

Nuts and seeds are a great source of healthy fats, but they contain phytic acid, which binds to minerals such as iron, zinc, calcium, potassium, and magnesium so that they can't be readily absorbed. Activating nuts and seeds lessens the phytates, so we absorb as many of the good things as possible. Activated nuts and seeds are available from health-food stores. Or, to save money and make your own, simply soak the nuts in filtered water (hard nuts, like almonds, need to soak for 12 hours; softer nuts, like cashews and macadamias, need only 4–6 hours). Rinse the nuts under running water, then spread out on a baking sheet and place in a 120°F oven or dehydrator to dry out. This will take anywhere from 6 to 24 hours, depending on the temperature and the kind of nuts or seeds. Store in an airtight container in the pantry for up to 3 months.

BITTER MELON

Bitter melon, also called bitter gourd, is a member of the gourd family. The cucumber-shaped fruit has soft, uneven skin with irregular lengthwise ridges and, as its name suggests, a bitter flavor. Bitter melon is great in stews, soups, stir-fries, and curries. It can be found in some large supermarkets and Asian grocers, and is best when firm and brightly colored.

BONITO FLAKES

Bonito flakes are made from the bonito fish, which is like a small tuna. The fish is smoked, fermented, dried, and shaved, and the end product looks similar to wood shavings. Bonito flakes are used to garnish Japanese dishes, to make sauces such as ponzu, soups such as miso, and to make the Japanese stock, dashi. You can find bonito flakes in Asian food stores.

CALENDULA

Calendula, better known as pot marigold, is a common garden flower. In naturopathy, calendula petals and flower extracts are used for wound healing, fever treatment, and as a natural skin care, as well in treating inflammation of internal organs and gastrointestinal ulcers. Dried calendula can be bought online, but it's very easy to grow, so why not adorn your garden with beauty and health benefits all in one?

CASSIA BARK

Cassia bark is a type of cinnamon that originates from southern China and is cultivated throughout Southeast Asia. Cassia is the most common type of cinnamon found on supermarket shelves, and varies from Ceylon or "true" cinnamon in a number of ways. Quills from cassia bark are thick and not easily broken, while Ceylon cinnamon sticks have thin, fibrous layers. Cassia also has a stronger and spicier taste. Both cassia and Ceylon cinnamon have been used medicinally for thousands of years to treat colds, arthritis, high blood pressure, and abdominal pain.

CAT'S CLAW BARK OR POWDER

Cat's claw is a woody vine found in Central and South America. Be careful not to confuse it with cat's foot. Cat's claw helps the body cleanse the entire intestinal tract. Do not use cat's claw if you are pregnant or planning to fall pregnant (see Note page 284). Cat's claw is found in health-food stores and online.

CHAMOMILE FLOWERS

Chamomile refers to a wide range of daisy-like plants from the Asteraceae family. Chamomile has been used for its anti-inflammatory and calming effects since ancient times. Although most commonly consumed as a tea, chamomile can be used both internally and externally and has been known to relieve cold symptoms, reduce inflammation, promote relaxation, and aid digestion. Dried chamomile flowers can be found in most health-food stores.

COCONUT AMINOS

Made from coconut sap, coconut aminos is similar in flavor to a light soy sauce. Because it is free of both soy and gluten, it makes a great paleo alternative to soy sauce and tamari. Coconut aminos is available at health-food stores.

COCONUT OIL

Coconut oil is extracted from the meat of mature coconuts. It has a high smoke point, making it great for cooking at high temperatures. The viscosity of coconut oil changes depending on the temperature, and ranges from liquid to solid. Although coconut oil is high in saturated fats, they are mainly medium-chain saturated fatty acids, which means the body can use them quickly and does not have to store them. Coconut oil is available from supermarkets and health-food stores. Look for virgin cold-pressed varieties as these have had the least amount of processing.

GELATIN

Gelatin is the cooked form of collagen, which is a protein found in bones, skin, and connective tissue. I always choose gelatin sourced from organic, grass-fed beef, such as Great Lakes Gelatin Company. Vegetarian substitutes for gelatin include agar agar and carrageen, which are made from two different types of seaweed. Sometimes these aren't as strong as regular gelatin, so you may need to increase the quantity. Some kosher gelatins are also vegan. You can buy gelatin made from organic, grass-fed beef, agar agar and carrageen from health-food stores or online.

GOOD-QUALITY ANIMAL FAT

I use either coconut oil or good-quality animal fats for cooking, as they have high smoke points (meaning they do not oxidize at high temperatures). Some of my favorite animal fats to use are lard (pork fat), tallow (rendered beef fat), rendered chicken fat, and duck fat. These may be hard to find – ask at your local butcher, look online or make your own when making bone broths (see pages 116–124).

JUNIPER BERRIES

Despite their name, juniper berries are actually cones rather than berries. They are purple in color and are most famous for lending their flavor to gin. Juniper berries are fabulous with meat dishes and sauerkrauts or other fermented vegetable dishes. You can buy fresh or dried juniper berries from some health-food stores, specialty food stores or online.

KOMBU SEAWEED

Kombu is a high-protein sea vegetable, rich in calcium, iron, iodine, and dietary fiber. It is salty and savory and plays a vital role in Japanese cuisine. Kombu can be used in a similar way to bay leaves – add them to a stew or curry for a flavor boost, and remove them after cooking. Kombu can be found in Asian grocers, and is mainly sold dried or pickled in vinegar. Dried kombu is often covered with a white powder from natural salts and starch. It is harmless, but can easily be removed with a damp cloth.

LEMON BALM

Lemon balm is a perennial plant in the mint family. It has been used medicinally for more than 2000 years to relieve cramps, gas, and nausea. Research suggests that lemon balm may help decrease stress and anxiety and can reduce the symptoms and recurrence of cold sores. It is a great addition to your herb garden, but you can also find dried lemon balm online and in health-food stores.

LICORICE ROOT POWDER

When ground into a powder, licorice root has a slightly sweet flavor and can be added to smoothies, drinks, and desserts. Licorice root has been used in Chinese medicine for many years, and is believed to help with a wide range of conditions, including digestive problems. You can find it in health-food stores.

MACA POWDER

Maca is a rainforest herb that is high in protein and other nutrients. It is believed to increase energy and support the immune system. Try adding a spoonful of maca powder to your smoothies for a protein boost.

NORI SEAWEED SHEETS

Nori is a dark green, paper-like, toasted seaweed used in Japanese dishes. Nori provides an abundance of essential nutrients and is rich in vitamins, iron, and other minerals, amino acids, omega-3 and omega-6, and antioxidants. Nori sheets are commonly used to roll sushi, but they can also be added to salads, soups, and many other dishes. You can buy nori sheets from Asian grocers and most supermarkets.

PAU D'ARCO POWDER

Pau d'arco powder is made from the dried bark of the South American pau d'arco tree. It adds a unique flavor to dishes, is high in antioxidants, and is said to boost immune function and help treat fungal infections. You can buy pau d'arco powder from health-food stores.

POMEGRANATE MOLASSES

Pomegranate molasses is a thick, tangy, and glossy reduction of pomegranate juice that is rich in antioxidants. Pomegranate molasses is used in Middle Eastern countries for glazing meat and chicken before roasting, and in sauces, salad dressings, and marinades. You can buy it from Middle Eastern grocers and some delis.

PROBIOTIC CAPSULES

Probiotic capsules contain live bacteria that can help to regulate digestion, clear up yeast infections, and assist with conditions such as irritable bowel syndrome. These capsules need to be kept in the fridge. They can be swallowed whole, or opened up and used to ferment drinks such as kefir. Probiotic capsules can be found at pharmacies and health-food stores.

SALT

I use sea salt or Himalayan salt in my cooking, as they are less processed than table salt, contain more minerals, and have a lovely crunchy texture. Himalayan salt is light pink in color due to the presence of a number of different minerals, including iron, magnesium, calcium, and copper. You can buy sea salt and Himalayan salt at supermarkets and health-food stores.

SLIPPERY ELM POWDER

Slippery elm powder comes from the inner bark of the slippery elm tree. It is believed to help the digestive system, and some people also take slippery elm to help with coughs and skin problems. Slippery elm doesn't have a particularly strong flavor, so it can be added to smoothies, juices, or sauces. You can buy it from heath-food stores and pharmacies.

SUMAC

Sumac is a spice made from red sumac berries that have been dried and crushed. It has antimicrobial properties and a tangy, lemony flavor, which makes it ideal for pairing with seafood. It's also delicious in salad dressings.

TAHINI

Tahini is a paste made from ground sesame seeds. It is an excellent source of protein, copper, and manganese, and a good source of calcium, magnesium, iron, phosphorus, vitamin B1, zinc, selenium, and essential fatty acids. Tahini is commonly used in North African, Greek, Turkish, and Middle Eastern cuisine. I prefer unhulled tahini, which has a stronger flavor, but there are hulled varieties available, as well as black tahini made from black sesame seeds. Buy it from supermarkets and heath-food stores.

TAPIOCA FLOUR

Tapioca flour is made by grinding up the dried root of the manioc (also known as cassava) plant. It can be used to thicken dishes or in gluten-free baking. You can find tapioca flour at health-food stores and some supermarkets.

VEGETABLE STARTER CULTURE

A vegetable starter culture is a preparation used to kickstart the fermentation process when culturing vegetables and yogurts. I use a broad-spectrum starter sourced from organic vegetables rather than one grown from dairy sources, as this ensures the highest number of living, active bacteria and produces consistently successful results free of pathogens. Vegetable starter culture usually comes in packets and can be purchased at health-food stores or online. You can also get fresh, nondairy starter cultures for yogurt and kefir (we recommend kulturedwellness.com).

WAKAME SEAWEED

Wakame is an edible seaweed used in Japanese, Korean, and Chinese cuisine. It's great in soups, salads, and stir-fries. Wakame contains iron, magnesium, iodine, calcium, and lignans. You can find it in Asian grocers and some supermarkets.

WATTLESEEDS

Wattleseeds are true bush tucker and have been a staple source of protein and carbohydrate for indigenous Australians for thousands of years. Wattleseeds are high in fiber and contain calcium, iron, zinc, and potassium in addition to most vitamins, except for B12, C, and riboflavin. Roasted ground wattleseeds have a nutty flavor and can be used in baking, beverages, sweets, confectionary, and marinades. Wattleseeds can be found in health-food stores and online.

WATER KEFIR GRAINS

Water kefir grains (also known as tibicos, sugar kefir grains, or Japanese water crystals) are used to make fermented drinks. These grains feed off sugar to produce lactic acid, acetic acid, various other acids, and carbon dioxide gas, which carbonates the drink. Water kefir grains can be cultured in a solution of sugar and water, but I like to use young coconut water. Drinks made from water kefir grains can help to balance the bacteria in your stomach, aiding digestion and fighting off harmful bacteria. You can purchase water kefir grains at health-food stores or online.

WOOD EAR FUNGUS

Wood ear fungus, also known as cloud ear, black fungus, or tree ear, is a high-protein, low-calorie mushroom. Wood ear is popular in Asian cooking and can be added to soups, stir-fries, and salads. It is sold fresh in Asian groceries, but is more commonly found in a dried form that needs to be reconstituted before eating.

YACON SYRUP

Extracted from the roots of the South American yacon plant, this sweetener is low in sugar and calories. Dark in color and with a caramel flavor, it can be found at health-food stores.

YOUNG COCONUTS

Young coconuts are harvested at around 5–7 months, and are usually white in color. To open one, cut a circle in the top using a large knife and then prise this circle off. There is usually about 1 cup of coconut water inside. You can then scoop out the soft flesh using a spoon. Look for young coconuts at Asian food stores, health-food stores, and supermarkets.

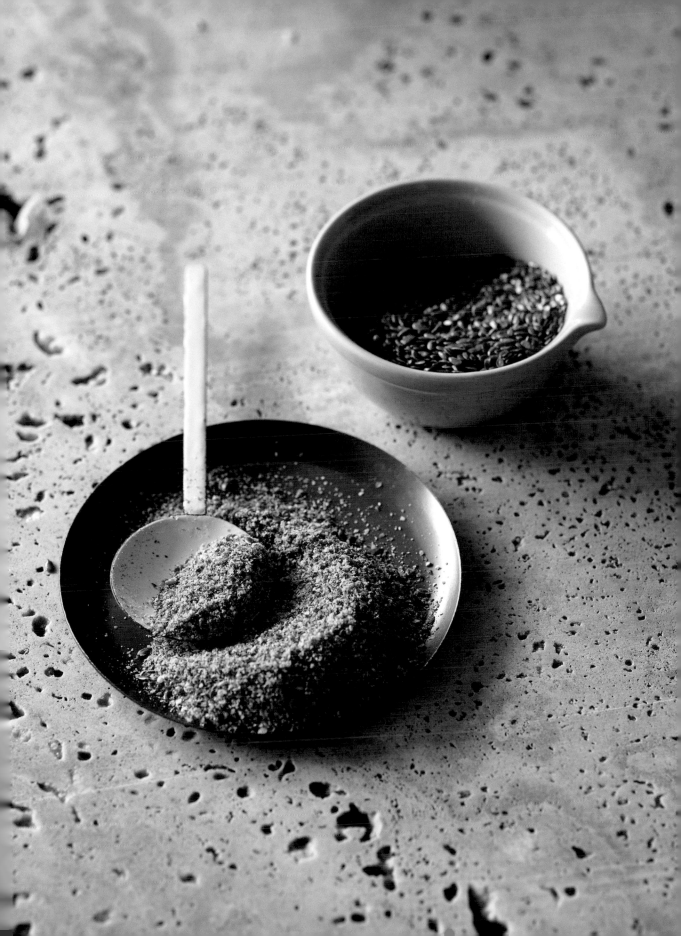

REFERENCES

Acne and gut health

Bowe, W. and Logan, A. (2011). Acne vulgaris, probiotics and the gut-brain-skin axis – back to the future? *Gut Pathogens*, 3(1), p.1.

Gueniche, A., Benyacoub, J., Philippe, D., Bastien, P., Kusy, N., Breton, L., Blum, S. and Castiel-Higounenc, I. (2010). Lactobacillus paracasei CNCM I-2116 (ST11) inhibits substance P-induced skin inflammation and accelerates skin barrier function recovery in vitro. *European Journal of Dermatology*, 20(6), pp.731–737.

Allergies (asthma, eczema) and gut health

Baviera, G., Leoni, M., Capra, L., Cipriani, F., Longo, G., Maiello, N., Ricci, G. and Galli, E. (2014). Microbiota in healthy skin and in atopic eczema. *BioMed Research International*, vol. 2014, Article ID 436921, 6 pages. doi: 10.1155/2014/436921

Cernadas, M. (2011). It takes a microbiome: commensals, immune regulation, and allergy. *American Journal of Respiratory and Critical Care Medicine*, 184(2), pp.149–150.

Hesselmar, B., Sjöberg, F., Saalman, R., Aberg, N., Adlerberth, I. and Wold, A. (2013). Pacifier cleaning practices and risk of allergy development. *Pediatrics*, 131(6), pp.e1829–e1837.

Hoskin-Parr, L., Teyhan, A., Blocker, A. and Henderson, A. (2013). Antibiotic exposure in the first two years of life and development of asthma and other allergic diseases by 7.5 yr: a dose-dependent relationship. *Pediatric Allergy Immunology*, 24(8), pp.762–771.

Jones, M., Walker, M., Ford, A. and Talley, N. (2014). The overlap of atopy and functional gastrointestinal disorders among 23,471 patients in primary care. *Alimentary Pharmacology & Therapeutics*, 40(4), pp.382–391.

Kobayashi, T., Glatz, M., Horiuchi, K., Kawasaki, H., Akiyama, H., Kaplan, D., Kong, H., Amagai, M. and Nagao, K. (2015). Dysbiosis and *Staphylococcus aureus* colonization drives inflammation in atopic dermatitis. *Immunity*, 42(4), pp.756–766.

Powell, N., Huntley, B., Beech, T., Knight, W., Knight, H. and Corrigan, C. (2007). Increased prevalence of gastrointestinal symptoms in patients with allergic disease. *Postgraduate Medical Journal*, 83(977), pp.182–186.

Yap, G., Loo, E., Aw, M., Lu, Q., Shek, L. and Lee, B. (2014). Molecular analysis of infant fecal microbiota in an Asian at-risk cohort-correlates with infant and childhood eczema. *BMC Research Notes*, 7(1), p.166.

Attention Deficit Hyperactivity Disorder (ADHD) and gut health

Bouchard, M., Bellinger, D., Wright, R. and Weisskopf, M. (2010). Attention-deficit/hyperactivity disorder and urinary metabolites of organophosphate pesticides. *Pediatrics*, 125(6), pp.e1270–e1277.

Bradstreet, J., Smith, S., Baral, M. and Rossignol, D. (2010). Biomarker-guided interventions of clinically relevant conditions associated with autism spectrum disorders and attention deficit hyperactivity disorder. *Alternative Medicine Review*, 15(1), pp.15–32.

Esparham, A., Evans, R., Wagner, L. and Drisko, J. (2014). Pediatric integrative medicine approaches to attention deficit hyperactivity disorder (ADHD). *Children*, 1(2), pp.186–207.

Knivsberg, A., Reichelt, K., Høien, T. and Nødland, M. (2002). A randomised, controlled study of dietary intervention in autistic syndromes. *Nutritional Neuroscience*, 5(4), pp.251–261.

Stevens, L., Kuczek, T., Burgess, J., Hurt, E. and Arnold, L. (2011). Dietary sensitivities and ADHD symptoms: thirty-five years of research. *Clinical Pediatrics*, 50(4), pp.279–293.

Autism and gut health

Li, Q. and Zhou, J. (2016). The microbiota–gut–brain axis and its potential therapeutic role in autism spectrum disorder. *Neuroscience*, 2(324), pp.131–139.

Reddy, B. and Saier, M. (2015). Autism and our intestinal microbiota. *Journal of Molecular Microbiology and Biotechnology*, 25(1), pp.51–55.

Autoimmunity and gut health

Fasano, A. (2012). Zonulin, regulation of tight junctions, and autoimmune diseases. *Annals of the New York Academy of Sciences*, 1258(1), pp.25–33.

Lin, R., Zhou, L., Zhang, J. and Wang, B. (2015). Abnormal intestinal permeability and microbiota in patients with autoimmune hepatitis. *International Journal of Clinical and Experimental Pathology*, 8(5), pp.5153–5160.

Luckey, D., Gomez, A., Murray, J., White, B. and Taneja, V. (2013). Bugs & us: the role of the gut in autoimmunity. *The Indian Journal of Medical Research*, 138(5), pp.732–743.

Versini, M., Jeandel, P., Bashi, T., Bizzaro, G., Blank, M. and Shoenfeld, Y. (2015). Unraveling the hygiene hypothesis of helminthes and autoimmunity: origins, pathophysiology, and clinical applications. *BMC Medicine*, 13, pp.81.

Blood–brain barrier

Daneman, R. and Rescigno, M. (2009). The gut immune barrier and the blood–brain barrier: are they so different?. *Immunity*, 31(5), pp.722–735.

Varatharaj, A. and Galea, I. (2016). The blood–brain barrier in systemic inflammation. *Brain, Behavior, and Immunity*. http://dx.doi.org/ 10.1016/j.bbi.2016.03.010

Bone broths and gut health

Barbul, A. (2008). Proline precursors to sustain Mammalian collagen synthesis. *The Journal of Nutrition*, 138(10), pp.2021S–2024S.

Soeters, P. and Grecu, I. (2012). Have we enough glutamine and how does it work? A clinician's view. *Annals of Nutrition and Metabolism*, 60, pp.17–26.

Wu, G., Bazer, F., Burghardt, R., Johnson, G., Kim, S., Knabe, D., Li, P., Li, X., McKnight, J., Satterfield, M. and Spencer, T. (2011). Proline and hydroxyproline metabolism: implications for animal and human nutrition. *Amino Acids*, 40(4), pp.1053–1063.

Brain, gut flora's influence on

Bauer, K., Huus, K. and Finlay, B. (2016). Microbes and the mind: emerging hallmarks of the gut microbiota-brain axis. *Cellular Microbiology*, 18(5), pp.632–644.

Cryan, J. and Dinan, T. (2012). Mind-altering microorganisms: the impact of the gut microbiota on brain and behaviour. *Nature Reviews Neuroscience*, 13(10), pp.701–712.

Farmer, A., Randall, H. and Aziz, Q. (2014). It's a gut feeling: How the gut microbiota affects the state of mind. *The Journal of Physiology*, 592(14), pp.2981-2988.

Galland, L. (2014). The gut microbiome and the brain. *Journal of Medicinal Food*, 17(12), pp.1261-1272.

Mayer, E., Knight, R., Mazmanian, S., Cryan, J. and Tillisch, K. (2014). Gut microbes and the brain: paradigm shift in neuroscience. *The Journal of Neuroscience*, 34(46), pp.15490-15496.

Broccoli and sulforaphane

Moon, J., Kim, J., Ahn, Y. and Shibamoto, T. (2010). Analysis and anti-Helicobacter activity of sulforaphane and related compounds present in broccoli (Brassica oleracea L.) sprouts. *Journal of Agricultural and Food Chemistry*, 58(11), pp.6672-6677.

Choline

Higdon, J., Drake, V. and Delage, B. (2003). *Choline | Linus Pauling Institute | Oregon State University*. [online] Lpi.oregonstate.edu. Available at: http://lpi.oregonstate.edu/mic/other-nutrients/choline [Accessed 1 Jan. 2016].

Depression and gut health

Berk, M., Williams, L., Jacka, F., O'Neil, A., Pasco, J., Moylan, S., Allen, N., Stuart, A., Hayley, A., Byrne, M. and Maes, M. (2013). So depression is an inflammatory disease, but where does the inflammation come from? *BMC Medicine*, 11(200).

Felger, J. and Lotrich, F. (2013). Inflammatory cytokines in depression: neurobiological mechanisms and therapeutic implications. *Neuroscience*, 246, pp.199-229.

Diabetes and gut health

Alkanani, A., Hara, N., Gottlieb, P., Ir, D., Robertson, C., Wagner, B., Frank, D and Zipris, D. (2015). Alterations in intestinal microbiota correlate with susceptibility to type 1 diabetes. *Diabetes*, 64(10), pp.3510-3520.

Boursi, B., Mamtani, R., Haynes, K. and Yang, Y. (2015). The effect of past antibiotic exposure on diabetes risk. *European Journal of Endocrinology*, 172(6), pp.639-648.

Geach, T. (2016). Diabetes: Gut microbiota improves dysglycaemia. *Nature Reviews Endocrinology*, 12, pp.310.

Kostic, A., Gevers, D., Siljander, H., Vatanen, T., Hyötyläinen, T., Hämäläinen, A., Peet, A., Tillmann, V., Pöhö, P., Mattila, I., Lähdesmäki, H., Franzosa, E., Vaarala, O., de Goffau, M., Harmsen, H., Ilonen, J., Virtanen, S., Clish, C., Orešič, M., Huttenhower, C., Knip, M. and Xavier, R. (2015). The dynamics of the human infant gut microbiome in development and in progression toward Type 1 diabetes. *Cell Host & Microbe*, 17(2), pp.260-273.

Romano-Keeler, J., Weitkamp, J. and Moore, D. (2012). Regulatory properties of the intestinal microbiome effecting the development and treatment of diabetes. *Current Opinion in Endocrinology & Diabetes and Obesity*, 19(2), pp.73-80.

Diet and gut health

Bischoff, S., Barbara, G., Buurman, W., Ockhuizen, T., Schulzke, J., Serino, M., Tilg, H., Watson, A. and Wells, J. (2014). Intestinal permeability – a new target for disease prevention and therapy. BMC *Gastroenterology*, 14, p.189.

Resnick, C. (2010). Nutritional protocol for the treatment of intestinal permeability defects and related conditions. *Natural Medicine Journal*, 2(3).

Walker, A., Ince, J., Duncan, S., Webster, L., Holtrop, G., Ze, X., Brown, D., Stares, M., Scott, P., Bergerat, A., Louis, P., McIntosh, F., Johnstone, A., Lobley, G., Parkhill, J. and Flint, H. (2010). Dominant and diet-responsive groups of bacteria within the human colonic microbiota. *The ISME Journal*, 5(2), pp.220-230.

Diverticulitis and gut health

Daniels, L., Budding, A., de Korte, N., Eck, A., Bogaards, J., Stockmann, H., Consten, E., Savelkoul, P. and Boermeester, M. (2014). Fecal microbiome analysis as a diagnostic test for diverticulitis. *European Journal of Clinical Microbiology & Infectious Diseases*, 33(11), pp.1927-1936.

Gueimonde, M., Ouwehand, A., Huhtinen, H., Salminen, E. and Salminen, S. (2007). Qualitative and quantitative analyses of the bifidobacterial microbiota in the colonic mucosa of patients with colorectal cancer, diverticulitis and inflammatory bowel disease. *World Journal of Gastroenterology*, 13(29), pp.3985-3989.

Exercise and gut health

O'Sullivan, O., Cronin, O., Clarke, S., Murphy, E., Molloy, M., Shanahan, F. and Cotter, P. (2015). Exercise and the microbiota. *Gut Microbes*, 6(2), pp.131-136.

Fibromyalgia and gut health

Goebel, A., Buhner, S., Schedel, R., Lochs, H. and Sprotte, G. (2008). Altered intestinal permeability in patients with primary fibromyalgia and in patients with complex regional pain syndrome. *Rheumatology* (Oxford), 47(8), pp.1223-1227.

Gluten, zonulin and leaky gut

Drago, S., El Asmar, R., Di Pierro, M., Grazia Clemente, M., Tripathi, A., Sapone, A., Thakar, M., Iacono, G., Carroccio, A., D'Agate, C., Not, T., Zampini, L., Catassi, C. and Fasano, A. (2006). Gliadin, zonulin and gut permeability: Effects on celiac and non-celiac intestinal mucosa and intestinal cell lines. *Scandinavian Journal of Gastroenterology*, 41(4), pp.408-419.

Lammers, K., Lu, R., Brownley, J., Lu, B., Gerard, C., Thomas, K., Rallabhandi, P., Shea-Donohue, T., Tamiz, A., Alkan, S., Netzel-Arnett, S., Antalis, T., Vogel, S. and Fasano, A. (2008). Gliadin induces an increase in intestinal permeability and zonulin release by binding to the chemokine receptor CXCR3. *Gastroenterology*, 135(1), pp.194-204.e3.

Herbs and spices, antimicrobial activity of

Das, S., Anjeza, C. and Mandal, S. (2012). Synergistic or additive antimicrobial activities of Indian spice and herbal extracts against pathogenic, probiotic and food-spoiler micro-organisms. *International Food Research Journal*, 19(3), pp.1185-1191.

Roby, M., Sarhan, M., Selim, K. and Khalel, K. (2012). Antioxidant and antimicrobial activities of essential oil and extracts of fennel (*Foeniculum vulgare* L.) and chamomile (*Matricaria chamomilla* L.). *Industrial Crops and Products*, 44, pp.437-445. http://dx.doi.org/10.1016/j.indcrop.2012.10.012

Škrinjar, M. and Nemet, N. (2009). Antimicrobial effects of spices and herbs essential oils. *Acta Periodica Technologica*, (40), pp.195-209.

Immune system regulation and the gut

Myles, I. (2014). Fast food fever: reviewing the impacts of the Western diet on immunity. *Nutrition Journal*, 13, p.61.

Peterson, C., Sharma, V., Elmén, L. and Peterson, S. (2015). Immune homeostasis, dysbiosis and therapeutic modulation of the gut microbiota. *Clinical and Experimental Immunology*, 179(3), pp.363–377.

Wu, H. and Wu, E. (2012). The role of gut microbiota in immune homeostasis and autoimmunity. *Gut Microbes*, 3(1), pp.4–14.

Inflammatory Bowel Disease (IBD) and gut health

Antoni, L., Nuding, S., Wehkamp, J. and Strange, E. (2014). Intestinal barrier in inflammatory bowel disease. *World Journal of Gastroenterology*, 20(5), pp.1165–1179.

Gerova, V., Stoynov, S., Katsarov, D. and Svinarov, D. (2011). Increased intestinal permeability in inflammatory bowel diseases assessed by iohexol test. *World Journal of Gastroenterology*, 17(17), pp.2211–2215.

Marchesi, J., Adams, D., Fava, F., Hermes, G., Hirschfield, G., Hold, G., Quraishi, M., Kinross, J., Smidt, H., Tuohy, K., Thomas, L., Zoetendal, E. and Hart, A. (2015). The gut microbiota and host health: a new clinical frontier. *Gut*, 65(2), pp.330–339.

Matsuoka, K. and Kanai, T. (2015). The gut microbiota and inflammatory bowel disease. *Seminars in Immunopathology*, 37(1), pp.47–55.

Miele, L., Valenza, V., La Torre, G., Montalto, M., Cammarota, G., Ricci, R., Mascianà, R., Forgione, A., Gabrieli, M., Perotti, G., Vecchio, F., Rapaccini, G., Gasbarrini, G., Day, C. and Grieco, A. (2009). Increased intestinal permeability and tight junction alterations in nonalcoholic fatty liver disease. *Hepatology*, 49(6), pp.1877–1887.

Persborn, M., Gerritsen, J., Wallon, C., Carlsson, A., Akkermans, L. and Söderholm, J. (2013). The effects of probiotics on barrier function and mucosal pouch microbiota during maintenance treatment for severe pouchitis in patients with ulcerative colitis. *Alimentary Pharmacology & Therapeutics*, 38(7), pp.772–783.

Schicho, R., Marsche, G. and Storr, M. (2015). Cardiovascular complications in inflammatory bowel disease.

Current Drug Targets, 16(3), pp.181–188.

Wall, C., Day, A. and Gearry, R. (2013). Use of exclusive enteral nutrition in adults with Crohn's disease: A review. *World Journal of Gastroenterology*, 19(43), p.7652–7660.

Insulin sensitivity, foods to help improve

Arablou, T., Aryaeian, N., Valizadeh, M., Sharifi, F., Hosseini, A. and Djalali, M. (2014). The effect of ginger consumption on glycemic status, lipid profile and some inflammatory markers in patients with type 2 diabetes mellitus. *International Journal of Food Sciences and Nutrition*, 65(4), pp.515–520.

Davis, P. and Yokoyama, W. (2011). Cinnamon intake lowers fasting blood glucose: meta-analysis. *Journal of Medicinal Food*, 14(9), pp.884–889.

Hlebowicz, J., Darwiche, G., Björgell, O. and Almér, L. (2007). Effect of cinnamon on postprandial blood glucose, gastric emptying, and satiety in healthy subjects. *The American Journal of Clinical Nutrition*, 85(6), pp.1552–1556.

Kim, T., Davis, J., Zhang, A., He, X. and Mathews, S. (2009). Curcumin activates AMPK and suppresses gluconeogenic gene expression in hepatoma cells. *Biochemical and Biophysical Research Communications*, 388(2), pp.377–382.

Mozaffari-Khosravi, H., Talaei, B., Jalali, B., Najarzadeh, A. and Mozayan, M. (2014). The effect of ginger powder supplementation on insulin resistance and glycemic indices in patients with type 2 diabetes: a randomized, double-blind, placebo-controlled trial. *Complementary Therapies in Medicine*, 22(1), pp.9–16.

Sarkkinen, E., Poutanen, K., Mykkänen, H. and Niskanen, L. (2013). Berries reduce postprandial insulin responses to wheat and rye breads in healthy women. *Journal of Nutrition*, 143(4), pp.430–436.

Törrönen, R., Kolehmainen, M., Bamosa, A., Kaatabi, H., Lebdaa, F., Elq, A. and Al-Sultanb, A. (2010). Effect of Nigella sativa seeds on the glycemic control of patients with type 2 diabetes mellitus. *Indian Journal of Physiology and Pharmacology*, 54(4), pp.344–354.

Irritable Bowel Syndrome (IBS) and gut health

Hoveyda, N., Heneghan, C., Mahtani, K.,

Perera, R., Roberts, N. and Glasziou, P. (2009). A systematic review and meta-analysis: probiotics in the treatment of irritable bowel syndrome. *BMC Gastroenterology*, 9, p.15.

Lydiard, R. (2005). Increased prevalence of functional gastrointestinal disorders in panic disorder: clinical and theoretical implications. *CNS Spectrums*, 10(11), pp.899–908.

Moloney, R., O'Mahony, S., Dinan, T. and Cryan, J. (2015). Stress-induced visceral pain: toward animal models of irritable-bowel syndrome and associated comorbidities. *Frontiers in Psychiatry*, 6, pp.15.

Perona, M., Benasayag, R., Perelló, A., Santos, J., Zárate, N., Zárate, P. and Mearin, F. (2005). Prevalence of functional gastrointestinal disorders in women who report domestic violence to the police. *Clinical Gastroenterology and Hepatology*, 3(5), pp.436–441.

Kudzu and gut health

Zhang, R., Hu, Y., Yuan, J. and Wu, D. (2009). Effects of Puerariae radix extract on the increasing intestinal permeability in rat with alcohol-induced liver injury. *Journal of Ethnopharmacology*, 126(2), pp.207–214.

Leaky gut

Kelly, J., Kennedy, P., Cryan, J., Dinan, T., Clarke, G. and Hyland, N. (2015). Breaking down the barriers: the gut microbiome, intestinal permeability and stress-related psychiatric disorders. *Frontiers in Cellular Neuroscience*, 9, pp.392.

Ulluwishewa, D., Anderson, R., McNabb, W., Moughan, P., Wells, J. and Roy, N. (2011). Regulation of tight junction permeability by intestinal bacteria and dietary components. *The Journal of Nutrition*, 141(5), pp.769–776.

Mental health, impact of gut flora on

Bested, A., Logan, A. and Selhub, E. (2013). Intestinal microbiota, probiotics and mental health: from Metchnikoff to modern advances: Part I – autointoxication revisited. *Gut Pathogens*, 5, p.5.

Kiecolt-Glaser, J., Derry, H. and Fagundes, C. (2015). Inflammation: depression fans the flames and feasts on the heat. *The American Journal of Psychiatry*, 172(11), pp.1075–1091.

Saulnier, D., Ringel, Y., Heyman, M., Foster, J., Bercik, P., Shulman, R.,

Versalovic, J., Verdu, E., Dinan, T., Hecht, G. and Guarner, F. (2013). The intestinal microbiome, probiotics and prebiotics in neurogastroenterology. *Gut Microbes*, 4(1), pp.17–27.

Migraine and gut health

Bürk, K., Farecki, M., Lamprecht, G., Roth, G., Decker, P., Weller, M., Rammensee, H. and Oertel, W. (2009). Neurological symptoms in patients with biopsy proven celiac disease. *Movement Disorders*, 24(16), pp.2358–2362.

de Roos, N., Giezenaar, C., Rovers, J., Witteman, B., Smits, M. and van Hemert, S. (2015). The effects of the multispecies probiotic mixture Ecologic®Barrier on migraine: results of an open-label pilot study. *Beneficial Microbes*, 6(5), pp.641–646.

van Hemert, S., Breedveld, A., Rovers, J., Vermeiden, J., Witteman, B., Smits, M. and de Roos, N. (2014). Migraine associated with gastrointestinal disorders: review of the literature and clinical implications. *Frontiers in Neurology*, 5, p.241.

Multiple sclerosis and gut health

Berer, K., Boziki, M. and Krishnamoorthy, G. (2014). Selective accumulation of pro-inflammatory T cells in the intestine contributes to the resistance to autoimmune demyelinating disease. *PLoS ONE*, 9(2), p.e87876.

Berer, K., Mues, M., Koutrolos, M., Rasbi, Z., Boziki, M., Johner, C., Wekerle, H. and Krishnamoorthy, G. (2011). Commensal microbiota and myelin autoantigen cooperate to trigger autoimmune demyelination. *Nature*, 479(7374), pp.538–541.

Castillo-Álvarez, F. and Marzo-Sola, M. (2015). Role of intestinal microbiota in the development of multiple sclerosis. *Neurologia*, pii: S0213-4853(15), pp.180–182.

Dendrou, C., Fugger, L. and Friese, M. (2015). Immunopathology of multiple sclerosis. *Nature Reviews Immunology*, 15(9), pp 545–558.

Nouri, M., Bredberg, A., Weström, B. and Lavasani, S. (2014). Intestinal barrier dysfunction develops at the onset of experimental autoimmune encephalomyelitis, and can be induced by adoptive transfer of auto-reactive T cells. *PLoS ONE*, 9(9), p.e106335.

Stanisavljević, S., Lukić, J., Momčilović, M., Miljković, M., Jevtić, B., Kojić, M., Golić, N., Mostarica Stojković, M. and Miljković, D. (2016). Gut-associated lymphoid tissue, gut microbes and susceptibility to experimental autoimmune encephalomyelitis. *Beneficial Microbes*, 7(3), pp.363–373.

Number of cells in human body

Bianconi, E., Piovesan, A., Facchin, F., Beraudi, A., Casadei, R., Frabetti, F., Vitale, L., Pelleri, M., Tassani, S., Piva, F., Perez Amodio, S., Strippoli, P. and Canaider, S. (2013). An estimation of the number of cells in the human body. *Annals of Human Biology*, 40(6), pp.463–471.

Obesity and gut health

Ley, R., Turnbaugh, P., Klein, S. and Gordon, J. (2006). Microbial ecology: human gut microbes associated with obesity. Nature, 444(7122), pp.1022–1023.

Polycystic ovary syndrome (PCOS) and gut health

Akcalı, A., Bostanci, N., Özçaka, Ö., Öztürk-Ceyhan, B., Gümüş, P., Buduneli, N. and Belibasakis, G. (2014). Association between polycystic ovary syndrome, oral microbiota and systemic antibody responses. *PLoS ONE*, 9(9), p.e108074.

Kelley, S., Skarra, D., Rivera, A. and Thackray, V. (2016). The gut microbiome is altered in a letrozole-induced mouse model of polycystic ovary syndrome. *PLoS ONE*, 11(1), p.e0146509.

Zhang, D., Zhang, L., Yue, F., Zheng, Y. and Russell, R. (2015). Serum zonulin is elevated in women with polycystic ovary syndrome and correlates with insulin resistance and severity of anovulation. *European Journal of Endocrinology*, 172(1), pp.29–36.

Pomegranate and gut health

Faria, A. and Calhau, C. (2011). The bioactivity of pomegranate: impact on health and disease. *Critical Reviews in Food Science and Nutrition*, 51(7), pp.626–634.

Li, Z., Summanen, P., Komoriya, T., Henning, S., Lee, R., Carlson, E., Heber, D. and Finegold, S. (2015). Pomegranate ellagitannins stimulate growth of gut bacteria in vitro: Implications for prebiotic and metabolic effects. *Anaerobe*, 34, pp.164–168.

Viladomiu, M., Hontecillas, R., Yuan, L., Lu, P. and Bassaganya-Riera, J. (2013). Nutritional protective mechanisms against gut inflammation. *The Journal of Nutritional Biochemistry*, 24(6), pp.929–939.

Proton pump inhibitors (PPIs) and gut health

Fujimori, S. (2015). What are the effects of proton pump inhibitors on the small intestine? *World Journal of Gastroenterology*, 21(22), pp.6817–6819.

Psoriasis and gut health

Scher, J., Ubeda, C., Artacho, A., Attur, M., Isaac, S., Reddy, S., Marmon, S., Neimann, A., Brusca, S., Patel, T., Manasson, J., Pamer, E., Littman, D. and Abramson, S. (2015). Decreased bacterial diversity characterizes the altered gut microbiota in patients with psoriatic arthritis, resembling dysbiosis in inflammatory bowel disease. *Arthritis & Rheumatology*, 67(1), pp.128–139.

Rosacea and gut health

Parodi, A., Paolino, S., Greco, A., Drago, F., Mansi, C., Rebora, A., Parodi, A. and Savarino, V. (2008). Small intestinal bacterial overgrowth in rosacea: clinical effectiveness of its eradication. *Clinical Gastroenterology Hepatology*, 6(7), pp.759–764.

Stress and gut health

Kelly, J., Kennedy, P., Cryan, J., Dinan, T., Clarke, G. and Hyland, N. (2015). Breaking down the barriers: the gut microbiome, intestinal permeability and stress-related psychiatric disorders. *Frontiers in Cellular Neuroscience*, 9, pp.392.

Knowles, S., Nelson, E. and Palombo, E. (2008). Investigating the role of perceived stress on bacterial flora activity and salivary cortisol secretion: a possible mechanism underlying susceptibility to illness. *Biological Psychology*, 77(2), pp.132–137.

Konturek, P., Brzozowski, T. and Konturek, S. (2011). Stress and the gut: pathophysiology, clinical consequences, diagnostic approach and treatment options. *Journal of Physiology and Pharmacology*, 62(6), pp.591–599.

Surface area of the digestive tract

Helander, H. and Fändriks, L. (2014). Surface area of the digestive tract – revisited. *Scandinavian Journal of Gastroenterology*, 49(6), pp.681–689.

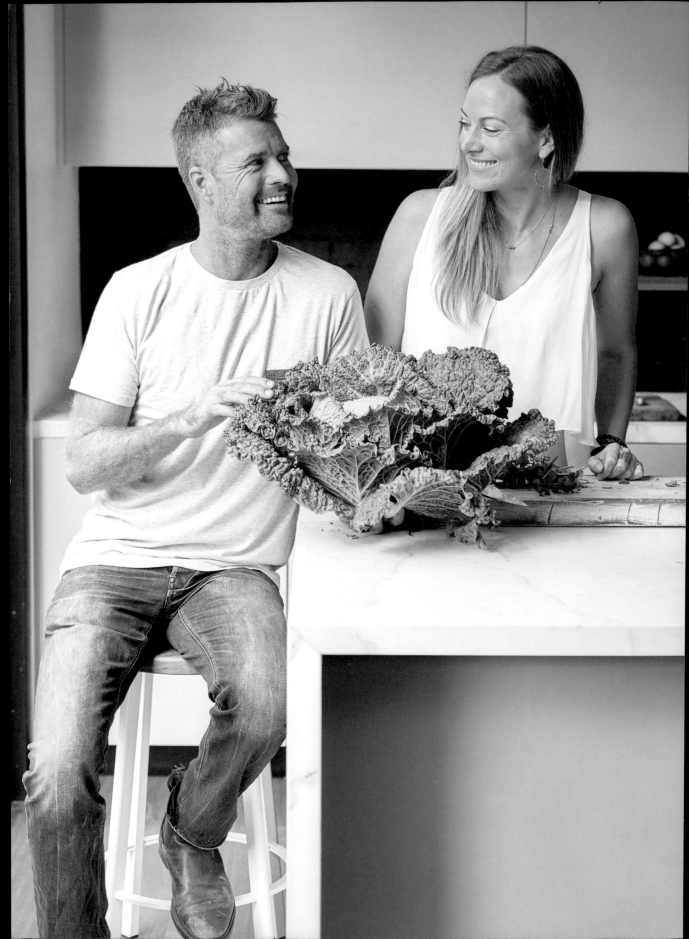

THANK YOU

Pete

Endless gratitude to my exquisite partner in life and love, Nicola. It is an honor to share this journey with you! Thank you for nurturing Chilli, Indii, Shikoba, Orlando, and me with your unconditional love and guidance and all of your deliciously nourishing food. I love you, angel!

To my bunnies, Indii and Chilli – you know this book wouldn't have come about if it weren't for the two of you. I love you both so much and you are both so unique in your own special ways. I hope that by the time your own children are at school this way of living will be considered normal and the current dietary guidelines considered extreme.

To Helen Padarin, I can't imagine collaborating with anyone else on this book. Your passion, dedication, and thirst for knowledge are constant sources of inspiration.

To photographers Mark Roper, Rob Palmer, and Steve Brown, and stylists Deb Kaloper and Lucy Tweed – thanks once again for making my food shine so brightly! And Steve, thanks for the extra lifestyle images for the book and the brilliant cover shots.

To Mary Small and Clare Marshall – once again, it was a pleasure working with you and creating another much-needed book.

To Megan Johnston – thank you for your careful and thorough editing.

To Emily O'Neill – thank you for creating such a gorgeous design for the book.

To Monica and Jacinta Cannataci – girls, I can't thank you enough, and I am so happy that you have discovered that food really is medicine.

To Charlotte Ree – thanks for being the best publicist any author could wish to work with.

To Mum – thanks for passing on your love of cooking.

And finally to my mentors and the trailblazers in health and nutrition, I couldn't have done it without you: Nora Gedgaudas and Lisa Collins, Dr. Libby, Trevor Hendy, Luke Hines, Pete Melov, Rudy Eckhardt, Pete Bablis, William (Bill) Davis, Tim Noakes, Gary Fettke, David Perlmutter, Gary Taubes, Frank Lipman, Wes and Charlotte Carr, Nahko Bear, Michael Franti, Trevor Hall, David Gillespie, Ben Balzer, Loren Cordain, Bruce Fife, Mat Lalonde, Martha Herbert, Joseph Mercola, Sally Fallon, Dr. Natasha Campbell-McBride, Kitsa Yanniotis, and Donna Gates.

Helen

Huge gratitude and appreciation to all my patients – you are my constant teachers. Each and every one of you helps me to help others (and myself) by giving me insights into the human body, mind, and soul. Thank you for choosing to share your journey with me.

A big thank you to my teachers, mentors, peers, friends, and inspirations in the healthcare, lifestyle, and research arenas: Dr. Alessio Fasano, Prof. Martha Herbert, Dr. Leila Masson, Dr. Debbie Fewtrell, Dr. Kelly Brogan, Dr. David Perlmutter, Dr. Natasha Campbell-McBride, Dr. Libby, Dr. Richard Schloeffel, Dr. Yuwen Lee, Dr. Antony Underwood, Dr. James Read, Prof. Tim Noakes, Anthony Milotic, Cyndi O'Meara, Heidi East, Charlotte Carr, Wes Carr, Willow Carr, Kim Morrison, Alice Nicholls, Therese Kerr, Luke Hines, Jeremy Princi, Nora Gedgaudas, Carl Hammington, and Ido Portal, to name but a few.

Thank you to my parents, Fay and Werner, my sister, Ann-maree, and my nieces and nephews, Alex, Emma, Sarah, and George, for all of your love and support and for sharing so many wonderful meals! I'm very lucky to have you all in my life.

Thank you to Leslie Embersits and the Mindd Foundation for helping to get integrative health information out to a community in such great need of it.

Monica and Jacinta Cannataci – the wonder twins. I am constantly in awe of your work, passion, and dedication. This book would not exist without you!

To photographers Steve Brown, Rob Palmer, and Mark Roper, and stylists Lucy Tweed and Deb Kaloper – thanks for making the food look so beautiful and for making me feel comfortable in front of the camera!

Thank you, Clare Marshall, for being my constant go-to and guide in the process of putting this project together. Thank you to Mary Small for believing in this project and to Charlotte Ree for getting the word out! Thanks to Emily O'Neill for a beautiful, clean design and Megan Johnston for editing.

And, of course, thank you, Pete, for being a force for good and for having such an impact on how Australians view food and how they eat. As Michael Pollan says, the first step to regaining health is to get back into the kitchen, and I admire your passion and resiliency in your mission to make this happen. We're blessed that you chose to spend some time in an earth suit, as beautiful Nic would say.

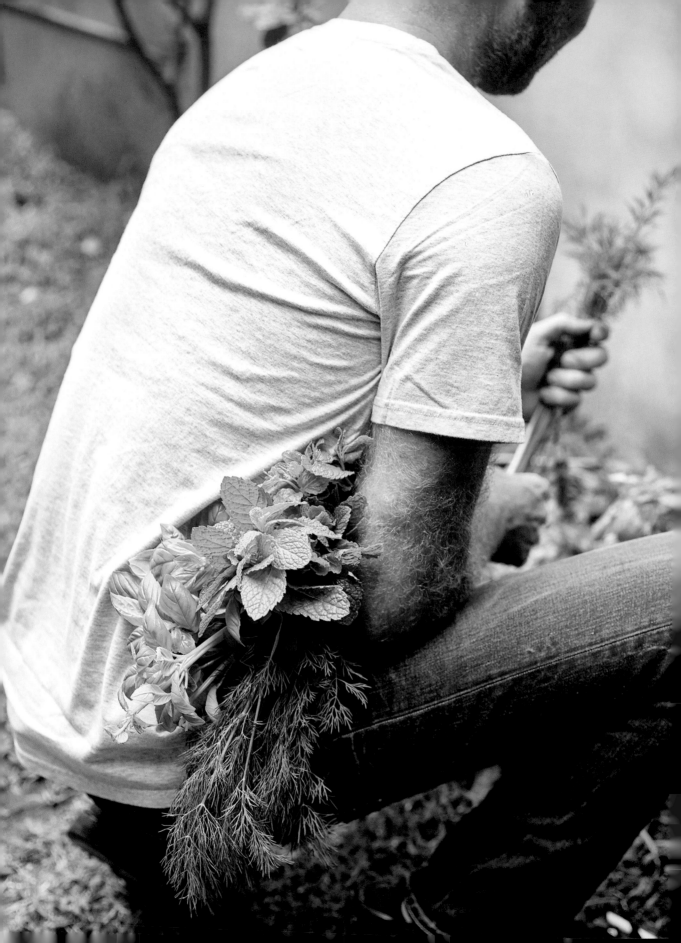

INDEX

weldonowen

Published in North America by Weldon Owen, Inc.
1045 Sansome Street, San Francisco, CA 94111
www.weldonowen.com
Weldon Owen is a division of Bonnier Publishing USA

This edition printed in 2016
First published in Australia in 2016
by Pan Macmillan Australia Pty Limited

Library of Congress Cataloging-in-Publication
data is available

ISBN 13: 978-1-68188-192-8
ISBN 10: 1-68188-192-6

Printed and bound in China
10 9 8 7 6 5 4 3 2 1

Photography by Mark Roper (with additional
photography by Steve Brown and Rob Palmer)
Prop and food styling by Deb Kaloper and Lucy Tweed